Ionic Transport in Hypertension: New Perspectives

Edited by

Antonio Coca, M.D., Ph.D.
Hypertension Unit
Department of General Internal Medicine
Hospital Clinic
University of Barcelona
Barcelona, Spain

Ricardo P. Garay, M.D., Ph.D.
INSERM Unit 2
Faculté de Médicine
Créteil, France

CRC Press
Boca Raton Ann Arbor London Tokyo

Library of Congress Cataloging-in-Publication Data

Ionic transport in hypertension : new perspectives / edited by Antonio
Coca, Ricardo Garay.
p. cm.
Includes bibliographical references and index.
ISBN 0-8493-5474-9
1. Essential hypertension--Pathophysiology.
2. Ions--Physiological transport. I. Coca, Antonio. II. Garay, Ricardo.
[DNLM: 1. Hypertension--metabolism. 2. Ion Transport--physiology.
WG 340 I635 1993]
RC685.H8I57 1993
616.1'3207--dc20
DNLM/DLC
for Library of Congress 93-7570
CIP

This book contains information obtained from authentic and highly regarded sources. Reprinted material is quoted with permission, and sources are indicated. A wide variety of references are listed. Reasonable efforts have been made to publish reliable data and information, but the author and the publisher cannot assume responsibility for the validity of all materials or for the consequences of their use.

Direct all inquiries to CRC Press, Inc., 2000 Corporate Blvd., N.W., Boca Raton, Florida 33431.

No claim to original U.S. Government works
International Standard Book Number 0-8493-5474-9
Library of Congress Card Number 93-7570
Printed in the United States of America 1 2 3 4 5 6 7 8 9 0
Printed on acid-free paper

PREFACE

There is increasing evidence that primary hypertension, both in animal models and humans, emerges as a result of a particular confluence of genetic and environmental factors. Among the latter, excess sodium intake, and low potassium or calcium intake have been proposed as pathogenetic factors in primary hypertension. Such ion-hypertension hypotheses assume that all subjects are similarly susceptible to diet. However, for a significant fraction of hypertensive patients, salt restriction or potassium- or calcium-rich diets do not lower blood pressure. Though the enthusiasts of the ion-hypertension hypothesis suggest that even these latter are subjects in whom high blood pressure was irreversibly induced by diet factors, what is undeniable is the existence of individual variations in ion sensitivity in relation to blood pressure.

The structural complexity of the vessel wall and other relevant organs for hypertension and the difficulty in obtaining blood vessel samples from patients has determined the use of circulating blood cells as a cellular model for the clinical investigation of membrane ion transport in hypertension. Therefore, red blood cells from essential hypertensive patients have been extensively investigated during the last fifteen years. The emerging picture has been extremely complex and frequently controversial. However, all authors seem to agree on at least two points: (1) red cell ion transport is *abnormal* in essential hypertension and (2) *different* ion transport abnormalities can be found in different subsets of essential hypertensive patients and strains of spontaneously hypertensive rats.

It took more than twenty years for Laragh and his colleagues to persuade the scientific community that measurement of plasma renin activity can distinguish two forms of essential hypertension i.e., low and normal (or high) renin hypertension. If instead of looking at the plasma we investigate the red cell membrane, we may detect at least seventeen ion transport abnormalities. Each of them should be integrated with other biochemical and clinical parameters in order to provide a clear, comprehensive picture of each form of essential hypertension, and they may indeed prove useful for identifying salt-sensitivity, or calcium-sensitivity, in subjects genetically predisposed to the development of hypertension. More importantly, easy and precise red cell tests should be introduced in the near future for the diagnosis and specific treatment of the different forms of essential hypertension.

Beyond our basic aim to present a "state-of-the-art" discussion of membrane transport in hypertension, the ambition of the present volume is to anticipate and set up the scientific background of what could be clear technological progress in the diagnosis and treatment of essential hypertension. We sincerely hope to see the accomplishment of such work in the coming years.

Antonio Coca
Barcelona, Spain
Ricardo P. Garay
Paris, France

THE EDITORS

Antonio Coca M.D., Ph.D., is Chief, Hypertension Unit, Department of General Internal Medicine, Hospital Clinico, School of Medicine, University of Barcelona, Spain.

Dr. Coca obtained his M.D. in 1974 from the School of Medicine at the University of Barcelona, Spain. In 1983 he obtained his Ph.D. *(summa cum laude)* from the University of Barcelona. He served as an Associate Professor at University of Barcelona from 1975 to 1986, as a Research Associate Professor at the Laboratory of Cardiovascular Physiology and Pharmacology (INSERM, CNRS, Hospital Necker, Paris, France) in 1986, and as a Professor of Medicine at the School of Medicine, University of Barcelona from 1986. It was in 1992 that he assumed his present position as Chief of the Hypertension Unit at the Hospital Clinico, University of Barcelona, Spain.

Dr. Coca is member of the International Society of Hypertension, American Society of Hypertension, European Society of Hypertension, Research Society on Alcoholism, and the International Society of Internal Medicine. He has served on the Spanish Society of Hypertension since 1992 and as President of the Hypertension Research Foundation of the Catalan Community Hospitals since 1992.

Dr. Coca has been the recipient of many research grants from the Spanish National Research Institutes (Fondo de Investigación Sanitaria, Comisión Asesora de Investigación Científica y Técnica) and private industry from 1982 to the present. He has published more than 100 papers and has presented over 40 invited lectures at national meetings and universities. His current research interests include the cellular pathogenesis of salt-induced hypertension and alcohol-induced hypertension and the molecular pathogenesis of left ventricular hypertrophy in essential hypertension.

Ricardo P. Garay, M.D., Ph.D., is Director of Research, INSERM Unit 2, School of Medicine of Créteil, France.

R. P. Garay was born in San Fernando, Argentina in 1943. He graduated with an M.D. degree from the University of Buenos Aires School of Medicine in 1966. In 1971 he graduated from the University of Buenos Aires School of Sciences with a Ph.D. in Chemistry. He then worked with Professor P. J. Garrahan in the Department of Biochemistry, School of Pharmacy at this university and studied the kinetics of the sodium pump in human red blood cells.

From 1974 through 1976, R. P. Garay worked with Professor R. Lefever in Belgium at the Service de Chimie Physique II (Faculte de Sciences, Universite Libre de Bruxelles) directed by Professor I. Prigogine, 1977 Nobel Prize winner in Chemistry. There he studied thermodynamics and kinetics of biochemical phenomenon, including membrane transport reactions.

In 1976, R. P. Garay was nominated Attaché de Recherche at CNRS (French National Council of Research) to investigate membrane sodium transport in primary hypertension at INSERM Unit 7/CNRS URA 318, Hôpital Necker, Paris. In 1978, he became Charge de Recherche and in 1982, Director of Research.

R. P. Garay published several scientific articles from 1979 to the present on membrane ion transport in erythrocytes from essential hypertensive patients. He has also published over 240 articles in various international scientific journals. He is a member of four scientific societies and the organizer of eight international scientific meetings. R. P. Garay has also been the editor of several books and special issues of scientific journals.

CONTRIBUTORS

Arantxa Arrázola, Sc.D.
Senior Researcher
Laboratory of Cellular Transport and Hypertension
Department of Internal Medicine
Center for Biomedical Research
School of Medicine
University of Navarra
Pamplona, Navarra, Spain

Abraham Aviv, M.D.
Professor and Director
Hypertension Research Center
University of Medicine and Dentistry of New Jersey
Newark, New Jersey

Giuseppe Bianchi, M.D., Ph.D.
Professor of Nephrology
Department of Nephrology, Dialysis, and Hypertension
S. Raffaele Hospital
Milan, Italy

Sylvie Cavalier, M.Sc.
INSERM Unit 2
Faculté de Médicine
Créteil, France

Josep Closas, M.D.
Attending Physician
Department of Internal Medicine
Hospital San Lorenzo
Viladecans, Spain

Antonio Coca, M.D., Ph.D.
Chief
Hypertension Unit
Department of General Internal Medicine
Hospital Clinic
School of Medicine
University of Barcelona
Barcelona, Spain

Jean R. Cusson, M.D., Ph.D., FRCPC
Senior Researcher
Centre de Recherche
Hôtel-Dieu de Montreal
Montreal, Canada
and Associate Researcher
Department of Pharmacology
Universite de Montreal
Montreal, Canada

Alejandro De la Sierra, M.D.
Attending Physician
Hypertension Unit
Department of General Internal Medicine
Hospital Clinic
School of Medicine
University of Barcelona
Barcelona, Spain

Javier Diez, M.D., Ph.D.
Chief
Laboratory of Internal Medicine
Professor of Internal Medicine
Department of Internal Medicine
Center for Biomedical Research
School of Medicine
University of Navarra
Pamplona, Navarra, Spain
and Professor of Medicine
Department of Medicine
University of Zaragoza
Zaragoza, Spain

Patrizia Ferrari, B.S., Ph.D.
Head of Cellular Pharmacology
Department of Cellular Pharmacology and Biology
Prassis Sigmatau Research Institute
Milano, Italy

Ricardo P. Garay, M.D., Ph.D.
Director of Research
INSERM Unit 2
Faculté de Médicine
Créteil, France

Kenneth A. Gruber, B.A., Ph.D.
Professor of Physiology
Department of Physiology and Biophysics
University of Puerto Rico
San Juan, Puerto Rico

Patrick A. Hannaert, Ph.D.
INSERM Unit 2
Faculté de Médicine
Créteil, France

Kent Hermsmeyer, Ph.D.
Professor
Oregon Regional Primate Research Center
Beaverton, Oregon

Steven C. Hunt, Ph.D.
Professor
Cardiovascular Genetics, Department of Internal Medicine
University of Utah School of Medicine
Salt Lake City, Utah

Pierre Larochelle, M.D., Ph.D., FRCPC
Director of Clinical Research
Centre de Recherche
Hôtel-Dieu de Montreal
and Professor
Department of Pharmacology
University of Montreal
Montreal, Canada

Jean-Pierre Ollivier
INSERM Unit 2
Faculté de Médicine
Créteil, France

Nancy J. Rusch, Ph.D.
Associate Professor
Departments of Physiology and Cardiothoracic Surgery
Medical College of Wisconsin
Milwaukee, Wisconsin

Andrea Semplicini, M.D.
Associate Professor of Therapeutics
Institute of Clinical Medicine
University of Padua
Padua, Italy

Nathalie Senn
INSERM Unit 2
Faculté de Médicine
Créteil, France

Javier Sobrino, M.D.
Attending Physician
Department of Internal Medicine
Hospital del Espiritu Santo
Santa Colona de Gramanet, Spain

Alvaro Urbano-Marquez, M.D., Ph.D.
Professor of Medicine
Department of Internal Medicine
School of Medicine
University of Barcelona
Barcelona, Spain
and Chairman
Hospital Clinic
Barcelona, Spain

Roger R. Williams, M.D.
Professor and Director
Cardiovascular Genetics, Department of Internal Medicine
University of Utah School of Medicine
Salt Lake City, Utah

Lily L. Wu, Ph.D.
Associate Professor
Cardiovascular Genetics, Department of Pathology
University of Utah School of Medicine
Salt Lake City, Utah

TABLE OF CONTENTS

Chapter 1
The Erythrocyte as a Cellular Model for the Clinical Investigation of Essential Hypertensive Patients 1
Antonio Coca and Ricardo P. Garay

Chapter 2
Genetic Abnormalities of the Na-K-Cl Cotransport in Experimental and Primary Hypertension 25
Patrizia Ferrari and Giuseppe Bianchi

Chapter 3
The [Na^+,K^+,Cl^-] Cotransport System: Relevance in Essential Hypertension 45
Ricardo P. Garay, Sylvie Cavalier, and Patrick A. Hannaert

Chapter 4
Kinetic Abnormalities of the Na^+,K^+ Pump in Essential Hypertension 57
Javier Diez and Arantxa Arrázola

Chapter 5
The Li^+/Na^+ Countertransport in Hypertension 89
Andrea Semplicini

Chapter 6
The Na^+/H^+ Antiport: Its Role in Cellular Metabolism and in the Pathophysiology of Essential Hypertension 119
Abraham Aviv

Chapter 7
The Cl^-/HCO_3^- Anion Exchanger in Hypertension 133
Javier Diez and Arantxa Arrázola

Chapter 8
Endogeneous Digitalis-Like Factors: Past Progress and Future Prospects 157
Kenneth A. Gruber

Chapter 9
Atrial Natriuretic Peptide, Sodium Transport Systems and Essential Hypertension 183
Josep Closas, Jean R. Cusson, and Pierre Larochelle

Chapter 10
Vascular Muscle Calcium Channels in Hypertension 197
Nancy J. Rusch and Kent Hermsmeyer

Chapter 11
Abnormalities of the Calcium Pump in Primary Hypertension.................229
Alejandro De la Sierra, Javier Sobrino, and Antonio Coca

Chapter 12
Ion Transport and Left Ventricular Hypertrophy in Essential
Hypertension 247
Antonio Coca, Alejandro De la Sierra, and Alvaro Urbano-Márquez

Chapter 13
Abnormalities of Ion Transport in Hypercholesterolemia and
Hypertriglyceridemia: A Link With Essential Hypertension? 273
Steven C. Hunt, Lily L. Wu, and Roger R. Williams

Chapter 14
Abnormalities of Ion Transport and the Pathophysiology of Essential
Hypertension: Therapeutic Implications and Future Perspectives 301
Ricardo P. Garay, Nathalie Senn, and Jean-Pierre Ollivier

Index 311

Ionic Transport in Hypertension: New Perspectives

Chapter 1

THE ERYTHROCYTE AS A CELLULAR MODEL FOR THE CLINICAL INVESTIGATION OF ESSENTIAL HYPERTENSIVE PATIENTS

Antonio Coca and Ricardo P. Garay

TABLE OF CONTENTS

I. Introduction 2

II. Ion Transport Systems in Cell Membranes 4
  A. General Aspects 4
  B. Ion Transport Systems in Epithelial Tissue 5
  C. Ion Transport Systems in Vascular Smooth Muscle 7
  D. Ion Transport Systems in Red Blood Cells 9

III. Rationale Underlying the Use of Red Blood Cells for the Clinical Investigation of Essential Hypertension 10
  A. Salt and Hypertension 10
  B. Increased Cell Sodium Content in Primary Hypertension 11
  C. Methodological Advantages of Ion Transport Studies in Red Blood Cells 11

IV. Preliminary Ion Flux Studies in Erythrocytes from Essential Hypertensive Patients 12

V. Kinetic Studies 12
  A. Changes in Erythrocyte Ion Transport Reflecting an Abnormal Compensatory Response to Excess Sodium Intake 12
  B. Genetic Changes in Red Cell Ion Transport Reflecting Increased Renal Sodium Reabsorption 14
  C. Genetic Changes in Red Cell Ion Transport Reflecting Increased Activity of Excitable Cells 16
  D. Other Genetic Changes in Red Cell Ion Transport 16
  E. Compensatory Erythrocyte Ion Transport Abnormalities 16
  F. Erythrocyte Ion Transport Abnormalities Unrelated to Hypertension 17

0-8493-5474-9/94/$0.00+$.50

VI. Clinical Aspects 17

VII. Perspectives 18

VIII. Summary and Conclusions 18

Acknowledgments 19

References 20

I. INTRODUCTION

Over the last 12 years an impressive amount of data has been accumulated concerning membrane sodium transport in erythrocytes from essential hypertensive patients. An overview of such data reveals that this field of investigation has evolved through four stages:

1. As early as 1960, Losse et al.[1] reported an increased sodium content in erythrocytes from essential hypertensive patients. Later, studies in the hypertensive offspring and rats with spontaneous hypertension suggested that the increased sodium content reflected the presence of an "inherited erythrocyte membrane abnormality".[2-5]
2. In 1980, flux studies revealed two "inherited erythrocyte membrane abnormalities", i.e., a defective [Na^+,K^+,Cl^-] cotransport system[6] and an increased Na^+:Li^+ countertransport.[7] Intriguingly, neither of these two abnormalities was able to induce an increased erythrocyte sodium content.
3. From 1980 to 1985, several authors tried to use co- and countertransport fluxes as "genetic markers" of essential hypertension. Unfortunately, the results were extremely variable from one laboratory to the other, and in some cases they were clearly controversial.[8-14]
4. Progress in fundamental knowledge of membrane ion transport allowed the development of sophisticated kinetic methods to measure molecular parameters of several ion transport systems (ion affinities, maximal translocation rates, and cooperativity coefficients). The use of such kinetic methods led to the discovery of a multiplicity of erythrocyte membrane abnormalities, characterizing different subsets of essential hypertensive patients and different strains of genetically hypertensive rats.[10,15-23] Interestingly, six different abnormalities were found in the [Na^+,K^+,Cl^-] cotransport system and two in the Na^+:Li^+ countertransport system (Table 1).

TABLE 1
Red Cell Ion Transport Abnormalities in Primary Hypertension

Transport abnormality	Pathological significance	Ref.
Na^+,K^+ pump		
Decreased V_{max}	Inhibition by endogenous "ouabain-like" factors	43–47
Increased V_{max}	Compensation of increased sodium content	66
Increased K_{Na}	Delayed recovery of basal Na_i in brain and heart	15, 65
$[Na^+,K^+,Cl^-]$ cotransport system		
Increased V_{max}	Increased renal sodium reabsorption	8, 10, 22, 57, 60
Decreased V_{max}	Inhibition by endogenous "bumetanide-like" factors	10, 44, 55
Increased K_{Na}	Lack of negative feedback on sodium influx	10, 15, 17, 18, 53
Decreased K_{Na}	Enhanced negative feedback on sodium influx	22
Increased K_K	?	68
Decreased K_K	?	68
$Na^+:Li^+$ countertransport		
Increased V_{max}	Increased renal sodium reabsorption	7–10, 16, 19, 48, 74
Increased K_{Na}	?	19
$Na^+:H^+$ exchange		
Increased V_{max}	Increased renal sodium reabsorption	23, 61
Low cooperativity index	?	23
Ca^{2+} pump		
Decreased calmodulin	Decreased cell calcium extrusion	76
Increased K_{Ca}	Delayed recovery of basal Ca_i	20
Na^+-dependent $[Cl^-/HCO_3^-]$ exchange		
Increased activity	Increased renal sodium reabsorption	63
Membrane sodium leak		
Increased k_{Na}	Increased sodium influx	2, 15, 66, 67

Note: About 30% of hypertensives have no red cell ion transport abnormality.

Ion transport studies in red blood cells are now providing a more profound understanding of the pathophysiology of primary hypertension. More importantly, they can be used for the diagnosis and specific treatment of different forms of essential hypertension. This chapter introduces the reader to basic aspects of membrane ion transport and summarizes recent data concerning the biochemistry, pathophysiology, and clinical interest of erythrocyte membrane abnormalities in primary hypertension. More detailed descriptions can be found in subsequent chapters.

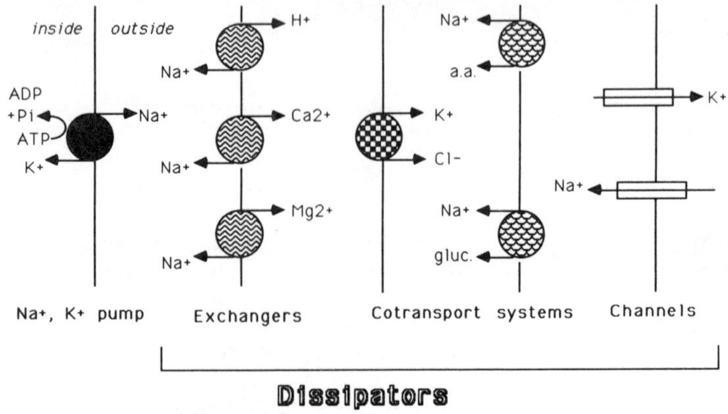

FIGURE 1. Na^+,K^+ pump and ion dissipators in cell membranes. A Na^+,K^+ pump exchanges internal sodium for external potassium using the energy supplied by ATP hydrolysis. Several sodium or potassium "ion dissipators" use the electrochemical energy stored in the sodium or potassium ion gradients in order to perform nonspontaneous thermodynamic work. These dissipators can be divided into channels, Na^+ "exchangers", Na^+ cotransport systems, and the [K^+,Cl^-] cotransport system.

II. ION TRANSPORT SYSTEMS IN CELL MEMBRANES

A. GENERAL ASPECTS

Generally speaking, ion transport proteins can be divided into two categories according to their physiological role (Figures 1 and 2):

1. Ion pumps, which generate electrochemical ion gradients across cell membranes by using the energy supplied by adenosine triphosphate (ATP) hydrolysis. Three of these ion pumps are well known: the Na^+,K^+ pump (Figure 1), which exchanges internal sodium for external potassium and is responsible for the low sodium/high potassium contents of most living cells; the Ca^{2+} pump (Figure 2), which extrudes calcium and decreases free cytosolic calcium contents to very low levels (about 10^{-4} times lower than in the extracellular space), and the H^+ pump, which is well characterized in parietal cells of the gastric mucose where it exchanges internal proton for external potassium.
2. Ion dissipators, which dissipate the electrochemical energy stored in the ion gradients in order to perform nonspontaneous thermodynamic work.

Figure 1 shows the dissipators of the sodium and potassium electrochemical gradients. These can be divided into:

1. The Na^+ and K^+ ion channels, which allow a very rapid and transient dissipation of the sodium and potassium ion gradients and which are responsible for the electrical activity of excitable cells

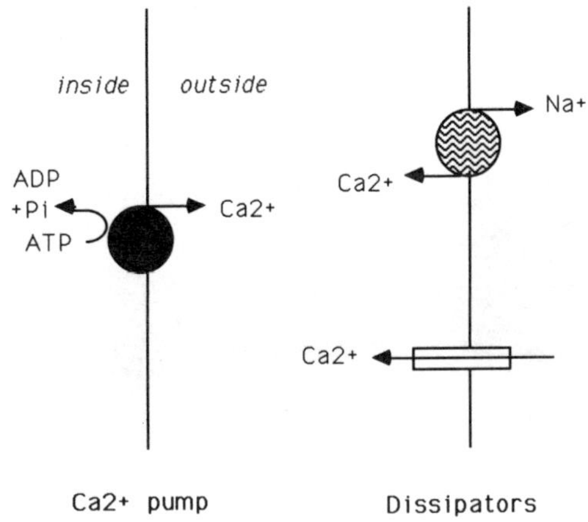

FIGURE 2. Ca^{2+} pump and calcium dissipators. A Ca^{2+} pump extrudes calcium using the energy supplied by ATP hydrolysis. The electrochemical calcium gradient is dissipated by the Ca^{2+} channels, which are responsible for the electrical activity of smooth muscle, and the Na^+:Ca^{2+} exchanger. Under basal conditions this transport protein is a sodium dissipator (exchanging internal calcium for external sodium). However, during the action potential it can work as a calcium dissipator (exchanging internal sodium for external calcium).

2. The Na^+ "exchangers", "antiports", or "countertransport systems", which use the energy supplied by sodium entry into the cell interior to extrude H^+, Ca^{2+}, or Mg^{2+} out of the cell
3. The Na^+ cotransport systems, which couple sodium influx to glucose or amino acid uptake (metabolic dissipators) or which catalyze NaCl entry into some epithelial cells (the [Na^+,K^+,Cl^-] cotransport system; Figures 3 and 4)
4. The [K^+,Cl^-] cotransport system, which couples potassium and chloride extrusion and regulates cell swelling

Figure 2 shows the dissipators of the calcium electrochemical gradient:

1. The Ca^{2+} channels are responsible for the electrical activity of smooth muscle.
2. The Na^+:Ca^{2+} exchanger is well represented in cardiocytes and neurons and to a lesser extent in smooth muscle. Under basal conditions this transport protein is a sodium dissipator (exchanging internal calcium for external sodium). However, during the action potential it can work as a calcium dissipator (exchanging internal sodium for external calcium).

B. ION TRANSPORT SYSTEMS IN EPITHELIAL TISSUE

A basic role of epithelial tissue is the net, vectorial transport of NaCl and water. According to the direction of the vectorial NaCl movements, the epithelia can be divided into absorptive epithelia (Figure 3), which catalyze NaCl absorption from the mucosal to the serosal side, and secretive epithelia (Figure 4), which catalyze

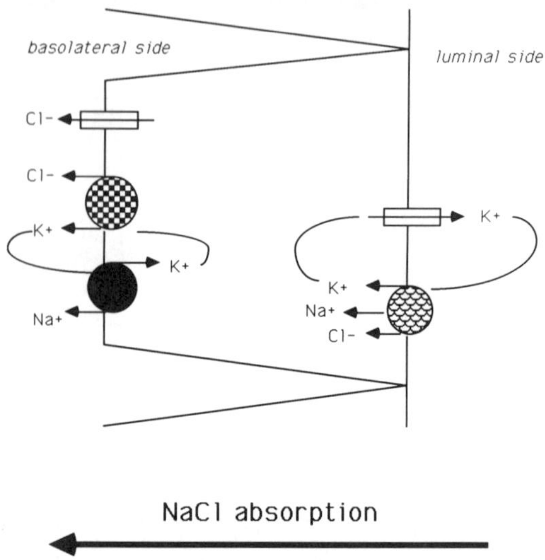

FIGURE 3. NaCl absorption in the ascending limb of Henle's loop of the nephron. On the luminal side, a [Na^+,K^+,Cl^-] cotransport system ensures NaCl entry into the cell interior. A K^+ channel allows continuous cycling of potassium ions across the luminal membrane. Basolateral cell membranes contain a Na^+,K^+ pump, a [K^+,Cl^-] cotransport system, and a Cl^- channel. Cycling of potassium ions across the basolateral border allows a net NaCl extrusion to the extracellular space.

NaCl secretion from the serosal to the mucosal side. Examples of absorptive epithelia are the intestine and the nephronic tubule, and examples of secretive epithelia are the choroid plexus and the epithelial glands.

NaCl absorption or secretion across epithelial tissue is ensured by an asymmetric distribution of ion transport systems in the plasma membrane of the cells. Figure 3 shows one example of asymmetric distribution in an absorptive epithelium: the ascending limb of Henle's loop of the nephron.[24]

On the luminal side of the ascending limb, cell membranes contain a furosemide-sensitive [Na^+,K^+,Cl^-] cotransport system and a K^+ channel (Figure 3). The [Na^+,K^+,Cl^-] cotransport system ensures NaCl entry into the cell interior, along with potassium uptake. The K^+ channel extrudes out of the cell all the excess in potassium ions that is continuously generated by the potassium influx through the [Na^+,K^+,Cl^-] cotransport system. Thus, potassium ions are continuously cycling across the luminal membrane (Figure 3).

Basolateral cell membranes contain a ouabain-sensitive Na^+,K^+ pump, a [K^+,Cl^-] cotransport system, and a Cl^- channel (Figure 3). The Na^+,K^+ pump is the only pump responsible for sodium extrusion to the extracellular space. Chloride extrusion is catalyzed by the [K^+,Cl^-] cotransport system and the Cl^- channel (Figure 3). Moreover, the [K^+,Cl^-] cotransport system extrudes out of the cell all excess potassium ions that are continuously generated by the potassium influx through the Na^+,K^+ pump. This cycling of potassium ions across the basolateral border allows a net NaCl extrusion to the extracellular space.

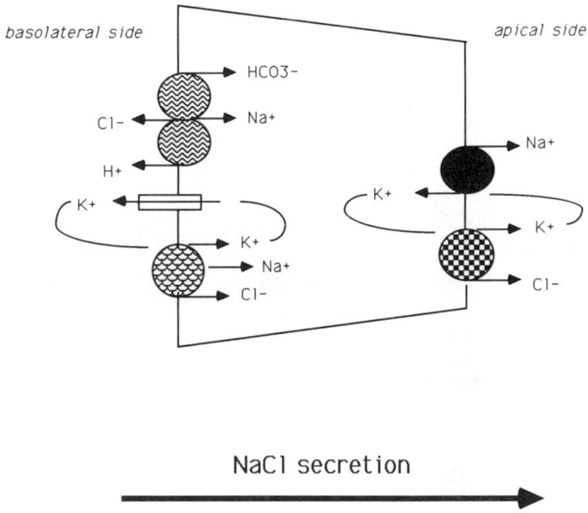

FIGURE 4. NaCl secretion across the choroid plexus. Generally speaking, the choroid plexus is like a Henle's loop with opposite polarity. However, one important difference is that in addition to the [Na^+,K^+,Cl^-] cotransport system, NaCl entry into the cell is ensured by an Na^+:H^+ exchanger coupled to a Cl^-:HCO_3^- exchanger (or a sodium-dependent Cl^-:HCO_3^- exchanger).

Figure 4 shows the ion transport pattern of a secretive epithelia, the choroid plexus. Generally speaking, the choroid plexus is like a Henle's loop with opposite polarity, i.e., the [Na^+,K^+,Cl^-] cotransport system is located on the basolateral side and the Na^+,K^+ pump is located on apical cell membranes (Figure 4). However, one important difference is that in addition to the [Na^+,K^+,Cl^-] cotransport system NaCl entry into the cell is ensured by an Na^+:H^+ exchanger coupled to a Cl^-:HCO_3^- exchanger (or sodium-dependent Cl^-:HCO_3^- exchanger). This difference is perhaps related to the higher water permeability of the choroid plexus compared with the ascending limb of Henle's loop.

C. ION TRANSPORT SYSTEMS IN VASCULAR SMOOTH MUSCLE

If membrane sodium translocation is the most important transport process in epithelial tissue, cardiovascular cell contraction is regulated by membrane calcium transport.

Figure 5 shows the pattern of ion transport mechanisms in vascular smooth muscle cell membranes. Under basal conditions, cytosolic free calcium content is extremely low due to the activity of (1) a sarcoplasmic membrane Ca^{2+} pump, which catalyzes calcium uptake into the sarcoplasmic reticulum, and (2) two plasma membrane transport proteins: the Ca^{2+} pump and the Na^+:Ca^{2+} exchanger, which extrudes calcium to the extracellular space (Figure 5).

The increase in free cytosolic calcium concentration is the unique, final trigger of the contractile apparatus. This calcium increase may result from two different types of cell calcium mobilization:

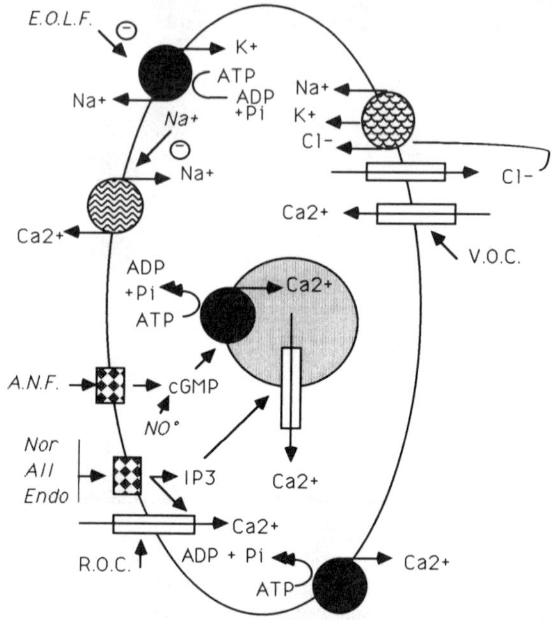

FIGURE 5. Ion transport mechanisms in vascular smooth muscle. Cytosolic free calcium content is extremely low due to the activity of a sarcoplasmic membrane Ca^{2+} pump, a plasma membrane Ca^{2+} pump, and a Na^+:Ca^{2+} exchanger. Vasoconstrictors (noradrenaline, angiotensin II, and endothelin) activate phospholipase C in a G protein-mediated fashion, resulting in IP_3 and diacylglycerol synthesis. IP_3 induces calcium extrusion from the sarcoplasmic reticulum. Mobilization of extracellular calcium results from the spontaneous opening of voltage-operated calcium channels in the plasma membrane or via the opening of receptor-operated calcium channels. Spontaneous membrane depolarization seems to take place via the loss of negative charges through Cl^- channels. A [Na^+,K^+,Cl^-] cotransport system catalyzes net chloride uptake into the cell interior.

1. Mobilization of intracellular calcium from internal stores. This phenomenon is responsible for the initial phase of the vascular contraction induced by vasoconstrictors (noradrenaline, angiotensin II, and endothelin, see Figure 5). All these agonists activate phospholipase C in a G protein-mediated fashion, resulting in inositol triphosphate (IP_3) and diacylglycerol synthesis. IP_3 induces calcium extrusion from the sarcoplasmic reticulum (Figure 5).
2. Mobilization of extracellular calcium. This results from the spontaneous opening of voltage-operated calcium channels in the plasma membrane (basal vascular tone) or via the opening of receptor-operated calcium channels during the late phase of vascular contraction induced by vasoconstrictors (Figure 5). The activation of voltage-operated calcium channels seems to be due to the spontaneous membrane depolarization that takes place via the loss of negative charges through Cl^- channels (Figure 5). The chloride ion loss is counterbalanced by the [Na^+,K^+,Cl^-] cotransport system which catalyzes net chloride uptake into the cell interior (Figure 5).

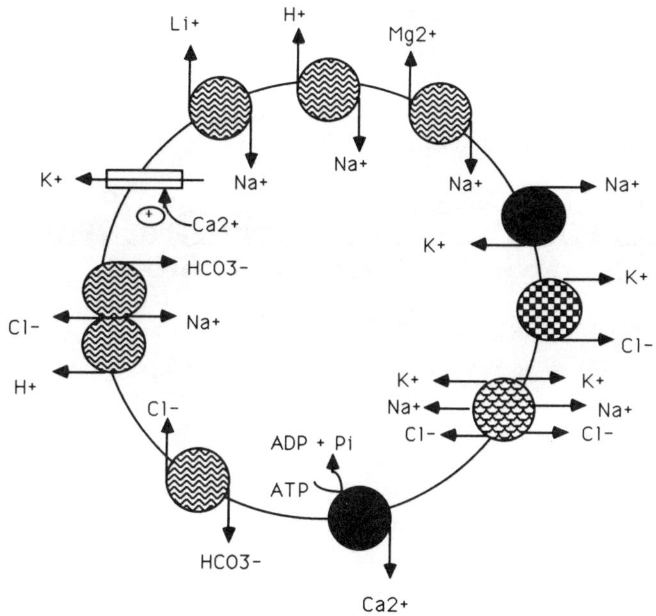

FIGURE 6. Ion transport systems in human red blood cells. Human erythrocyte membranes contain two pumps (the Na^+,K^+ pump and the Ca^{2+} pump) and several ion dissipators (the [Na^+,K^+,Cl^-] cotransport system, the Na^+:Li^+ countertransport, the Na^+:H^+ exchanger, the sodium-dependent Cl^-:HCO_3^- exchanger, the Na^+:Mg^{2+} exchanger, the Cl^-:HCO_3^- exchanger, and the [K^+,Cl^-] cotransport system).

D. ION TRANSPORT SYSTEMS IN RED BLOOD CELLS

The human erythrocyte has several ion transport systems which are qualitatively similar to those existing in nucleated cells, however, their membrane density is much lower than in excitable or epithelial cells.

Figure 6 shows six sodium transport systems that are present in red blood cell membranes: (1) the ouabain-sensitive Na^+,K^+ pump, which maintains and regulates low sodium/high potassium cell contents, (2) the bumetanide (or furosemide)-sensitive [Na^+,K^+,Cl^-] cotransport system, which, in contrast to other cells, is close to equilibrium (outward and inward sodium fluxes have similar magnitude), (3) the Na^+:Li^+ countertransport, (4) the Na^+:H^+ exchanger, (5) the sodium-dependent Cl^-:HCO_3^- exchanger, and (6) the Na^+:Mg^{2+} exchanger. Whether the Na^+:Li^+ countertransport is a transport modality of the Na^+:H^+ exchanger or a different ion transport system is still a matter of investigation.

The only calcium transport protein well characterized in red cell membranes is the Ca^{2+} pump. This Ca^{2+} pump maintains and regulates extremely low cytosolic free calcium contents (Figure 6).

In contrast to other cells, the erythrocyte membrane has an unusually high anion:cation permeability ratio. This is due to the presence of a very active Cl^-:HCO_3^- exchanger (Figure 6) which plays an important role in blood CO_2 dilution and transport.

Another important transport protein of red cell membranes is the $[K^+,Cl^-]$ cotransport system (Figure 6). This membrane carrier is the unique cell volume regulator in human red blood cells.

Under basal conditions, Na^+ and Ca^{2+} entry in erythrocytes is essentially mediated by passive ion permeability (or Na^+ or Ca^{2+} "leak").

III. RATIONALE UNDERLYING THE USE OF RED BLOOD CELLS FOR THE CLINICAL INVESTIGATION OF ESSENTIAL HYPERTENSION

A. SALT AND HYPERTENSION

Several authors suggested that the tendency for blood pressure to rise with age was a phylogenetically recent event, directly attributable to the use of salt as a food additive.[25] Indeed, the major metabolic, enzymatic, and neurohumoral pathways of homo sapiens evolved to their present state 50,000 years ago, a time where our ancestors had a basic diet of plant foods irregularly supplemented with meat.[26] The technology used to obtain salt from rock salt or seawater, dating from about the last 5000 years, enables the preservation of food by salting. Salt preserves food only in high concentrations by inhibiting bacterial and fungal growth. Palates that have adjusted to the salt levels in preservative contents also require it as a condiment, leading to a consumption of between 10 and 30 times greater than the physiological need for sodium chloride.[25]

The notion that high salt intake plays a role in the development of essential hypertension was first suggested more than 80 years ago.[27] Since then numerous epidemiological[28-30] and experimental observations[31,32] and therapeutic maneuvers including low sodium diets[33-35] and treatment with salidiuretic agents have supported the hypothesis that sodium chloride plays a role in the etiology and pathophysiology of hypertension.

The "salt saga" has been controversial due to several important issues which are not readily apparent in individuals studies. The salt-hypertension hypothesis holds that the majority of humans are susceptible to exposure to salt. However, some subjects respond well to salt restriction, whereas others do not, which may be due to an individual salt sensitivity[36] similar to responses found in rats.[32] Salt-induced hypertension in the Sprague-Dawley rat resembles human essential hypertension in that it is only partially reversible by diet. As many as 40% of these rats had no decrease in blood pressure on return to the standard laboratory diet.[32] The enthusiasts of the salt-hypertension hypothesis have suggested that human cases of essential hypertension that are irreversible by diet could have been induced by salt originally, similar to that in the Sprague-Dawley rat. In any case salt sensitivity in humans and rats is not a general attribute but an individual characteristic exhibited by approximately 50% of essential hypertensives.

B. INCREASED CELL SODIUM CONTENT IN PRIMARY HYPERTENSION

Based on the above evidence, Dahl and others[32,37] postulated that hypertension was due to the presence of an "inborn error of sodium metabolism" in susceptible subjects.

In contrast to many other metabolites, sodium does not undergo chemical reactions in the body (redox or acid-base). Thus, sodium metabolism is devoid from enzymes. Indeed, the only functional proteins involved in sodium metabolism are membrane transport proteins.

Evidence for an abnormal membrane sodium transport was first suggested by Tobian and Binion in 1952. These authors reported that the Na^+ content of renal arteries, as measured during postmortem examination, was increased in hypertensive subjects as compared to normotensive controls.[38] Unfortunately, several factors hampered the investigation of sodium transport in vascular cells. First, samples of blood vessels can rarely be obtained during clinical investigation of hypertensive patients. Second, the structural complexity of the vessel wall (interstitial space, cell heterogeneity) and the small amount of available tissue makes it difficult to perform and/or interpret membrane ion fluxes. Third, larger vessels such as the aorta and its main branches differ both anatomically and functionally from the smaller resistance vessels.[39] Finally, because vessel walls undergo structural changes when hypertension is developed, it is difficult to ensure that any alterations in ion composition are a consequence or cause of these structural changes.

C. METHODOLOGICAL ADVANTAGES OF ION TRANSPORT STUDIES IN RED BLOOD CELLS

Membrane transport proteins were supposed to be more or less the same in different cells, including red blood cells. Therefore, it seemed reasonable to expect that either genetic or acquired defects in membrane electrolyte transport might be present in many cell types. This hypothesis was supported early on by the observation of an increased erythrocyte sodium content in essential hypertensive patients,[1,2] thus confirming the findings of Tobian and Binion in vascular tissue. Moreover, the increased erythrocyte sodium content was found to be transmitted to the normotensive offspring, further supporting the genetic hypothesis.[1,2]

In contrast to vascular cells, erythrocytes are accessible to clinical investigation and have unique methodological advantages for molecular studies of ion transport (pure cell population, available in high amounts, with only one ion compartment, slow cation fluxes, and easy to manipulate). Indeed, red blood cells were classically used by several investigators for molecular studies of membrane ion transport.

In the late 1970s, all the above reasons strongly stimulated the search for a genetic defect in red blood cells from essential hypertensive patients.

IV. PRELIMINARY ION FLUX STUDIES IN ERYTHROCYTES FROM ESSENTIAL HYPERTENSIVE PATIENTS

Ion transport studies in primary hypertension were first carried out by using simple flux techniques and by considering this disease as an homogeneous entity. This led to an initial wave of numerous, frequently controversial results, with different genetic abnormalities being proposed — or discarded — as the etiological agent of primary hypertension.[8-14]

However, the aforementioned homogenous approach went against all current clinical evidence. Indeed, besides high blood pressure, no other clinical sign or laboratory abnormality is common to all essential hypertensive patients. Thus, only half of the hypertensive subjects increase blood pressure after excess sodium intake. Some hypertensives are obese, others hyperreactive to stress; some hypertensives have increased plasma catecholamines, other increased plasma renin activity, or even a decreased urinary excretion of prostacyclin metabolites. This heterogeneity of essential hypertension is certainly involved in the variability of the therapeutical response to weight reduction, to low salt diet, or to antihypertensive drugs.

It is important to mention that not all authors used homogenous approaches for biochemical studies of essential hypertension. In this respect, the pioneering classification by Laragh et al.[40] of essential hypertensive patients according to their plasma renin activity appears as a precursor study of the molecular heterogeneity of primary hypertension.

V. KINETIC STUDIES

Since 1987, several authors have measured apparent affinities (K_m) and maximal translocation rates (V_{max}) of the different erythrocyte sodium and calcium transport systems in primary hypertension. These kinetic studies have clearly shown that no unique red cell ion transport defect characterizes the whole population of essential hypertensive patients.[15-23] Conversely, several complex patterns of ion transport abnormalities may be present in different subsets of essential hypertensive patients. Table 1 summarizes the most relevant ion transport abnormalities described in red blood cells from human and rats with primary hypertension.

A. CHANGES IN ERYTHROCYTE ION TRANSPORT REFLECTING AN ABNORMAL COMPENSATORY RESPONSE TO EXCESS SODIUM INTAKE

In spite of decades of investigation, the mechanism by which excess sodium intake leads to hypertension in animals or humans remains poorly understood. Most investigators assume that the presence of high blood pressure reflects a failure in some adaptive mechanism to compensate the excess sodium intake, in particular the natriuretic response that follows excess sodium intake.

Part of the natriuretic response to sodium loading is mediated by the atrial natriuretic factor (ANF). This is a 28-amino acid circulating peptide secreted by the heart in response to the increase in atrial stretch or wall tension that follows acute volume expansion, excess sodium intake, and other experimental maneuvers.[41]

Glomerular receptors for ANF represent about 80% of the total renal ANF receptors, and one main renal action of ANF is an increase in glomerular filtration rate. This seems to take place via the stimulation of a membrane-bound guanylate cyclase, cyclic guanosine monophosphate (cGMP) synthesis and inhibition of calcium mobilization in mesangial cells.

ANF does not seem to be a physiological regulator of vascular resistance under normal circumstances. Moreover, there is no conclusive evidence that ANF deficiency of refractoriness to ANF is involved in the pathogenic mechanism of essential hypertension. Conversely, plasma levels of ANF tend to be increased in humans and rats with primary hypertension, suggesting that it can act as a compensatory mechanism against blood pressure increase.

Red blood cell membranes do not contain functional ANF receptors and ANF has no direct action on membrane ion transport in human erythrocytes.[42] Therefore, it seems unlikely that the increased plasma ANF levels in hypertension may provoke per se any modification of erythrocyte ion transport *in vivo*.

DeWardener and Clarkson[43] and several others[44-47] have found that in addition to ANF, excess sodium intake may evoke increases in other circulating natriuretic factors, enabling the inhibition of tubular sodium reabsorption. The best characterized of these circulating factors is the "endogenous ouabain-like factor" (EOLF), which is able to inhibit the Na^+,K^+ pump in basolateral cell membranes of the nephron and other cell membrane preparations.

EOLF is secreted by acute volume expansion, excess sodium intake, and other experimental maneuvers which are able to increase ANF levels. However, the significance of EOLF as natriuretic factor, together with its chemical structure and site of production, remain to be elucidated.

Red blood cell membranes contain the functional receptor for EOLF; i.e., the membrane Na^+,K^+ pump. Indeed, acute volume expansion or excess sodium intake induce a clear inhibition of Na^+,K^+ pump activity in red blood cells.[44] However, such inhibition is less evident under chronic conditions, due perhaps to the presence of compensatory mechanisms such as the synthesis of new pump units (in erythroblasts), as previously seen during the treatment of chronic digitalis.[48]

In contrast to ANF, EOLF is an hypertensinogenic factor. EOLF is able to increase peripheral vascular resistance via two mechanisms:

1. Increases in cytosolic free calcium contents of vascular smooth muscle cells; EOLF inhibits the Na^+,K^+ pump, slightly depolarizes the cell membrane (by 5 to 10 mV), and opens voltage-dependent calcium channels[49] and/or slightly increases internal Na^+ contents, which in turn inhibits cell calcium extrusion by the $Na^+:Ca^{2+}$ exchanger[47]

2. Increased noradrenergic output by inhibition of the Na^+,K^+ pump in noradrenergic endings[50]

In primary hypertension, plasma levels of EOLF tend to be increased, particularly in those hypertensive conditions associated with volume expansion and low plasma renin activity.[43,47]

In erythrocytes from spontaneously hypertensive rats (SHR), the maximal rate of the Na^+,K^+ pump decreases with the onset of hypertension, and in adult rats it reaches values 50% lower than in Wistar Kyoto (WKY) normotensive rats.[51] Interestingly, this pump inhibition is associated with the appearance of endogenous "digitalis-like" factors in the circulation.[46]

Therefore, decreased erythrocyte Na^+,K^+ pump activity and/or increased internal sodium contents seem to be markers of those forms of high blood pressure associated with increased EOLF. Further investigations are required to establish if such abnormalities are markers of "salt-sensitive" hypertension.

EOLF does not seem to be a potent natriuretic agent *in vivo*. Indeed, diuretic drugs act on luminal sodium reabsorption and not on the basolateral Na^+,K^+ pump. Moreover, recent evidence in the literature suggests the existence of "diuretic-like" endogenous factors that are different than EOLF. In particular, excess Na^+ intake induces a decrease in the maximal rate of the erythrocyte $[Na^+,K^+,Cl^-]$ cotransport system, suggesting the release into the circulation of endogenous "bumetanide-like" factors.[44]

A causal relationship between volume expansion and endogenous "bumetanide-like" factors was further suggested by the correlation between low plasma renin activity and low V_{max} for cotransport.[13,52-54] Moreover, vascular smooth muscle from SHR exhibits a decreased V_{max} of the $[Na^+,K^+,Cl^-]$ cotransport system.[55]

Another erythrocyte cotransport abnormality, frequently seen in essential hypertensive patients and particularly in blacks, is an increased K_m for internal sodium.[10,53] Canessa et al.[53] have found that in the case of young blacks, those with high K_m for cotransport showed a salt-sensitive increase in blood pressure. Moreover, Canessa et al.[18] recently reported that high sodium intake induced an increase in K_m for cotransport, but only in the hypertensive subjects.

Therefore, the results suggest that decreased V_{max} and/or increased K_m of the erythrocyte $[Na^+,K^+,Cl^-]$ cotransport system may be markers of "salt-sensitive" hypertension.

B. GENETIC CHANGES IN RED CELL ION TRANSPORT REFLECTING INCREASED RENAL SODIUM REABSORPTION

Dahl et al.[56] and Bianchi et al.[57] have shown that hypertension can be "transplanted" from hypertensive or prehypertensive rats with genetic hypertension by kidney transplantation. Retrospective studies of kidney transplantation suggest that the same is true for humans.[57]

The transplanted kidney seems to increase blood pressure through an enhanced renal sodium reabsorption.[57] This in turn seems to reflect a genetic disturbance in some ion transport system catalyzing luminal sodium reabsorption. In the prehypertensive stage, renal function is preserved by an increased glomerular filtration rate, which compensates for the increased luminal sodium transport.[57] Later in life, a failure in the compensatory glomerular mechanism unmasks a negative sodium balance and announces the onset of hypertension.

In the Milan strain of spontaneously hypertensive rat (MSH), the ion transport system responsible, at least in part, for the increased renal sodium reabsorption seems to be the $[Na^+,K^+,Cl^-]$ cotransport system of the ascending limb of Henle's loop.[22,57] In human hypertensives, it has been proposed that the increased renal sodium reabsorption is due to the activation of the $Na^+:H^+$ exchanger in the luminal border of the proximal tubule.[58,59]

As we have previously seen, most sodium transport systems involved in renal sodium reabsorption are also present in the red cell membrane. Moreover, genetic disturbances in membrane sodium transport proteins are likely generalized to all cell types. This was clearly confirmed in erythrocytes from MSH rats, which exhibit high $[Na^+,K^+,Cl^-]$ cotransport fluxes.[22,57] A similar increased V_{max} for cotransport was observed in erythrocytes from SHR rats (60). In humans, an increased V_{max} for cotransport was observed in erythrocytes from about 35% of Caucasian essential hypertensive patients.[10,15,17]

Another biochemical marker of increased renal sodium reabsorption seems to be the red cell $Na^+:Li^+$ countertransport system. Increased V_{max} of the $Na^+:Li^+$ countertransport was observed in erythrocytes from 25 to 50% of (Caucasian) hypertensives,[7,10,15,17] and it appears to be absent in black hypertensives. Weder[58] and others (see for instance Reference 57) have found that increased erythrocyte $Na^+:Li^+$ countertransport was correlated with high lithium fractional reabsorption. Therefore, the increased red cell $Na^+:Li^+$ countertransport perhaps reflects an enhanced proximal sodium reabsorption.

Other erythrocyte ion transport abnormalities that have been described in primary hypertension and which can reflect an enhanced renal sodium reabsorption are increased V_{max} of the $Na^+:H^+$ exchanger[23,61,62] and increased sodium-dependent $Cl^-:HCO_3^-$ exchanger.[63] Increased V_{max} of the $Na^+:H^+$ exchanger was detected in erythrocytes from 20 to 60% of essential hypertensive patients.[23,61,62] In a recent study Canessa et al.[23] reported that hypertensive patients with elevated $Na^+:H^+$ exchange represented 21% of all untreated hypertensives and displayed normal $Na^+:Li^+$ countertransport. Finally, increased sodium-dependent $Cl^-:HCO_3^-$ exchanger has been recently reported in erythrocytes from 23% of (Caucasian) essential hypertensive patients.[63]

All these are erythrocyte abnormalities that precede (and are not modified by) the development of high blood pressure; they are present in adult hypertensives and in some of their normotensive offspring. They can also be present during the whole life of a given strain of genetically hypertensive rats. Moreover, these abnormalities not only tend to increase sodium movements in the kidney tubule but also in other epithelia such as the choroid plexus.[64]

C. GENETIC CHANGES IN RED CELL ION TRANSPORT REFLECTING INCREASED ACTIVITY OF EXCITABLE CELLS

Increased peripheral resistance is the common denominator of all forms of hypertension. In some cases, this seems to be the final manifestation of an increased activity of excitable cells: enhanced vascular smooth muscle contractility, increased cardiac output followed by vascular changes, and/or increased noradrenergic output.

Some of the ion transport abnormalities described in erythrocytes from essential hypertensive patients may reflect an increased membrane activity of excitable cells. In particular, this can be the case for two regulatory abnormalities: increased K_m of the sodium pump for internal sodium, found in 10% of Caucasian essential hypertensive patients[15,17,65] and increased K_m of the calcium pump for internal calcium, found in 25% of Caucasian essential hypertensive patients.[20]

In noradrenergic neurons and/or in cardiocytes, the high K_m for the sodium pump may led to transitory increases in cell Na^+ contents after the action potential. This in turn may increase noradrenergic and/or cardiac output. In vascular smooth muscle, the high K_m for the calcium pump may induce a delayed recovery of basal cytosolic calcium levels after muscle contraction.

D. OTHER GENETIC CHANGES IN RED CELL ION TRANSPORT

There are five erythrocyte abnormalities that are difficult to classify: increased membrane sodium leak,[2,15,17,66,67] low Hill coefficient for pH activation of the Na^+:H^+ exchanger,[23] increased K_m of the Na^+:Li^+ countertransport for internal sodium,[19] and increased or decreased K_m of the [Na^+,K^+,Cl^-] cotransport system for external potassium.[68]

The increased sodium leak is a well-recognized genetic disturbance which is present in about 10 to 25% of Caucasian essential hypertensive patients[2,15,17,66,67] and in the hypertension-prone substrain (HPS) of Sabra rats.[69] A cell membrane with increased sodium leak has a tendency to dissipate the sodium gradient and increase the internal sodium contents. This may disturb membrane function in all kinds of cells, including excitable cells and epithelia. Therefore, it is for the moment difficult to hypothesize about the target organ in which the increased sodium leak may act as hypertensive pathogenic factor.

Several observations have suggested that the Na^+:H^+ exchanger is involved in cell replication.[70] On the other hand, vascular hypertrophy is a well-recognized component of the increased peripheral resistance in hypertension.[71] Therefore, the low cooperativity index of the Na^+:H^+ exchanger for internal H^+ perhaps reflects some membrane abnormality involved in vascular hypertrophy.

E. COMPENSATORY ERYTHROCYTE ION TRANSPORT ABNORMALITIES

Hypertensive subjects with increased erythrocyte sodium leak have an increased net Na^+ entry by passive permeability. In some of them, this defect tends to be compensated for by an increased sodium extrusion by the Na^+,K^+ pump (increased V_{max}), allowing the erythrocyte Na^+ contents to remain within the normal range.[66]

Interestingly, 10% of the total population of essential hypertensives have a clear increase in erythrocyte sodium content.[66] These are hypertensive subjects with increased sodium leak, not compensated for by an increased V_{max} of the Na^+,K^+ pump.[66]

A compensatory increase in V_{max} was also observed in the sodium pump of all hypertensive patients, with increased K_m for internal sodium.[15] Moreover, those calcium pumps with increased K_m for internal calcium frequently present a compensatory increase in V_{max}.[20] Again, these V_{max} changes may help the cells to prevent transitory or permanent increases in cell sodium or calcium contents.

Another erythrocyte abnormality which seems to be compensatory is the decreased K_m for internal sodium of the $[Na^+,K^+,Cl^-]$ cotransport system in MSH rats.[22] In the Henle's loop, this decreased K_m for cotransport may exert negative feedback on the increased luminal sodium entry.

F. ERYTHROCYTE ION TRANSPORT ABNORMALITIES UNRELATED TO HYPERTENSION

There is at least one membrane abnormality found in SHR erythrocytes which is clearly unrelated to high blood pressure, increased $[K^+,Cl^-]$ cotransport activity.[72]

In adult rats, $[K^+,Cl^-]$ cotransport activity is fully repressed under isotonic conditions. Cell swelling (in hypoosmotic media) activates the $[K^+,Cl^-]$ cotransport system which extrudes KCl and water, thus counterbalancing the increase in cell volume. In SHR erythrocytes, the $[K^+,Cl^-]$ cotransport system is partially derepressed under isotonic conditions.[72] This induces cell dehydration and explains the lower cell volume of SHR erythrocytes.

Studies in the F2 (WKY × SHR) generation have shown that the derepressed $[K^+,Cl^-]$ cotransport does not cosegregate with high blood pressure.[72] Indeed, the derepressed $[K^+,Cl^-]$ cotransport seems to be a manifestation of the erythrocytosis seen in adult SHR, with appearance of high numbers of young red cells in the circulation.[73]

VI. CLINICAL ASPECTS

Whether ion transport abnormalities are etiological factors of different forms of primary hypertension is a matter of discussion. Nevertheless, the high heterogeneity of these abnormalities strongly supports the idea[40] that high blood pressure is a common denominator of multiple diseases regrouped for convenience (and ignorance) under the term "essential hypertension".

Unfortunately, we know very little concerning the clinical aspects of the different forms of hypertension associated with each erythrocyte sodium transport abnormality. Nevertheless, it appears that hypertension with increased Na^+:Li^+ countertransport is more severe and requires control by a higher number of antihypertensive drugs than that with increased K_m for cotransport.[8,10,74] Furthermore, hypertension with increased Na^+:Li^+ countertransport is characterized by a tendency to increased plasma renin activity, increased low density lipoprotein (LDL) cholesterol levels, and left ventricular hypertrophy.[9,19,74] Conversely, hypertension with increased K_m for cotransport seems to be associated with increased plasma catecholamines.[75]

VII. PERSPECTIVES

In the 1970s, all forms of "essential" hypertension were considered to be associated to a not well-defined, but simple, "increase in membrane sodium permeability". Ten years of intensive research were necessary to reveal the stable ion transport abnormalities reviewed here. This is perhaps a preliminary description, however, because an even higher multiplicity of molecular abnormalities was shown in genetic disorders of hemoglobin and others. Therefore, we suspect that the study of the molecular heterogeneity of essential hypertension is only beginning. Indeed, important ion transport systems such as the Na^+:Ca^{2+} exchanger still requires kinetic studies in hypertensive patients. On the other hand, studies of potential abnormalities in endogenous regulators of ion transport activity require previous definition of their chemical structures.

In conclusion, we expect that the 1990s will see the development of simple assays, allowing large-scale screening of ion transport abnormalities in circulating cells of essential hypertensive patients. This typology of membrane transport defects will help the clinician to diagnose different forms of "essential" hypertension, and more importantly, it can help to select the antihypertensive drug to be prescribed in first intention.

VIII. SUMMARY AND CONCLUSIONS

Since 1987, several authors measured apparent affinities and maximal translocation rates of the different Na^+ and Ca^{2+} transport systems in erythrocytes from essential hypertensive patients. These kinetic studies have clearly shown that no unique red cell ion transport defect characterizes the whole population of essential hypertensive patients. Conversely, several complex patterns of ion transport abnormalities may be present in different subsets of essential hypertensive patients. Kinetic studies are now providing a more profound biochemical insight into the molecular heterogeneity of primary hypertension. In particular, they may permit the diagnosis and specific treatment of different forms of primary hypertension in the 1990s.

We reviewed the abnormalities described in red blood cells from essential hypertensive patients and rats with primary hypertension. From a physiopathological point of view these can be divided into:

1. Changes in erythrocyte ion transport reflecting an abnormal compensatory response to excess sodium intake: decreased V_{max} of the sodium pump and increased internal sodium content (due to "endogenous ouabain-like fac-

tors''), decreased V_{max} of the $[Na^+,K^+,Cl^-]$ cotransport system (due to endogenous ''bumetanide-like'' factors), and increased K_m for cotransport (marker of ''salt-sensitive'' hypertension).

2. Genetic changes in red cell ion transport reflecting increased renal sodium reabsorption: increased V_{max} for the $[Na^+,K^+,Cl^-]$ cotransport system, Na^+:Li^+ countertransport and/or the Na^+:H^+ exchanger, and increased sodium-dependent Cl^-:HCO_3^- exchanger.
3. Genetic changes in red cell ion transport reflecting increased activity of excitable cells: increased K_m of the sodium pump for internal sodium and increased K_m of the calcium pump for internal calcium.
4. Other genetic changes in red cell ion transport: increased membrane sodium leak, low Hill coefficient for pH activation of the Na^+:H^+ exchanger, increased K_m of the Na^+:Li^+ countertransport for internal sodium, and increased or decreased K_m of the $[Na^+,K^+,Cl^-]$ cotransport system for external potassium.
5. Compensatory erythrocyte ion transport abnormalities: increased V_{max} of the Na^+,K^+ pump, increased V_{max} of the calcium pump, and decreased K_m for internal sodium of the $[Na^+,K^+,Cl^-]$ cotransport system.
6. Erythrocyte ion transport abnormalities unrelated to hypertension: increased $[K^+,Cl^-]$ cotransport activity.

Whether ion transport abnormalities are etiological factors of different forms of primary hypertension is a matter of discussion. Nevertheless, the high heterogeneity of these ion transport abnormalities strongly supports the idea that high blood pressure is a common denominator of multiple diseases regrouped under the term ''essential hypertension''.

ACKNOWLEDGMENTS

We are greatly indebted to all the colleagues and friends who worked in the laboratory of INSERM U7: Pharmacologie des Régulations Cardiovasculaires, Hôpital Necker, Paris (France) in the last 12 years. We are particularly indebted to Corinne Nazaret, Patrick Hannaert, Celia Rosati, Nathalie Senn (INSERM U2, Faculté de Médicine, Créteil, France), Jean-Pierre Ollivier (Hôpital du Val-de-Grâce, Paris), Daniele Cusi (Università di Milano, Milan), Jean-Guy Mongeau (St. Justine Hospital, Montreal), Michael Tuck (UCLA, Los Angeles), Michael Price (Baylor College of Medicine, Houston), Javier Diez (Universidad de Zaragoza, Zaragoza, Spain), Alejandro de la Sierra (Hospital Clínico, Barcelona, Spain), Agatangelo Soler (Universidad de Granada, Granada, Spain), Armando Lindner (Veterans Administration Hospital, Seattle), and to our wives Montse and Elizabeth.

REFERENCES

1. **Losse, H., Wehmeyer, H., and Wessels, F.,** Der Wasser- und Elektrolytgehalt von Erythrocyten bei arterieller Hypertonie, *Klin. Woschenschr.,* 1960; 38: 393–395.
2. **Wessels, F., Junge-Hülsing, G., and Losse, H.,** Untersuchungen zur Natriumpermeabilität der Erythrozyten bei Hypertonikern mit familiärer Hochdruckbelastung, *Z. Kreislaufforsch.,* 1967; 56: 374–380.
3. **Friedman, S., Nakashima, M., McIndoe, R., and Friedman, C.,** Increased permeability to Li^+ in spontaneously hypertensive rats, *Experientia,* 1976; 32: 476–478.
4. **Postnov, Y., Orlov, S., Gulak, P., and Shevchenko, A.,** Altered permeability of the erythrocyte membrane for sodium and potassium ions in spontaneously hypertensive rats, *Pfluegers Arch.,* 1976; 365: 257–263.
5. **Yamori, Y., Nara, Y., Horrie, R., and Ohtaka, M.,** Ion permeability of erythrocyte membrane in SHR, *Jpn. Heart J.,* 1977; 18: 604–608.
6. **Garay, R. P., Dagher, G., Pernollet, M. G., Devynck, M. A., and Meyer, P.,** Inherited defect in a Na^+-K^+ cotransport system in erythrocytes from essential hypertensive patients, *Nature,* 1980; 284: 281–283.
7. **Canessa, M., Adragna, N., Solomon, H. S., Connolly, T. M., and Tosteson, D. C.,** Increased sodium-lithium countertransport in red cells of patients with essential hypertension, *N. Engl. J. Med.,* 1980; 302: 772–776.
8. **Adragna, N., Canessa, M., Solomon, H., Slater, E., and Tosteson, D. C.,** Red cell lithium-sodium countertransport and sodium-potassium cotransport in patients with essential hypertension, *Hypertension,* 1982; 4: 795–804.
9. **Brugnara, C., Corrocher, R., Foroni, L., Steinmayr, M., Bonfanti, F., and De Sandre, G.,** Lithium-sodium countertransport in erythrocytes of normal and hypertensive subjects: relationship with age and plasma renin activity, *Hypertension,* 1983; 5: 529–534.
10. **Garay, R. P., Nazaret, C., Hannaert, P., and Price, M.,** Abnormal Na^+,K^+ cotransport function in a group of patients with essential hypertension, *Eur. J. Clin. Invest.,* 1983; 13: 311–320.
11. **Cusi, D., Barlassina, C., Ferrari, P., Ferrandi, M., and Bianchi, G.,** Cation transport abnormalities in human and rat essential hypertension, in *Topics in Pathophysiology of Hypertension,* Villareal, H. and Sambhi, M. P., Eds., Boston: Martinus-Nijhoff, 1984; 136–146.
12. **Montanari, A., Sani, E., Canali, M., Simon, I., Schianchi, P., Borghetti, A., and Novarini, A.,** Low sodium cotransport in red cells with physiological internal sodium concentration in essential hypertension, *Hypertension,* 1984; 6: 826–831.
13. **Canessa, M., Spalvins, A., Adragna, N., and Falkner, B.,** Red cell sodium countertransport and cotransport in normotensive and hypertensive blacks, *Hypertension,* 1984; 6: 344–351.
14. **Behr, J., Witzgall, H., Lorenz, R., Weber, P. C., and Duhm, J.,** Red cell Na^+,K^+ transport in various forms of human hypertension. Role of cardiovascular risk factors and plasma potassium, *Klin. Wochenschr.,* 1985; 63(Suppl. III): 63–65.
15. **Diez, J., Hannaert, P., and Garay, R.,** A kinetic study of the Na^+,K^+ pump in erythrocytes from essential hypertensive patients, *Am. J. Physiol.,* 1987; 252: H1–H6.
16. **Canessa, M., Brugnara, C., and Escobales, N.,** The Li^+-Na^+ exchange and Na^+,K^+,Cl^- cotransport systems in essential hypertension, *Hypertension,* 1987; 10(Suppl. 1): 4–10.
17. **De la Sierra, A., Coca, A., Aguilera, M. T., Ingelmo, M., and Urbano-Márquez, A.,** Clinical profiles and erythrocyte Na^+ transport of four major types of essential hypertension in Spain, *Kidney Int.,* 1989; 36: 114–119.
18. **Canessa, M., Redgrave, J., Laski, C., and Williams, G. H.,** Does sodium intake modify red cell Na^+ transporters in normal and hypertensive subjects?, *Am. J. Hypertension,* 1989; 2: 515–523.
19. **Yap, L., Arrazola, A., Soria, F., and Diez, J.,** Is there increased cardiovascular risk in essential hypertensive patients with abnormal kinetics of red blood cell sodium-lithium countertransport, *J. Hypertension,* 1989; 7: 667–673.

20. **De la Sierra, A., Hannaert, P., Ollivier, J. P., Senn, N., and Garay, R.,** Kinetic study of the Ca^{2+} pump in erythrocytes from essential hypertensive patients, *J. Hypertension,* 1990; 8: 285–293.
21. **Mongeau, J. G., Mauran, P., Poirot, G., and Davignon, A.,** Longitudinal study of various transport abnormalities as an index of severity in children and adolescents suffering from essential hypertension, *J. Hypertension,* 1990; 8: 657–662.
22. **Ferrari, P., Torielli, L., Cirillo, M., Salardi, S., and Bianchi, G.,** Sodium transport kinetics in erythrocytes and inside-out vesicles from Milan rats, *J. Hypertension,* in press.
23. **Canessa, M., Morgan, K., Goldszer, R., Moore, T. J., and Spalvins, A.,** Kinetic abnormalities of the red blood cell sodium-proton exchange in hypertensive patients, *Hypertension,* 1991; 17: 340–348.
24. **Greger R.,** Ion transport mechanisms in the thick ascending limb of Henle's loop of mammalian nephron, *Physiol. Rev.,* 1985; 65: 760–797.
25. **Beard, T. C.,** A salt-hypertension hypothesis, *J. Cardiovasc. Pharmacol.,* 1990; 16(Suppl. 7): 35–38.
26. **Blackburn, H. and Prineas, R.,** Diet and hypertension: anthropology, epidemiology and public health implications, in *Progress in Biochemical Pharmacology,* Vol. 9, Paoletti, R., Ed., Basel: S. Karger, 1983: 31–79.
27. **Ambard, L. and Beaujard, E.,** Causes de l'hypertension artérielle, *Arch. Gen. Med.,* 1904; 1: 520–533.
28. **Page, L. B.,** Epidemiologic evidence on the etiology of human hypertension and its possible prevention, *Am. Heart J.,* 1976; 91: 527–534.
29. **Hunt, J. C.,** Sodium intake and hypertension: a cause for concern, *Ann. Intern. Med.,* 1983; 98: 724–728.
30. **Intersalt Cooperative Research Group,** Intersalt: an international study of electrolyte excretion and blood pressure. Results for 24 hour urinary sodium and potassium excretion, *Br. Med. J.,* 1988; 297: 319–328.
31. **Grollman, A., Harrison, T. R., and Williams, J. R.,** Effect of various sterol derivatives on blood pressure of rat, *J. Pharmacol. Exp. Ther.,* 1940; 69: 149–155.
32. **Dahl, L. K.,** Effects of chronic excess salt feeding. Induction of self-sustained hypertension in rats, *J. Exp. Med.,* 1961; 114: 231–236.
33. Medical Research Council, The rice diet in the treatment of hypertension, *Lancet,* 1950; 2: 509–513.
34. **Hatch, F. T., Wertheim, A. R., Eurman, G. H. et al.,** Effects of diet in essential hypertension. III. Alterations in sodium chloride, protein and fat intake, *Am. J. Med.,* 1954; 17: 499–513.
35. **Morgan, T. O. and Myers, J. B.,** Hypertension treated by sodium restriction, *Med. J. Aust.,* 1981; 2: 396–397.
36. **Luft, F. C., Miller, J. Z., Weinberger, M. H., Christian, J. C., and Skrabal, F.,** Genetic influences on the response to dietary salt reduction, acute salt loading or salt depletion in humans, *J. Cardiovasc. Pharmacol.,* 1988; 12(Suppl. 13): 549–555.
37. **Dahl, L. K., Heine, M., and Tassinari, L.,** Role of genetic factors in susceptibility to experimental hypertension due to chronic excess salt ingestion, *Nature,* 1962; 194: 480–482.
38. **Tobian, L. and Binion, J. T.,** Tissue cations and water in arterial hypertension, *Circulation,* 1952; 5: 754–758.
39. **Hilton, P. J.,** Cellular sodium transport in essential hypertension, *N. Engl. J. Med.* 1986; 314: 222–229.
40. **Laragh, J.,** Personal views on the mechanisms of hypertension, in *Hypertension,* Genest, J., Kuchel, O., Hamet, P., and Cantin, M., Eds., New York: McGraw-Hill, 1983: 615–631.
41. **De Bold, A.,** Atrial natriuretic factor: a hormone produced by the heart, *Science,* 1985; 230: 767–770.
42. **Garay, R. P., Hannaert, P., Rodrigue, F., Longchamps, M. O., Féray, J. C., Rosati, C., Dunham, B., Nazaret, C., Cantin, M., Genest, J., Meyer, P., and Braquet, P.,** Involvement of cytosolic free calcium in the action mechanism of atrial natriuretic factor (ANF), *Regul. Peptides,* 1985; Suppl 4: 97–100.

43. **DeWardener, H. E. and Clarkson, E. M.,** Concept of natriuretic hormone, *Physiol. Rev.,* 1985; 65: 658–759.
44. **Dagher, G., Brossard, M., Féray, J. C., and Garay, R.,** Modulation of erythrocyte Na transport pathway(s) by excess Na intake, *Life Sci.,* 1985; 37: 243–253.
45. **Gruber, K. A., Whitaker, J. M., and Buckalew, V. M., Jr.,** Endogenous digitalis-like substance in plasma of volume expanded dogs, *Nature,* 1980; 287: 743–745.
46. **Wauquier, I., Pernollet, M. G., Grichois, M. L., Lacour, B., Meyer, P., and Devynck, M. A.,** Endogenous digitalis like circulating substances in spontaneously hypertensive rats, *Hypertension,* 1988; 12: 108–116.
47. **Blaustein, M. P. and Hamlyn, J. M.,** Sodium transport inhibition, cell calcium, and hypertension: the natriuretic hormone/Na^+-Ca^{2+} exchange/hypertension hypothesis, *Am. J. Med.,* 1984; 77: 45–59.
48. **Aronson, J. K., Ford, A. R., and Grahame-Smith, D. G.,** Techniques for studying the pharmacodynamic effects of cardiac glycosides on patients' own erythrocytes during glycoside therapy, *Klin. Wochenschr.,* 1981; 59: 1323–1332.
49. **Hermsmeyer, K.,** Electrogenesis of increased norepinephrine sensitivity of arterial vascular smooth muscle in hypertension, *Circ. Res.,* 1976; 38: 362–367.
50. **Nakazato, Y., Ohga, A., and Onoda, Y.,** The effect of ouabain on noradrenaline output from peripheral adrenergic neurons of isolated guinea pig vas deferens, *J. Physiol.,* 1978; 278: 45–54.
51. **Rosati, C., Meyer, P., and Garay, R.,** Sodium transport kinetics in erythrocytes from spontaneously hypertensive rats, *Hypertension,* 1988; 11: 41–48.
52. **Garay, R., Nazaret, C., Dagher, G., Marc, J. C., Bertrand, E., and Meyer, P.,** Approche génétique de l'épidémiologie géographique de l'hypertension artérielle: étude du cotransport Na^+,K^+ chez des africans, *Cardiol. Trop.,* 1982; 8: 49–54.
53. **Canessa, M., Laski, C., and Falkner, B.,** Red blood cell Na^+ transport as a predictor of blood pressure response to Na^+ load in young blacks and whites, *Hypertension,* 1990; 16: 508–514.
54. **Tuck, M. L., Gross, C., Maxwell, M. H., Brickman, A. S., Krasnoshtein, G., and Mayes, D.,** Erythrocyte Na^+,K^+ cotransport and Na^+,K^+ pump in black and Caucasian hypertensive patients, *Hypertension,* 1984; 6: 536–544.
55. **O'Donnell, M. E. and Owen, N. E.,** Reduced Na-K-Cl cotransport in vascular smooth muscle from spontaneously hypertensive rats, *Am. J. Physiol.,* 1988; 255: C169–C180.
56. **Dahl, K., Heine, M., and Thompson, K.,** Genetic influence of the kidneys on blood pressure. Evidence from chronic renal homografts in rats with opposite predispositions to hypertension, *Circ. Res.,* 1974; 34: 94–102.
57. **Bianchi, G., Niutta, E., Ferrari, P., Salvati, P., Salardi, S., Cusi, D., Colombo, R., Cesana, B., Tripodi, G., Pati, P., and Alberghini, E.,** A possible primary role for the kidney in essential hypertension, *Am. J. Hypertension,* 1989; 2(Suppl. 2): 2S–6S.
58. **Weder A. B.,** Red cell lithium countertransport and renal lithium clearance in hypertension, *N. Engl. J. Med.,* 1986; 314: 198–201.
59. **Aronson, P. S.,** Red cell sodium-lithium countertransport and essential hypertension, *N. Engl. J. Med.,* 1983; 307: 313.
60. **Saitta, M., Hannaert, P., Rosati, C., Meyer, P., and Garay, R.,** A kinetic analysis of inward Na^+,K^+ cotransport in erythrocytes from spontaneously hypertensive rats, *J. Hypertension,* 1987; 5(Suppl. 5): S285–S286.
61. **Semplicini, A., Canessa, M., Mozzato, M. G., Ceolotto, G., Marzola, M., Buzzaccarini, F., Casolino, P., and Pessina, A. C.,** Red blood cell Na^+/H^+ and Na^+/Li^+ exchange in patients with essential hypertension, *Am. J. Hypertension,* 1989; 2: 903–908.
62. **De la Sierra, A., Coca, A., Paré, J. C. et al.,** Clinical profiles of essential hypertensives based on their ion transport abnormalities: preliminary results, *J. Hypertension,* in press.
63. **Diez, J., Arrazola, A., Castiella, J., Iñigo, B., and Cía, P.,** Increased activity of the Na^+-dependent Cl^-/HCO_3^- anion exchanger in red cells of patients with essential hypertension, *J. Hypertension,* 1991; 9(Suppl. 6): s308–s309.

64. **Rosati, C., Ruchoux, M. M., Gruber, K., and Garay, R. P.,** Na^+,K^+,Cl^- cotransport system in primary hypertension: studies in red cells and in the choroid plexus of spontaneously hypertensive rats, in *Cellular Aspects of Hypertension,* Bruschi, G. and Borghetti, A., Eds., Heidelberg: Springer-Verlag, 1991: 257–262.
65. **De la Sierra, A., Coca, A., Aguilera, M. T., and Urbano, A.,** Na^+,K^+ ATPase kinetics in a subset of essential hypertensive patients, *Eur. J. Clin. Invest.,* 1988; 18: 337–342.
66. **Garay, R. P. and Nazaret, C.,** Na^+ leak in erythrocytes from essential hypertensive patients, *Clin. Sci.,* 1985; 69: 613–624.
67. **De la Sierra, A., Coca, A., Aguilera, M. T., and Urbano, A.,** Abnormal erythrocyte sodium leak in a subset of essential hypertensive patients, *Klin. Wochenschr.,* 1989; 67: 31–37.
68. **Price, M., Hannaert, P., Dagher, G., and Garay, R. P.** The interaction of internal Na^+ and external K^+ with the erythrocyte Na^+,K^+ cotransport system in essential hypertension, *Hypertension,* 1984; 6: 352–359.
69. **De Mendonça, M., Knorr, A., Grichois, M. L., Ben-Ishay, D., Garay, R., and Meyer, P.,** Erythrocytic sodium ion transport systems in primary and secondary hypertension of the rat, *Kidney Int.,* 1982; 21(Suppl. 11): S69–S75.
70. **L'Allemain, G., Franchi, A., Cragoe, E., Jr., and Pouysségur, J.,** Blockade of the Na^+/H^+ antiport abolishes growth factor-induced DNA synthesis in fibroblasts. Structure activity relationships in the amiloride series, *J. Biol. Chem.,* 1984; 259; 4313–4319.
71. **Folkow, B.,** The structural cardiovascular factor in primary hypertension-pressure dependence and genetic reinforcement, *J. Hypertension,* 1986; Suppl. 3: S51–S56.
72. **Rota, R., Nazaret, C., Henrotte, J. G., Garay, R. P., and Guicheney, P.,** Dissociation between derepressed $[K^+,Cl^-]$ cotransport system and high blood pressure in the F2 hybrid generation (SHR × WKY), *J. Hypertension,* 1991; 9(Suppl. 6): s298–s299.
73. **Pavlovic-Kentera, V., Basara, N., Jerkic, M., Biljanovic-Paunovic, Clemons, G. K., Milenkovic, P., and Susic, D.,** Erythrocytosis in spontaneously hypertensive rats, *Exp. Hematol.,* 1988; 16: 950–953.
74. **De la Sierra, A., Coca, A., Aguilera, M. T., and Urbano-Márquez, A.,** Na^+-Li^+ countertransport in essential hypertension, *J. Hypertension,* 1988; 6: 931–937.
75. **Mongeau, J. G.,** Erythrocyte cation fluxes in essential hypertension of children and adolescents, *Int. J. Pediatr. Nephrol.,* 1985; 6: 41–46.
76. **Postnov, Y. V. and Orlov, S. N.,** Calmodulin-dependent Ca^{2+} transport across plasma membranes in primary hypertension, *Hypertension,* 1983; 1(Suppl. 2): 9–10.

Chapter 2

GENETIC ABNORMALITIES OF THE Na-K-Cl COTRANSPORT IN EXPERIMENTAL AND PRIMARY HYPERTENSION

Patrizia Ferrari and Giuseppe Bianchi

TABLE OF CONTENTS

I. Introduction 26

II. Na-K-Cl Cotransport Characteristics 27

III. Rat Studies 28
- A. Spontaneously Hypertensive Rats 28
- B. Dahl 31
- C. Milan Hypertensive Strain 32

IV. Experimental Hypertension 36

V. Humans 37

VI. Conclusions 39

References 40

0-8493-5474-9/94/$0.00 + $.50

I. INTRODUCTION

Blood pressure (BP) is a quantitative trait which is under genetic and environmental control.[1,2] In Western populations the genetic component accounts for approximately 50% of the BP variability. Essential hypertension (EH) can be considered a familial condition in which polygenes and both individual and shared family environment contribute to the set point of the abnormal BP levels.

Over the last 20 years, many attempts have been made to identify some functional, hormonal, and cellular abnormalities that could be specifically recognized in patients with EH and in the offspring of hypertensive parents as compared to the offspring of normotensive parents.

The aim of these extensive studies was to search for one or more genetic marker(s) to be used either for early diagnosis or, more significantly, to identify the primary molecular mechanisms leading to EH. Among the many alterations observed, a special focus has been pointed toward the alterations of Na handling both at organ (kidney, vasculature, adrenals) and cellular levels. In fact, the evidence that Na handling, especially at kidney level, is altered in a portion of EH and in genetic animal models of hypertension, is widely documented.[3,4] These observations, together with the demonstration that hypertension can be "transplanted" in normotensive rats and humans with the kidney from a hypertensive donor,[5,6] well support the notion of the primary role of the kidney in determining this disease.

As ion transport systems across the cell membrane are the principal determinants of renal Na handling and are involved in vascular and nervous activities, these systems have been extensively studied in human essential hypertensives, normotensive offspring with familiality for hypertension, and rat models of genetic hypertension in an attempt to find some intermediate phenotypes related to the primary genetic mechanisms of hypertension. Research in this direction has been carried out mainly on red or white blood cells (RBC, WBC) under the assumption that these cells could be suitable models for studying generalized abnormalities of cells more directly involved in BP regulation (renal, vasal, nervous).

In this chapter we discuss the problems involved when evaluating the role of one of these transport systems, namely the Na-K-Cl cotransport, in the pathogenesis of hypertension. In particular, we will take into account studies on animal models of genetic hypertension, since the homogeneity of genetic background combined with well-controlled environmental and experimental conditions makes it possible to verify the validity of human studies without interference due to the genetic and environmental heterogeneity of the human population. Furthermore, the use of genetic animal models gives us the opportunity of fixing discrete portions of the parental genotype (hypertensive or normotensive) via selective breeding in recombinant and congenic substrains.[7] The study of these substrains, together with the F2 hybrid population, allows the evaluation of genetic associations between the "pressure level" phenotype and the cellular or biochemical phenotype, identified as abnormal in the parental strain (for instance, faster Na-K-Cl cotransport). These studies represent the preliminary approach for the identification, through a functional cell abnormality, of the molecular, and consequently, genetic abnormality(ies), related to high blood pressure, avoiding the interferences due to the environment and the heterogenous genetic background.

According to these provisos, we summarize and comment on the principal results of the alterations of the Na-K-Cl cotransport reported in genetically hypertensive rats of the spontaneously hypertensive rat (SHR), Dahl, and the Milan strains and in some forms of secondary experimental hypertension. Special reference is made to the Milan strain, in which we have accumulated much evidence of a genetic link between Na-K-Cl cotransport abnormality and the pathogenesis of hypertension. Finally, we attempt to fit the data concerning rats in with those reported by different authors and ourselves in essential hypertensive patients and their offspring in order to understand the meaning of such a membrane ion transport abnormality for human EH.

II. Na-K-Cl COTRANSPORT CHARACTERISTICS

Na-K-Cl cotransport is a system present in different cell types, which couples the movements of Na outside the cell, against its gradient, with that of K along its gradient and vice versa. This system does not require energy, even though adenosine triphosphate (ATP) is important for its maximal efficiency,[8] but it is neutral from the electrochemical point of view because the transport of one Na and one K ion is coupled with that of two Cl ions.[9] Na-K-Cl cotransport is also defined as a furosemide- and bumetanide-sensitive and Cl-dependent pathway, is stimulated by cell shrinkage,[10] and in avian red cells is under control of cyclic adenosine monophosphate (cAMP) stimulation[11] as a consequence of the β-adrenergic receptor activation.[12] An important role of Na-K-Cl cotransport is that of maintaining the Cl ion concentration far from equilibrium, as happens in vascular smooth muscle cells,[13,14] while in epithelial cells, such as those of secretory organs or kidney tubular cells, it mediates the polarized movements of ions leading to net ion extrusion (glands)[15,16] or reabsorption (kidney).[17-19] It is therefore evident that an alteration of this system can play a key role in BP regulation because it can affect vascular contractility and renal Na reabsorption.

As previously reported, the Na-K-Cl cotransport properties in EH and genetic hypertension have been studied mainly in red cells, often giving conflicting results. Some discrepancies among different laboratories can arise from methodological differences in the cotransport measurement. Many authors have examined the outward cotransport mode measuring the furosemide- or bumetanide-sensitive Na or K efflux in Na- and K-free media (''0-trans method''). This system can be applied both to fresh cells with their ''physiological'' intracellular Na concentration and to Na loaded cells in which intracellular Na is artificially raised. Under the 0-trans conditions the cotransporter has a higher rate of translocation and this is a suitable method for measuring the kinetic parameters as a function of the substrate concentrations (cell Na or K). However, considering that the ''physiological'' intracellular Na concentration is a variable function, among the different species, of the experimental and environmental conditions (diet, hormonal status, physical, status, etc.), an alteration of the cotransport activity observed in intact cells does not make it possible to distinguish between a primary abnormal affinity for the substrates or a difference in the number of transport sites from a secondary alteration due to some extracellular factor. Moreover, because cotransport activity is differently stimulated or inhibited by the ion distributions across the cell membrane,[20-22] other relevant information on the characteristics of cotransport in hypertension can be obtained by studying ion influx (usually K or Rb uptake) as a function of the intracellular Na concentrations. These methodological aspects are considered in the following sections when commenting on the results obtained by different authors.

III. RAT STUDIES

The general problem when dealing with a comparison of a phenotypical trait among different strains of SHR is that the possible genetic variability of the same strain produced by different breeders and the methodological variability due to the different procedures applied by different laboratories must be taken into consideration. In particular, it should be noticed that SHR and its control Wistar Kyoto (WKY) rats, bred by different institutions and commercial suppliers, are not genetically homogenous among themselves, and should be considered to be different substrains.[23] Also, the Dahl strain of Brookhaven origin showed some degree of heterozygosis, at least for the renin gene locus.[24] Bearing in mind these provisos, and by selecting those results which have been obtained under comparable experimental conditions, the following attempts to find some common background in order to describe and comment on the Na-K-Cl cotransport alterations in these strains.

A summary of the results obtained in these strains is reported in Table 1, in which for each genetic hypertensive strain and experimental model we have indicated the principal characteristics of RBC in terms of intracellular Na concentration, cotransport rate (at physiological Na_i or V_{max}), and experimental procedure adopted for the ion transport measurements. For comparison with RBC the cotransport rate of other cell types have also been reported. The reference numbers relative to each result are indicated, as explained in more detail in the following paragraphs.

A. SPONTANEOUSLY HYPERTENSIVE RATS

After the first report by Garay et al.[25] of a defect of the RBC Na-K-Cl cotransport in essential hypertension, many studies have been conducted on the RBC of the SHR strain in order to confirm and better understand the functional alterations of the Na-K-Cl cotransport in hypertension in this animal model. The first studies reported a decreased net Na extrusion from Na loaded RBC of both young prehypertensive and adult SHR, without distinguishing between cotransport and other ion transport systems[26] (summarized in Table 1). Afterward, De Mendoca et al.[27] confirmed that at high intracellular Na concentration (70 mmol/l RBC), obtained by loading the cells using PCMBS as the ionophore, the RBC bumetanide-sensitive

TABLE 1
Intracellular Na [Na_i] and Na-K Cotransport Characteristics in RBC of Different Rat Strains With Either Genetic or Experimental Hypertension

Genetic hypertension rat strain	RBC [Na_i]	RBC manipulation	Measurement method	RBC cotransport rate (Km)	Other cells cotransport rate
SHR					
Young	—	Na loaded	Na efflux	↓ (26, 27) ↑ (28)	
Adult	= ↑ (26, 28, 33)	Fresh	Rb uptake	↑ (31–35)	VSMC ↑ (36, 37)
Dahl					
LS young	↑ (41)	Fresh	Rb uptake	↑ (cotr + p.p) (41)	—
HS adult	—	Na loaded	Na efflux	↑ (27)	—
Dahl/JR					
LS young	= (42)	Fresh	Rb uptake	= (42)	—
LS adult	= (42)	Fresh	Rb uptake	= (42)	—
HS young	= (42)	Fresh	Rb uptake	= (42)	—
HS adult	↑ (42)	Fresh	Rb uptake	↑ (42)	—
MHS					
Young	↓ (55)	Fresh	Na efflux	↑ (55,56)	—
Adult	↓ (55)	Na loaded	Na efflux	↑ = (35,55,56) ↓ (56)	VSMC ↑ (88) TAHL ↑ (49)
Experimental hypertension					
2K − 1C	= (32)	Fresh	Rb uptake	= ↑ (32)	—
DOC + Na	↑ (32)	Fresh	Rb uptake	↑ (32)	—
RRM + Na	= (66)	Fresh	Rb uptake	= (66)	—

Note: RBC intracellular Na [(Na_i)], manipulation and methodologies for the measurement of the rate and affinity for internal Na_i (Km) of the RBC Na-K-Cl cotransport in four strains of genetically hypertensive rats and three forms of animal experimental hypertension. 2K-IC = 2 kidney, 1 clip hypertension; DOC + Na = deoxycorticosterone + high Na intake hypertension; RRM + Na = reduced renal mass plus high Na intake hypertension; ↑ ↓ = increased, reduced or equal as compared to the respective normotensive controls; VSMC = vascular smooth muscle cells; TAHL = thick ascending limb of Henle's loop; ( ) = relevant reference numbers, (as explained in text).

Na efflux, measured in Mg-sucrose medium in adult SHR rats, was half that of normotensive WKY rats. More recently, Rosati et al.[28] performed a more complete study on the kinetics of the RBC Na-K-Cl cotransport in both young and adult SHR and WKY rats by measuring both the V_{max} and the K_m for intracellular Na using a less disruptive technique than 2,5-chloromercuribenzoate (PCMBS) for Na loading. In this study, in which the bumetanide-sensitive Na efflux was detected in Mg-sucrose medium (0-trans), Na-K-Cl cotransport of SHR, as compared to WKY rats, showed a decreased affinity for internal Na and a similar V_{max} both at the prehypertensive and hypertensive stages[28] (Table 1). This difference in the cotransport kinetics was also paralleled by a significant increase of the basal intracellular Na concentration in SHR RBC. It seems, therefore, that rather than an abnormality in the maximal rate of Na translocation, the SHR cotransport has a reduced ability to extrude Na in a physiological range of intracellular Na concentrations. This defect could be due either to a primary modification of the internal site for Na (the defect being present before the development of hypertension) or to a different regulatory mechanism of the cotransport carrier, which in turn is due either to a difference in the proteic or lipidic membrane composition or to a second messenger pathway, such as the cAMP-dependent kinase activity.[29] The discrepancy with the first reports, which pointed to a defect in the V_{max} rather than the K_m, may be explained on a methodological basis; in fact, the PCMBS procedure for cation loading can cause important damage to the cell membrane, as verified by a certain degree of hemolysis, and is poorly reproducible. Moreover, the use of a 75 m*M* Mg-sucrose medium for the efflux measurement is not recommended for cotransport analysis, being as this ion transport system is drastically inhibited by a high concentration of extracellular Mg.[30] It is possible, therefore, that in this experimental condition the frequency of low cotransport rate was, in some way, overestimated. Further studies on RBC cotransport in SHR and WKY rats revealed that under physiological conditions, i.e., incubating fresh, nonloaded cells in the presence of Na and K at physiological concentrations, the rate of the bumetanide-sensitive Rb uptake, taken as a congener of K, is increased more in adult SHR than in WKY[31-35] (Table 1). In similar incubating conditions Feig et al.[31] confirmed that the Na efflux, also mediated by the cotransport, is higher in SHR.

The relevance of these results for the characterization of the cotransport alterations in SHR can be better understood bearing in mind the following considerations: (1) under physiological conditions it has been demonstrated that the RBC Na-K-Cl cotransport mediates a net Na extrusion;[21] (2) the net Na extrusion is stimulated by intracellular Na;[21] and (3) the inward K cotransport (i.e., the bumetanide-sensitive Rb uptake) is stimulated by increasing concentrations of intracellular Na;[20] mainly because of an increase in the K/K exchange cotransport mode of operation.[20] Because the intracellular Na concentration in SHR RBC has usually been found to be increased,[26,28,33] probably because of a higher Na passive permeability,[27,31,32] the faster Na-K-Cl cotransport in fresh SHR cells may be secondary to the higher Na content. Furthermore, another possible explanation for the higher Na_i concentration under physiological conditions may be that of a primary abnormality at the intracellular

Na site of the cotransporter. This affects the affinity for ion substrate, and in turn causes the extrusion of Na through the carrier to be defective.

According to the original hypothesis that RBC can represent a cell model for ion transport abnormalities that is also present in other cells which are more directly involved in BP regulation, similar alterations of the Na-K-Cl cotransport have also been found in vascular smooth muscle cells (VSMC) of SHR rats. In particular, two studies from Tokushige et al.[36] and from Kuriyama et al.[37] reported an increased Na-K-Cl cotransport in cultured SHR VSMC (measured in physiological medium) as compared to WKY (Table 1). Because the involvement of cotransport in VSMC and in endothelial cells is mainly in that of reestablishing the Cl and K gradients[13,14] when dissipated, and it is differently modulated by vasoactive hormones such as angiotensin II and atrial natriuretic factor (ANF),[38,39] its alteration in SHR vascular cells can affect vascular contractility or relaxation in this strain.

From a functional point of view, the alterations of Na-K-Cl cotransport in SHR rats are in keeping with an altered cellular Na metabolism, which in turn can affect vascular reactivity or salt and fluid homeostasis in the different tissues. However, no precise indications of a possible genetic link between the BP levels and the phenotypic characteristics of cotransport in SHR have been furnished. The demonstration of such a link, in fact, should be valid proof that the altered Na-K-Cl cotransport is not only functionally but also genetically related to the development of hypertension in this strain. The only study which to our knowledge has approached this problem was conducted by the Postnov group.[34] They studied the cosegregation of c-*src* alleles (coding for the *src* oncogene) with the intermediate phenotype RBC Na-K-Cl cotransport in the two parental strains SHR and WKY and in the F2 hybrids. The results showed that WKY rats with the homozygous genotype WW for the c-*src* locus have a Na-K-Cl cotransport similar to F2 hybrids with the same genotype and statistically lower than those with WS (heterozygous) and SS genotypes, the latter being a characteristic of SHR rats. It seems, therefore, that c-*src* locus cosegregates with the genome locus, determining the Na-K cotransport activity. No further studies have been conducted that could better clarify the possible link between the locus coding for the c-*src* oncogene and cotransport. Moreover, the number of rat hybrids studied was too low and their BP levels were not furnished; thus, a statistically significant conclusion could not be drawn. This remains a possible direction for further studies of genetic cosegregation.

B. DAHL

This strain is characterized by its predisposition to develop hypertension under high Na intake (DS), whereas its control (DR) remains normotensive with the same diet.[41] There are two strains of Dahl rats, one (DS/Jr) which is fully inbred and the other (DS) which does not seem to be fully inbred.[24] This distinction is important in order to understand the genetic meaning of a phenotypic difference between two strains without a completely homogeneous genetic background.

The ion transports have been studied both in DS/Jr and DS rats as a function of the Na diet. De Mendoca et al.[27] measured the Na efflux from Na loaded RBC in DS and DR rats maintained on a high Na diet and found an increased rate of the Na-K-Cl cotransport in DS (Table 1). McCormick et al.[42] found a faster ouabain-insensitive Rb uptake in fresh RBC from prehypertensive DS rats on a low Na diet, without discriminating between the two components of this transport, the passive permeability and the cotransport. A more detailed and complete study was performed by Zicha and Duhm[43] on DS/Jr and DR/Jr rats before and after the development of hypertension using both high and low Na diets (Table 1). The RBC were loaded with a mild procedure to obtain an intracellular Na concentration between 1 and 10 m*M;* the furosemide-sensitive Na and Rb uptake in physiological medium was also measured. Both strains showed an age-dependent increase of the cotransport V_{max}, and only a high Na diet significantly augmented the V_{max} of DS rats without influencing the affinity for extracellular Rb, which did not differ in the two strains. Because adult DS rats that are maintained on a high Na diet showed an increased intracellular Na concentration paralleled by an increased Na leak, the faster rate of cotransport might be secondary to this imbalance of the intracellular Na homeostasis,[43] as also previously seen in SHR rats. It seems, therefore, that in DS and DS/Jr rats the alteration of Na-K-Cl cotransport, when present, is not consistent with a primary defect responsible for the development of hypertension, but is secondary to the effect of the Na load and may represent a compensatory mechanism.

C. MILAN HYPERTENSIVE STRAIN

Milan hypertensive strain (MHS) rats and their normotensive controls, the Milan normotensive strain (MNS), represent an example of two strains maintained for 70 generations by brother-sister mating under inbred conditions.[44] Therefore, from a genetic point of view they represent a suitable model for studying the possible genetic relationship between a functional and a biochemical alteration and the development of high BP. Furthermore, the different methodological approaches of different research groups often responsible for conflicting results on the same subject are avoided when considering the MHS rats, because all the most relevant findings concerning the role of ion transport alterations have been obtained in our own laboratories under well-controlled and comparable conditions.

The study on cell ion transport alterations in MHS rats was the natural successor of the original studies on the organic dysfunctions involved in the pathogenesis of hypertension in Milan rats. In fact, much evidence pointed toward the possibility that an alteration of the cell Na transport at the renal level could be responsible for the key role played by the kidney in MHS hypertension.[45] This evidence can be summarized as follows. In MHS rats hypertension can be transplanted with the kidney;[46,47] therefore, the genetic message responsible for the malfunction may be transmitted through a modification of renal function. When studied *in vitro* MHS kidney showed a faster Na reabsorption and greater oxygen consumption than MNS kidneys.[48] Sodium transport across the luminal tubular membrane was also faster in vesicles from both proximal[49] and ascending portions of the tubule.[50] In the brush border membrane from proximal tubuli the faster Na transport seems to be mediated by the Na-H countertransport,[49] while in the thick ascending limb vesicles it is the

Na-K-Cl cotransport which is responsible for the faster Na transport[50] (Table 1). The latter conclusion was also supported by the results of studies comparing the diuretic effect of bumetanide, hydrochlorothiazide, and amiloride in isolated kidneys from MHS and MNS rats. Sodium excretion after bumetanide treatment was higher in MHS than in either MNS kidney or in MHS kidney receiving the other two diuretics.[51]

That the cotransport system has a key role in transmitting the signal into the macula densa cells that generate the tubuloglomerular feedback (TGF) mechanism is supported by much experimental evidence.[52] As compared to MNS, MHS rats showed a depressed TGF mechanism at the prehypertensive stage, although it was more active during the development of hypertension.[53] This TGF depression in MHS at the prehypertensive stage is most likely due to an increased renal interstitial pressure, which disappears during the development of hypertension,[53] thus unmasking the underlying greater sensitivity of the feedback in the MHS rats. Na-K-Cl adenosine triphosphatase (ATPase) activity was also greater in isolated proximal tubuli[54] and in purified enzyme from the kidney cortex of MHS as compared to MNS.[55] Taken together, these findings are consistent with the notion that faster Na transport across the tubular epithelium is an important cause of hypertension in MHS rats and that an abnormality of the Na-K-Cl cotransport may well be linked to the primary defect responsible for the renal dysfunction. The studies were then extended to RBC under the provisos that they can represent a model for more generalized defects and also because they are easily handled.

Because hypertension develops in MHS rats at 1 month of age, age-dependent RBC characteristics have been studied[56] and three principal differences present before and during the development of hypertension have been recognized in MHS as compared to MNS rats (Table 1): (1) a smaller RBC volume, (2) a lower intracellular Na concentration, and (3) a faster outward Na-K-Cl cotransport measured as 0-trans in fresh, nonloaded cells. Kinetic analysis, performed according to the method applied by Rosati et al.[28] for SHR studies, revealed that the faster RBC cotransport of MHS, measured at physiological intracellular Na concentration, was due to a higher affinity for Na_i than in MNS RBC[57] (Table 1). From this point of view it can also be speculated that the lower Na_i of MHS RBC, present before the development of hypertension, is actually due to the faster rate of cotransport at "physiological" Na content level, because the Na-K pump is the same in the two groups.[56] These results on MHS RBC have also been confirmed by other groups,[35,90] in particular by Orlov et al.,[35] who found an increased cotransport in MHS RBC, measured also as furosemide-sensitive Rb uptake.

A biochemical abnormality in a plasma membrane may have three different causes: genetic, environmental, or secondary readjustment to an extracellular or intracellular mechanism (for instance, hormonal or humoral factors). In order to differentiate among these possibilities, we transplanted bone marrow from MHS and MNS rats into F1 hybrids that had been previously irradiated to destroy their own bone marrow.[58] The RBC volume was measured 3 months after transplantation and found to be smaller in the recipients of MHS bone marrow as compared to the volume in recipients of MNS bone marrow. The intracellular Na concentration was lower and the rate of the Na-K-Cl cotransport was also faster.[58] This clearly demonstrated that the genetic message responsible for the faster Na-K-Cl cotransport and the smaller RBC volume of MHS was present in the stem cell, and that environmental factors or secondary readjustment through extracellular mechanisms were not responsible for these differences between MHS and MNS rats. Moreover, in F2 hybrids, obtained by crossing (MHS × MNS) F1 hybrids, the rate of RBC Na-K-Cl cotransport was correlated with the level of BP, suggesting a genetic association between these two traits.[58] More recently, we have confirmed this result using a different experimental approach. Starting from the F2 population, by selective crosses, we fixed different portions of the genetic background of the two parental strains into recombinant substrains (MHN) that are phenotypically characterized by different levels of BP.[59] In these strains we measured some RBC characteristics such as the volume, the cotransport rate, and the activity of a cytosolic Ca-dependent protease, calpain, previously found to be more active in MHS rats,[60] and therefore possibly involved in a secondary readjustment of the ion transport activity. The aim of this experiment was to verify if these cellular phenotypic traits were maintained according to the BP levels or dissociated in the recombinants and, therefore, whether they were related to each other. The results showed that only the RBC cotransport rate paralleled the levels of BP in the different recombinant strains, while the cell volume and the calpain activity were similar to those of the MNS rats, despite the high BP levels of the MHNE strain.[61] However, these experiments do not exclude that the faster Na-K-Cl cotransport may be due to a secondary modification aimed at reestablishing the cell homeostasis otherwise altered by a gene mutation, the product of which is not strictly related to the proteins involved in the Na-K-Cl cotransport control.

To evaluate this possibility we carried out the following series of experiments. To verify whether the faster Na-K-Cl cotransport was influenced by the membrane protein composition or by some cytosolic factor, we compared the cotransport kinetics both in intact RBC and in inside-out vesicles (IOV) prepared from MHS and MNS erythrocytes.[57]

In these vesicles the transmembrane proteins responsible for ion translocation across the cell membrane were preserved, while the cytosol and the membrane skeleton proteins were removed. In contrast to intact RBC, Na-K-Cl cotransport rate and the affinity for internal Na were similar in IOV from both strains.[57] This excludes the possibility that the transmembrane protein itself causes the differences in intact RBC, but neither does it prove the possible influence of a cytosolic factor. To exclude the last hypothesis, we characterized the Na-K-Cl cotransport (measured as bumetanide-, K-, and Cl-sensitive Na efflux) in resealed ghosts, in which the membrane skeleton is preserved without the cytosolic component.[62] Resealed ghosts of MHS still showed a faster Na-K-Cl cotransport at physiological Na_i concentrations and a smaller volume than those from MNS rats.[62] Therefore, the results from IOV and resealed ghosts support the hypothesis that the primary alteration of the cotransport system in MHS is in some way related to a membrane skeletal component, probably having a modulatory role, rather than to an integral protein or a cytosolic factor.

With the aim of discovering possible structural protein differences between MHS and MNS, we then injected erythrocyte membrane or membrane skeleton extracts from MNS into MHS and vice versa. After two immunizations MHS recipients treated with MNS extract selectively produced an antibody against a 105-kDa membrane skeleton protein.[63] This protein was later identified as adducin.[64] In human erythrocytes this protein is an α-β heterodimer with subunit of M_r 103,000 α and 97,000 β. In the beginning, the MHS antisera was used to screen a cDNA expression library; a positive clone coding for a portion of the rat β adducin subunit was identified. Then, the polymerase chain reaction (PCR) techniques were used to isolate the full-length cDNA coding for the β adducin subunit. Degenerate primers PCR amplification allowed us to obtain 90% of the coding region for the rat α adducin subunit. The comparison between MHS and MNS nucleotide sequences revealed a point mutation in the thus far known α subunit sequence leading to a tyrosine (MHS) and phenylalanine (MNS) substitution. A second point mutation was found in the coding sequence of the β subunit resulting in an arginine-glutamine substitution. We had already noticed some degree of polymorphism in MNS when studying the antibody response of the two strains after the antigen injection. The evaluation of the genotypes confirmed this phenomenon, at least for the β sequence. Namely, all the MHS rats studied were arg/arg, while in the MNS strains three genotypes were present: arg/arg, arg/gln, and gln/gln,[64,65] suggesting that in spite of the close inbreeding, for more than 50 generations something prevented the achievement of homozygosis at the β adducin locus in the normotensive strain. It should be noted that when tested for 15 other loci, homozygosis was present in all.[91] Studies to complete the cDNA sequence of the α adducin subunit and to investigate tissue and strain specific expression of adducin genes are still in progress. In accordance with present knowledge, we proposed four possible reasons for this selective heterozygosis at the β adducin locus in the MNS inbred strain of rats:[66]

1. Homozygosis is lethal
2. Homozygosis reduces biological fitness
3. Selection for lower blood pressure favors heterozygosis
4. Mutations occur

The first two reasons are not likely because we have animals with homozygosis at the β adducin locus without differences in the body growth as compared to the heterozygotic animal. The fourth possibility is also unlikely because the difference in the antibody response was detected for the first time in 1989,[63] and since then more than 10 generations have been obtained, although the heterozygosis was maintained throughout these generations. Therefore, if a point mutation occurred without being related to the process of selection, it would be expected to disappear during the following generations. All things considered, therefore, we tend to favor the third hypothesis, which is currently under experimental evaluation. This series of experiments can be taken as one attempt to establish a cause-effect relationship from a given alteration of a gene through a membrane ion transport abnormality to the renal dysfunction responsible for the increase in BP, at least in this rat model.

IV. EXPERIMENTAL HYPERTENSION

The analysis of the ion transport pathways in animals which have been made hypertensives by an experimental maneuver could be particularly useful to discriminate primary alterations from a secondary readjustment or alteration caused by the hypertensive maneuver. Unfortunately, to our knowledge only two reports approached the problem of the cotransport modifications in experimental hypertension (Table 1). In 1983 Duhm et al.[32] measured the RBC volume, intracellular Na concentration, and the principal ion transport systems both in rats with a 2K-1C and DOC or DOC + salt hypertension. The 2K-1C rats did not show significant modifications of the cotransport system, measured in fresh RBC as furosemide-sensitive Rb uptake, as compared to controls. However, a tendency to an increased rate was observed, but the low number of rats studied did not allow any further speculation. In DOC and DOC + salt hypertension, the Na-K-Cl cotransport was greatly increased (respectively, two and three times more than in controls).[32] This effect did not seem due to a direct effect of DOC on RBC, because *in vitro* preincubation of the RBC with DOC did not alter the Na and K transports.[32] However, the alteration of cotransport should be due to a secondary effect of DOC on plasma K concentration and cell volume. In fact, rats treated with DOC or DOC + salt showed an important hypokalemia and parallel reduction of RBC volume. In experimental conditions in which Na-K-Cl cotransport was studied both in RBC from rat with hypokalemia induced by a low K diet or in rat RBC whose volume was osmotically altered, the furosemide-sensitive Rb uptake rose according to the level of hypokalemia and shrinking, suggesting that the increase of cotransport observed in DOC + salt hypertension was at least partially due to the K deficiency.[32]

The second study concerns rats made hypertensives by a subtotal nephrectomy with high Na diet.[67] Severe hypertension developed when the renal mass reduction and the Na load was performed in young Sprague-Dawley rats and was characterized by an increase of heart rate and reduction of hematocrit compatible with a volume-dependent hypertension.[67] The furosemide-sensitive Rb uptake, measured in a physiological range of intracellular Na concentrations, did not show any significant differences in the kinetic parameter as compared to normotensive controls (sub-nephrectomized rats at low Na diet). The same was true for the Na and K passive permeability, while the Na-K-Cl pump showed a lower affinity for intracellular Na responsible for a decreased rate at physiological Na concentration level (around 3 m*M*).[67] Therefore, these findings question the hypothesis that in secondary forms of hypertension alterations of the Na-K-Cl cotransport may be responsible for the development or maintenance of high BP.

V. HUMANS

The implications of the Na-K-Cl cotransport alterations in human essential hypertension are arguments dealt with in Chapter 3 of this book. However, here we attempt to draw some parallels between the most relevant results obtained in humans, in particular, those obtained by our group, and rat studies, with an aim to explaining some of the discrepancies in the human studies and to developing new approaches for understanding the molecular basis of the cell dysfunction responsible for the essential hypertension.

Historically, interest in the alterations of the ion transport systems as possible causes or genetic markers for essential hypertension arose from human studies that described a defect of the net Na and K transport in RBC from Caucasian essential hypertensives and some of their descendants.[68] This was later recognized as being due to a deficiency of the Na-K-Cl cotransport.[25] Since those studies, dozens of papers have been published on the existence of other ion transport defects in EH and, in particular, for the Na-K-Cl cotransport; either normal,[69-72] reduced,[73-76] or increased[77-80] activities have been reported. As previously stated, many of these conflicting results can be interpreted in terms of methodological differences of the assay and, more relevantly, the different criteria adopted for sampling the human population for these studies. Na-K-Cl cotransport has been measured mostly in fresh RBC as furosemide-sensitive Na efflux in Na-free medium (0-trans method); although this method of measurement gives the ''physiological'' rate of this transport, it does not furnish any information on its kinetic characteristics and in particular on its ability to respond, in different subjects, to different intracellular Na challenge. The main findings obtained in studying the K_m and the V_{max} of the system in RBC loaded with increasing Na contents are

1. The V_{max} is a family aggregate,[73] and is under genetic control. Lewitter and Canessa[81] calculated from twin studies that heritability can account for 84% of the general variability.
2. The V_{max} in EH as compared to normotensives is highly variable, being either higher, lower, or equal.[69-80]
3. The regulatory ability to handle Na_i was found to be decreased (lower affinity for Na_i) in 20 to 40% EH, according to Price et al.[82]

To understand the apparent discrepancy of the results on V_{max}, at point (2), we studied the distribution of the RBC Na-K-Cl cotransport in 209 EH rats that were either never treated with hypotensive drugs or were under washout from at least 4 months old, and 123 normotensive controls without familiality for hypertension.[83] All the subjects were healthy, nonobese, and nondislipidemic. By adjusting the results for the confounding variables such as sex, weight, age, and height, we found that the distribution models that best fit in with the experimental data were unimodal in normotensives and bimodal in EH (Figure 1). The finding that cotransport is distributed bimodally only in EH can be interpreted in terms of a genetic

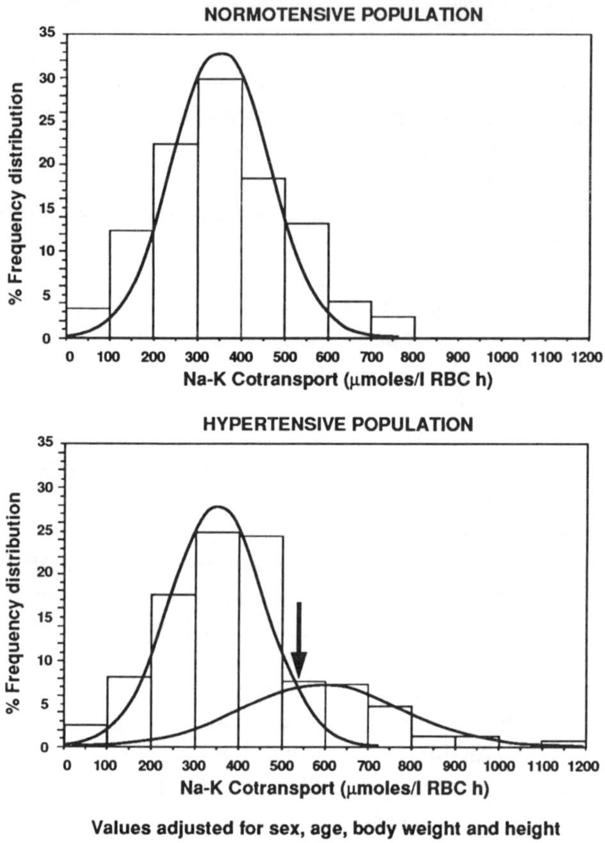

FIGURE 1. Distribution of adjusted Na-K-Cl cotransport values in hypertensive and normotensive groups of patients. The arrow indicates the nadir of the two distributions, corresponding to 530 μmol/l RBC h^{-1}, the arbitrary dividing point between "normal" and "high" Na-K-Cl cotransport hypertensive patients. (From Cusi, D. et al., *Am. J. Hypertension,* 4, 729, 1991. With permission.)

polymorphism of the cotransport only in EH; i.e., some major gene may influence the phenotypic expression of this ion transport in hypertensives.

In a second study,[83] we also considered the interfamilial correlation of different RBC transport systems and Na_i between spouses and between midparent (mean of the two parents) and offspring values in 47 families with at least one hypertensive parent and 39 families with both normotensive parents. This kind of study allows the dissection of the genetic from the environmental component of the variance of a phenotypic trait. Na_i and Na-K-Cl pump were found highly and significantly correlated between spouses, suggesting a strong influence of environment on these parameters. Conversely, Na-K-Cl cotransport was found to correlate between mid-parents and offspring only in hypertensive families ($r = 0.42$ hypertensives, $r = 0.09$ normotensives) and not between spouses of the two family groups, indicating that only in the hypertensive subset of population does this phenotypic trait have greater genetic polymorphism. According to the bimodal distribution in EH, an arbitrary cutoff for the high and low cotransport activity was put at 530 μmol/l RBC/h^{-1}, and a simple segregation analysis was performed on the total of the families to verify the hypothesis that Na-K-Cl cotransport is transmitted as a recessive character for the high phenotype. The results were compatible with such a hypothesis, suggesting that cotransport can be partly determined by a recessive major gene coding for the "high" phenotype, and this gene effect is present only in hypertensive families, because the "high" phenotype is absent in normotensives with a negative family history.[83]

When patients with high cotransport were compared to those with either normal cotransport or with normotensive controls, the former showed lower plasma renin, increased diuretic response to a furosemide injection,[84] greater BP fall with diuretic treatment as compared to angiotensin-converting enzyme (ACE) inhibitor or beta-blocker treatments,[85] and a lower fractional excretion of urate[86] than normotensive subjects (taken as an index of proximal tubular reabsorption). This suggests that as in MHS, patients with high cotransport may also have a faster proximal tubular reabsorption. Moreover, according to the bimodal distribution of cotransport in EH, it is conceivable that animal models other than MHS might represent other subsets of hypertensive patients with different phenotypic expressions of the cotransport. For instance, Dahl rats show a faster Na-K-Cl cotransport when undergoing a high Na diet.[43] Recently, Canessa et al.[87] showed that both the K_m and the V_{max} of the RBC Na-K-Cl cotransport were significantly influenced by the level of the Na diet only in hypertensive subjects. It is possible that the low intracellular Na affinity of the cotransport in EH[88] or the reduced activity[73-76] reported by some authors are, in part, linked to a variable salt intake.

VI. CONCLUSIONS

From all the rat and human study findings collected, it is logical to suggest the existence, among the overall EH population, of a defined nosological entity with its own pathogenetic mechanism(s). However, in order to prove the existence of this new clinical entity we need to demonstrate that these biochemical, cell, or organic dysfunctions are accompanied by precise genetic-molecular abnormality(ies) which may explain such dysfunctions. Only by measuring all these factors (or the most important of them) in the individual patients or subjects within a family tree can we evaluate the genetic mode of transmission of a given ion transport system abnormality and its relevance for the BP set point. Indeed, the complexity of the interactions between genetic and environmental factors, which may also influence the level of BP, hampers the attempt to study the mode of genetic transmission of their variables in the individual member of a family tree. We may reduce the complexity of these factors by studying the genetics of ion transport systems as an intermediate phenotype. However, we must recognize that we are only at the beginning of new research which will give meaningful results only if we are aware of the requirements to be fulfilled in order to identify the genetic-molecular mechanisms of a complex disease such as arterial hypertension. The most important of these requirements is the appropriate genetic characterization of the strain of animals we are going to use as genetic models for these experiments. Only when the sequence of events going from a given genetic abnormality to arterial hypertension is clarified in animal models of primary hypertension shall we have the theoretical background to be able to approach in man, with the appropriate tools, the huge complexity of the relationship between the ion transport systems and both the primary genetic-molecular abnormality and the cell dysfunction responsible for arterial hypertension.

REFERENCES

1. **Mialle, W. E., Heneage, P., Kholsa, T., Lovell, H. G., and Moore, P.,** Factors influencing the degree of resemblance in arterial pressure of close relatives, *Clin. Sci.,* 33, 271, 1967.
2. **Mongeau, J., Byron, P., and Sing, C. F.,** The influence of genetics and household environment upon the variability of normal blood pressure: the Montreal adoption study, *Clin. Exp. Hypertension,* 8, 653, 1986.
3. **DeWardener, H. E.,** The primary role of the kidney and salt intake in the aetiology of essential hypertension. I., *Clin. Sci.,* 79, 193, 1990.
4. **DeWardener, H. E.,** The primary role of the kidney and salt intake in the aetiology of essential hypertension. II., *Clin. Sci.,* 79, 289, 1990.
5. **Bianchi, G., Fox, U., Di Francesco, G. F., Giovanetti, A. M., and Pagetti, D.,** Blood pressure changes produced by kidney cross-transplantation between spontaneously hypertensive rats and normotensive rats, *Clin. Sci. Mol. Med.,* 47, 435, 1974.
6. **Guidi, E., Bianchi, G., and Rivolta, E.,** Hypertension in man with a kidney transplant: role of familial versus other factors, *Nephron,* 41, 14, 1985.
7. **Green, E. L.,** Mating systems, in *Biology of the Laboratory Mouse,* Green, E. L., Ed., McGraw-Hill, New York, 1966, 11.
8. **Dagher, G., Brugnara, C., and Canessa, M.,** Effect of metabolic depletion on the furosemide-sensitive Na and K fluxes in human red blood cells, *Membr. Biol.,* 86, 145, 1985.
9. **Haas, M.,** Properties and diversity of (Na-K-Cl) cotransporters, *Annu. Rev. Physiol.,* 51, 443, 1989.
10. **Lauf, P. K., McManus, T. J., Haas, M. et al.,** Physiology and biophysics of chloride and cation cotransport across the cell membrane, *Fed. Proc.,* 46, 2377, 1987.
11. **Palfrey, H. C., Feit, P. W., and Greencard, P.,** cAMP-stimulated cation cotransport in avian erythrocytes: inhibition by "loop" diuretics, *Am. J. Physiol.,* 238(Cell Physiol. 7), C139, 1980.
12. **Haas, M., Schmidt, W. F., III, and McManus, T. J.,** Catecholamine-stimulated ion transport in duck red cells. Gradient effects in electrically neutral (Na^+K^+2Cl) cotransport, *J. Gen. Physiol.,* 80, 125, 1982.
13. **Owen, N. E.,** Regulation of Na/K/Cl cotransport in vascular smooth muscle, *Biochem. Biophys. Res. Commun.,* 125, 500, 1985.
14. **Brock, T. A., Brugnara, C., Canessa, M., and Gimbrone, M. A.,** Bradykinin and vasopressin stimulate Na-K-Cl cotransport in cultured endothelial cells, *Am. J. Physiol.,* 250, C888, 1986.
15. **Hannafin, J., Kinne-Saffran, E., Friedman, D., and Kinne, R.,** Presence of a sodium-potassium-chloride cotransport system in the rectal gland of *Squalus acanthias, J. Membr. Biol.,* 75, 73, 1983.

16. **Turner, R. J., George, J. N., and Baum, B. J.,** Evidence for a Na/K/Cl cotransport system in basolateral membrane vesicles from rabbit parotid, *J. Membr. Biol.*, 94, 143, 1986.
17. **Greger, R.,** Ion transport mechanisms in thick ascending limb of Henle's loop mammalian nephrons, *Physiol. Rev.*, 65, 760, 1985.
18. **Greger, R. and Schlatter, E.,** Properties of the basolateral membrane of cortical thick ascending limb of Henle's loop of rabbit kidney, *Pfluegers' Arch.*, 396, 325, 1983.
19. **Molony, D. A., Reeves, W. B., and Andreoli, T. E.,** Na^+:K^+:$2Cl^-$ cotransport and the thick ascending limb, *Kidney Int.*, 36, 418, 1989.
20. **Canessa, M., Brugnara, C., Cusi, D., and Tosteson, D. C.,** Modes of operation and variable stoichemetry of the furosemide-sensitive Na and K fluxes in human red cells, *J. Gen. Physiol.*, 87, 113, 1986.
21. **Brugnara, C., Canessa, M., Cusi, D., and Tosteson, D. C.,** Furosemide-sensitive Na and K fluxes in human red cells. Net uphill Na extrusion and equilibration properties, *J. Gen. Physiol.*, 87, 91, 1986.
22. **Duhm, J.,** Furosemide-sensitive K^+ (Rb^+) transport in human erythrocytes: modes of operation, dependence on extracellular and intracellular Na^+, kinetics, pH dependency and the effect of cell volume and N-ethylmaleimide, *J. Membr. Biol.*, 98, 15, 1987.
23. **Nabika, T., Nara, Y., Ikeda, K., Endo, J., and Yamori, Y.,** Genetic heterogeneity of the spontaneously hypertensive rat, *Hypertension,* 18, 12, 1991.
24. **O'Dowd, B. F. and Rapp, J. P.,** Heterogeneity of renin alleles in outbred Dahl salt-sensitive (Brookhaven) rats, *Hypertension,* 18, 9, 1991.
25. **Garay, R. P., Dagher, G., Pernollet, M. G., Devynck, M. A., and Meyer, P.,** Inherited defect in Na^+,K^+-cotransport system in erythrocytes from essential hypertensive patients, *Nature,* 284, 281, 1980.
26. **DeMendoca, M., Garay, R. P., Ben-Ishay, D., and Meyer, P.,** Abnormal erythrocyte cation transport in primary hypertension. Clinical and experimental studies, *Hypertension,* 3(Suppl. I), 179, 1981.
27. **DeMendoca, M., Knorr, A., Grichois, M. L., Brossard, M., Garay, R. P., Ben-Ishay, D., and Meyer, P.,** Erythrocyte Na^+ transport systems in three strains of genetically hypertensive rats, *Klin. Wochenschr.*, 63 (Suppl. III), 66, 1985.
28. **Rosati, C., Meyer, P., and Garay, R.,** Sodium transport kinetics in erythrocytes from spontaneously hypertensive rats, *Hypertension,* 11, 41, 1988.
29. **Garay, R. P.,** Inhibition of the Na^+,K^+ cotransport system by cyclic AMP and intracellular Ca^{2+} in human red cells, *Biochem. Biophys. Acta,* 688, 786, 1984.
30. **Ellory, J. C., Flatman, P. W., and Stewart, G. W.,** Inhibition of human red cell Na and K transport by divalent ions, *J. Gen. Physiol.*, 340, 1983.
31. **Feig, P. U., Mitchell, P. P., and Boylan, J. W.,** Erythrocyte membrane transport in hypertensive humans and rats. Effect of sodium depletion and excess, *Hypertension,* 7, 423, 1985.
32. **Duhm, J., Göbel, B. O., and Beck, F. X.,** Sodium and potassium ion transport accelerations in erythrocytes of DOC, DOC-Salt, two-kidney, one clip and spontaneously hypertensive rats. Role of hypokalemia and cell volume, *Hypertension,* 5, 642, 1983.
33. **Saitta, M. N., Hannaert, P. A., Rosati, C., Meyer, P., and Garay, R. P.,** A kinetic analysis of inward Na^+,K^+ cotransport in erythrocytes from spontaneously hypertensive rats, *J. Hypertension,* 5(Suppl. 5), S285, 1987.
34. **Kotelevtsev, Y. V., Spitkovski, D. D., Orlov, S. N., and Postnov, Y. V.,** Interstrain restriction fragment length polymorphism in the c-src correlates with Na,K cotransport and calcium content in hybrid rat erythrocytes, *J. Hypertension,* 7(Suppl. 6), S112, 1989.
35. **Orlov, S. N., Postnov, I. Y., Pokudin, N. I., Kukharenko, V. Y., and Postnov, Y. V.,** Na^+-H^+ exchange and other ion-transport systems in erythrocytes of essential hypertensives and spontaneously hypertensive rats: a comparative analysis, *J. Hypertension,* 7, 781, 1989.
36. **Tokushige, A., Kino, M., Tamura, H., Hopp, L., Searle, B. M., and Aviv, A.,** Bumetanide-sensitive sodium-22 transport in vascular smooth muscle cell of the spontaneously hypertensive rat, *Hypertension,* 8, 379, 1986.

37. **Kuriyama, S., Denny, T. N., and Aviv, A.,** $^{22}Na^+$ and $^{86}Rb^+$ transport in vascular smooth muscle of SHR, Wistar Kyoto, and Wistar rats, *J. Cardiovasc. Pharmacol.*, 11, 722, 1988.
38. **O'Donnell, M. E.,** Endothelial cell sodium-potassium-cloride cotransport. Evidence of regulation by Ca^{2+} and protein kinase C, *J. Biol. Chem.*, 266, 11559, 1991.
39. **Owen, N. E. and Ridge, K. M.,** Mechanism of angiotensin II stimulation of Na-K-Cl cotransport of vascular smooth muscle cells, *Am. J. Physiol.*, 257(Cell Physiol. 26), C629, 1989.
40. **O'Donnell, M. E. and Owen, N. E.,** Reduced Na-K-Cl cotransport in vascular smooth muscle cells from spontaneously hypertensive rats, *Am. J. Physiol.*, 255(Cell Physiol. 24), C169, 1988.
41. **Dahl, L. K., Knudsen, K. D., and Heine, M.,** Effects of chronic excess salt ingestion: modification of experimental hypertension in the rat by variations in the diet, *Circ. Res.*, 22, 11, 1968.
42. **McCormick, C. P., Hennessy, J. F., Rauch, A. L., and Buckalew, V. M., Jr.,** Erythrocyte sodium concentration and ^{86}Rb uptake in weanling Dahl rats, *Am. J. Hypertension*, 2, 604, 1989.
43. **Zicha, J. and Duhm, J.,** Kinetics of Na^+ and K^+ transport in red blood cells of Dahls rats. Effects of age and salt, *Hypertension*, 15, 612, 1990.
44. **Bianchi, G., Barber, B. R., Ferrari, P., and Duzzi, L.,** The Milan hypertensive strain of rats and its control normotensive strain, *Hypertension*, 9(Suppl. I), 30, 1987.
45. **Bianchi, G., Ferrari, P., and Barber, B. R.,** Lessons from experimental genetic hypertension, in *Hypertension: Pathophysiology, Diagnosis and Management*, Laragh, J. H. and Brenner, B. M., Eds., Raven Press, New York, 1990, chap. 58.
46. **Bianchi, G., Fox, U., Di Francesco, G. F., Giovanetti, A. M., and Pagetti, D.,** Blood pressure changes produced by kidney cross-transplantation between spontaneously hypertensive rats and normotensive rats, *Clin. Sci. Mol. Med.*, 47, 435, 1974.
47. **Fox, U. and Bianchi, G.,** The primary role of the kidney in causing the blood pressure difference between the Milan hypertensive strain (MHS) and normotensive rats (MNS), in *Proc. Symp. Spontaneous Genetic Hypertension in Rats, Clin. Exp. Pharm. Physiol.*, Suppl. 3, 71, 1976.
48. **Salvati, P., Ferrario, R. G., Parenti, P., and Bianchi, G.,** Renal function of isolated perfused kidneys from hypertensive (MHS) and normotensive (MNS) rats of the Milan strain: role of calcium, *J. Hypertension*, 5, 31, 1987.
49. **Hanozet, G., Parenti, P., and Salvati, P.,** Presence of a potential sensitive Na transport across renal brush-border membrane vesicles from rats of the Milan hypertensive strain, *Biochem. Biophys. Acta*, 819, 179, 1985.
50. **Ferrandi, M., Salardi, S., Parenti, P., Ferrari, P., Bianchi, G., Braw, R., and Karlish, S. J. D.,** $Na^+/K^+/Cl^-$-cotransporter mediated Rb^+ fluxes in membrane vesicles from kidneys of normotensive and hypertensive rats, *Biochim. Biophys. Acta Biomembr.*, 1021, 13, 1990.
51. **Salvati, P., Ferrario, R. G., and Bianchi, G.,** Diuretic effect of bumetanide in isolated perfused kidneys of Milan hypertensive rats, *Kidney Int.*, 37, 1084, 1990.
52. **Lapoint, J. Y., Bell, P. D., and Cardinal, J.,** Direct evidence for apical Na^+:$2Cl^-$:K^+ cotransport in macular densa cells, *Am. J. Physiol.*, 258, F1469, 1990.
53. **Boberg, U. and Persson, E. G.,** Increased tubuloglomerular feedback activity in Milan hypertensive rats, *Am. J. Physiol.*, 250, F967, 1986.
54. **Melzi, M. L., Bertorello, A., Fukuda, Y., Muldin, I., Sereni, F., and Aperia, A.,** Na,K-ATPase activity in renal tubule cells from Milan hypertensive rats, *Am. J. Hypertension*, 2, 563, 1989.
55. **Parenti, P., Villa, M., Hanozet, G. M., Ferrandi, M., and Ferrari, P.,** Increased Na pump activity in the kidney cortex of the Milan hypertensive rat strain, *FEBS Lett.*, 290, 200, 1991.
56. **Ferrari, P., Ferrandi, M., Torielli, L., Canessa, M., and Bianchi, G.,** Relationship between erythrocyte volume and sodium transport in the Milan hypertensive rat and age-dependent changes, *J. Hypertension*, 5, 199, 1987.
57. **Ferrari, P., Torielli, L., Cirillo, M., Salardi, S., and Bianchi, G.,** Sodium transport kinetics in erythrocytes and inside-out vesicles from Milan rats, *J. Hypertension*, 9, 703, 1991.
58. **Bianchi, G., Ferrari, P., Trizio, D., Ferrandi, M., Torielli, L., Barber, B. R., and Polli, E.,** Red blood cell abnormalities and spontaneous hypertension in the rat: a genetically determined link, *Hypertension*, 7, 319, 1985.

59. **Barber, B. R.,** *Rat News Lett.,* 22, 16, 1989.
60. **Pontremoli, S., Melloni, E., Salamino, F., Sparatore, B., Viotti, P., Michetti, M., Duzzi, L., and Bianchi, G.,** Decreased level of Calpain inhibitor activity in kidney from Milan hypertensive rats, *Biochem. Biophysical. Res. Commun.,* 145, 1287, 1987.
61. **Ferrari, P., Torielli, L., Barber, B. R., Soldati, L., Duzzi, L., and Bianchi, G.,** Characteristics of Recombinant Strains of Milan Rats, abstract submitted to the 14th Meet. Int. Soc. Hypertension, Madrid, 1992.
62. **Ferrari, P., Torielli, L., Salardi, S., Rizzo, A., and Bianchi, G.,** Na-K-Cl cotransport in resealed ghosts from erythrocytes of the Milan hypertensive rats, *Biochem. Biophys. Acta,* 1111, 111, 1992.
63. **Salardi, S., Saccardo, B., Borsani, G., Modica, R., Ferrandi, M., Tripodi, M. G., Soria, M., Ferrari, P., Baralle, F. E., Sidoli, A., and Bianchi, G.,** Erythrocyte adducin differential properties in normotensive and hypertensive rats of the Milan strain (characterization of spleen adducin m-RNA), *Am. J. Hypertension,* 2, 229, 1989.
64. **Joshi, R., Gilligan, D. M., Otto, E., McLaughlin, T., and Bennett, V.,** Primary structure and domain organization of human alpha and beta adducin, *J. Cell Biol.,* 115, 665, 1991.
65. **Tripodi, G., Piscone, A., Borsani, G., Tisminietzky, S., Salardi, S., Sidoli, A., James, P., Pongor, S., Bianchi, G., and Baralle, F. E.,** Molecular cloning of an adducin-like protein: evidence of a polymorphism in the normotensive and hypertensive rats of the Milan strain, *Biochem. Biophys. Res. Commun.,* 177, 939, 1991.
66. **Bianchi, G., Ferrari, P., Cusi, D., Tripodi, G., and Barber, B.,** Genetic aspects of ion transport systems in hypertension, *J. Hypertension,* 8(Suppl. 7), S213, 1990.
67. **Zicha, J., Kronauer, J., and Duhm, J.,** Effects of a chronic high salt intake on blood pressure and the kinetics of sodium and potassium transport in erythrocytes of young and adult subtotally nephrectomized Sprague-Dawley rats, *J. Hypertension,* 8, 207, 1990.
68. **Garay, R. P. and Meyer, P.,** A new test showing abnormal net Na^+ and K^+ fluxes in erythrocytes of essential hypertensive patients, *Lancet,* 1, 349, 1979.
69. **Weder, A. B., Torretti, B. A., and Julius, S.,** Racial differences in erythrocyte cation transport, *Hypertension,* 6, 115, 1984.
70. **Delva, P., De Gaspari, M., Degan, M., Covi, G., and Lechi, A.,** Kinetics of bumetanide-sensitive Na-K cotransport in erythrocytes of essential hypertensive patients, *Clin. Sci.,* 69, 607, 1985.
71. **Ringel, R. E., Hamlyn J. M., Schaeffer, J., Hamilton, B. P., Kowarski, A. A., Blaustein, M. P., and Berman, M. A.,** Red cell cotransport activity and sodium content in black men: relationship to essential hypertension, *Hypertension,* 6, 724, 1984.
72. **Krzesinski, J. M. and Rorive, G. L.,** The erythrocyte sodium-potassium cotransport in hypertensive patients: advantages and limitations, *Clin. Exp. Hypertension,* A7, 553, 1985.
73. **Cusi, D., Barlassina, C., Ferrandi, M., Lupi, P., Ferrari, P., and Bianchi, G.,** Familial aggregation of cation transport abnormalities and essential hypertension, *Clin. Exp. Hypertension,* 3, 871, 1981.
74. **Ghione, S., Buzzigoli, G., Bartolini, V., Balzan, S., and Donato, L.,** Comparison of outward and inward Na/K cotransport-mediated fluxes in erythrocytes of essential hypertensive patients. Preliminary results, *Clin. Exp. Hypertension,* 3, 809, 1981.
75. **Davidson, J. S., Opie, L. H., and Kedig, B.,** Sodium-potassium cotransport activity as a genetic marker in essential hypertension, *Br. Med. J.,* 284, 539, 1982.
76. **Andrews, D. I., Evans, J. I., Waal-Manning, H. J., and Simpson F. O.,** Hypertension: an association with cellular transport of sodium, *Proc. Univ. Otago Med. J.,* 59, 67, 1982.
77. **Adragna, N. C., Canessa, M. L., Solomon, H., Slater, E., and Tosteson, D. C.,** Red cell sodium-lithium countertransport in patients with essential hypertension, *Hypertension,* 4, 795, 1982.
78. **Smith, J. B., Ash, K. O., Hunt, S. C., Hentschel, W. M., Sprowell, W., Dadone, M. M., and Williams, R. R.,** Three red cell Na transport systems in hypertensive and normotensive Utah adults, *Hypertension,* 6, 159, 1984.

79. **Tuck, M. L., Gross, C., Maxwell, L. H., Brickman, A. S., Krasnoshtein, G., and Mayes, D.,** Erythrocyte Na,K cotransport and Na,K pump in black and Caucasian hypertensive patients, *Hypertension,* 6, 536, 1984.
80. **Tuck, M. L., Correy, D. B., Maxwell, M., and Stern, N.,** Kinetic analysis of erythrocyte Na-K pump and cotransport in essential hypertension, *Hypertension,* 10, 204, 1987.
81. **Lewitter, F. I. and Canessa, M.,** Red cell cotransport studies in adult twins, *Am. J. Human Gen.,* Suppl. 136, 172s, 1985.
82. **Price, M., Hannaert, P., Dagher, G., and Garay, R. P.,** Interaction of internal Na^+ and external K^+ with erythrocyte Na^+,K^+ cotransport system in essential hypertension, *Hypertension,* 6, 352, 1984.
83. **Cusi, D., Fossali, E., Piazza, A. et al.,** Heritability estimate of erythrocyte Na-K-Cl cotransport in normotensive and hypertensive families, *Am. J. Hypertension,* 4, 1, 1991.
84. **Manunta, P., Melis, M. G., Cusi, D. et al.,** Differential effects of furosemide on sodium and water excretion in relation to erythrocyte Na-K-Cl cotransport in essential hypertensive patients, *J. Hypertension,* submitted.
85. **Niutta, E., Cusi, D., Colombo, R. et al.,** Antihypertensive effect of captopril, canreonate potassium, and atenolol; relations with red blood cell sodium transport and renin, *Am. J. Hypertension,* 1, 364, 1988.
86. **Cusi, D., Barlassina, C., Tripodi, M. G. et al.,** Genetic factors involved in ion transport abnormalities in essential hypertension, *J. Hypertension,* 5(Suppl. 5), S255, 1987.
87. **Canessa, M., Redgrave, J., Laski, C., and Williams, G. H.,** Does sodium intake modify red cell Na^+ transporters in normal and hypertensive subjects?, *Am. J. Hypertension,* 2, 515, 1989.
88. **Garay, R. P., Nazaret, C., Hannaert, P., and Price, M.** Abnormal Na^+,K^+ cotransport function in a group of patients with essential hypertension, *Eur. J. Clin. Invest.,* 13, 311, 1983.
89. **Vallega, G., Atkinson, W., Tsai, E., Torielli, L., and Canessa, M.,** Milan hypertensive (MHS) rat vascular smooth muscle cells in culture exhibit increased growth and Na-K-Cl cotransport, abstract presented at FASEB Meeting, *FASEB J,* 3, A1187, 1989.
90. **Garay, R. P.,** personal communication.
91. **Barber, B. R.,** personal communication.

Chapter 3

THE $[Na^+,K^+,Cl^-]$ COTRANSPORT SYSTEM: RELEVANCE IN ESSENTIAL HYPERTENSION

Ricardo P. Garay, Sylvie Cavalier, and Patrick A. Hannaert

TABLE OF CONTENTS

I. Introduction 46

II. Physiological Role of the $[Na^+,K^+,Cl^-]$ Cotransport System 46
- A. Epithelial Cells 47
- B. Red Blood Cells 48
- C. Vascular Smooth Muscle Cells 49

III. $[Na^+,K^+,Cl^-]$ Cotransport in Primary Hypertension 50
- A. Red Blood Cells 50
- B. Epithelial Cells 51
- C. Vascular Smooth Muscle Cells 52

IV. Summary and Conclusions 53

References 54

0-8493-5474-9/94/$0.00+$.50

I. INTRODUCTION

Although excess salt intake has been identified as a major pathogenic factor in many patients with primary hypertension, the intrinsic mechanism of this relationship remains obscure.

In the early 1980s, different sodium transport abnormalities were found in erythrocytes from humans and rats with primary hypertension (see Chapter 1), and were proposed to reflect a disorder in the sodium handling by the kidney, the cardiovascular system, or other relevant organs in hypertension (for review, see References 1 and 2). For instance, the increased erythrocyte Na^+:Li^+ countertransport was suggested to reflect increased renal sodium reabsorption.[3] Moreover, the increased K_m of the erythrocyte Na^+,K^+ pump for internal sodium was proposed to reflect a delayed recovery of basal cell sodium contents in excitable cells after electrical or contractile activity (due to the opening of sodium channels or the activation of sodium "dissipators" such as the Na^+:H^+ and Na^+:Ca^{2+} exchangers[2]). Conversely, no simple mechanistic extrapolation was proposed for the [Na^+,K^+,Cl^-]-cotransport system, a very complex transport protein that was poorly known at the time when an erythrocyte cotransport abnormality was first reported in essential hypertension.[4] This finding raised much interest in the characterization of the cotransport system and its homeostatic regulation by hormonal, genetic, and environmental factors, particularly in cells relevant to blood pressure regulation. Such fundamental studies allowed a better understanding of the physiopathological relevance of the erythrocyte cotransport abnormalities in primary hypertension.

II. PHYSIOLOGICAL ROLE OF THE [Na^+,K^+,Cl^-] COTRANSPORT SYSTEM

The [Na^+,K^+,Cl^-]-cotransport system is a membrane transport protein which exists in almost every cell in which it has been investigated.[5-7] The cotransport system is perhaps the most complex ion transport protein because under physiological conditions it moves six translocating substrates; i.e., it catalyzes coupled fluxes of sodium, potassium, and chloride in both inward and outward directions across the cell membrane (Figure 1).

[Na^+,K^+,Cl^-] cotransport fluxes are usually characterized by their sensitivity to loop diuretics, particularly bumetanide. The inhibitory action of loop diuretics is due to the interaction of their negatively charged carboxylic acid group with the chloride receptor site of the cotransport system. Bumetanide is a potent cotransport inhibitor, with IC_{50} between 10^{-7} and 5×10^{-6} *M*, and is rather specific for cotransport; i.e., it inhibits other chloride transport systems at concentrations at least 50 times higher than those required to inhibit the [Na^+,K^+,Cl^-] cotransport system.

The cotransport system is electroneutral, and it is usually assumed that its stoichiometry is $1Na^+$:$1K^+$:$2Cl^-$. However, a K^+ to Na^+ stoichiometry higher than 1 was found in human erythrocytes[8] and in peritoneal mouse macrophages.[9]

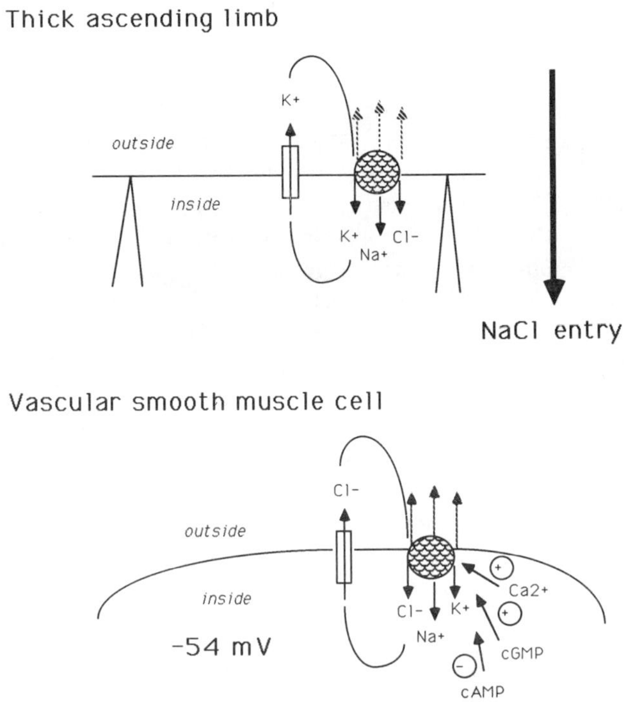

FIGURE 1. [Na^+,K^+,Cl^-]-cotransport system in the thick ascending limb of Henle's loop and in vascular smooth muscle cells. In the thick ascending limb and other epithelial tissue, the cotransport system catalyzes net NaCl entry into the cell interior. A K^+ channel extrudes out of the cell all the excess in potassium ions that is continuously generated by the cotransport system. In vascular smooth muscle, the cotransport system seems to counterbalance cell chloride loss by chloride channels. Cell chloride loss tends to depolarize the cell membrane (by the loss of negatively charged ions; −54 mV is the resting membrane potential of A10 vascular smooth muscle cells).[45]

Moreover, a $2Na^+$:$1K^+$:$3Cl^-$ stoichiometry has been found in the squid giant axon.[10]

A. EPITHELIAL CELLS

The [Na^+,K^+,Cl^-] cotransport system is present in several epithelial cell membranes. In absorptive epithelia, the cotransport system is apically located, whereas in secretive epithelia it is present in basolateral cell membranes.

The physiological role of the cotransport system in epithelial tissue is to allow net NaCl entry into the cell interior. For instance, in the thick ascending limb of Henle's loop, an apical cotransport system catalyzes net uptake of $1Na^+$, $1K^+$, and $2Cl^-$ into the cell interior. Moreover, an apical K^+ channel extrudes out of the cell all the excess in potassium ions that is continuously generated by the cotransport system. The final consequence is net NaCl entry inside the cell (see Chapter 1).

It is important to note that in the medullary thick ascending limb, the cotransport system accounts for almost all luminal sodium reabsorption.[7] However, in other epithelia it often catalyzes net NaCl uptake along with the Na^+:H^+ exchanger and the Na^+-dependent [Cl^-/HCO_3^-] exchanger (see Chapter 1).

Hormonal regulation of the [Na^+,K^+,Cl^-] cotransport system has been reported for several epithelia.[11,12] Thus, in the flounder small intestine, cyclic guanosine monophosphate (cGMP) and elevated cytosolic calcium levels inhibit the cotransport system, apparently through phosphorylation of a brush border membrane protein. In human airway epithelium, α_1-adrenergic stimulation of [Na^+,K^+,Cl^-]-cotransport fluxes seems to take place via elevated intracellular calcium.[12]

B. RED BLOOD CELLS

In contrast to epithelial cells, little was known about the physiological role of the [Na^+,K^+,Cl^-] cotransport system in nonepithelial cells.

The first nonepithelial cell in which the cotransport system was well characterized was the avian red blood cell (RBC), particularly turkey and duck erythrocytes.[5] The turkey erythrocyte responds to β-adrenergic stimulation by increases in cotransport activity and phosphorylation by cyclic adenosine monophosphate (cAMP) -dependent and of distinct sites in goblin, a high molecular weight protein (230,000 Da) of the plasma membrane.[13] This regulatory pathway seems to play a very important physiological role in avians; i.e., catecholamine-mediated stimulation of inward erythrocyte [Na^+,K^+,Cl^-] cotransport seems to counterbalance the hyperkalemia resulting from flight.

Another cotransport stimulatory agent is cell shrinkage. Thus, cell shrinkage stimulates net NaCl influx via the cotransport system, with the simultaneous entry of osmotic equivalents of water (''regulatory volume increase'').

A [Na^+,K^+,Cl^-] cotransport system has been described in mammal erythrocytes, although its activity is much lower than in nucleated avian erythrocytes. Moreover, in contrast with avian erythrocytes, cAMP inhibits the cotransport system in human erythrocytes.[14] Indeed, plasma K^+ in mammals is regulated by the Na^+,K^+ pump of skeletal muscle[15] and by the kidney.

One unusual property of the cotransport system in human erythrocytes is that it is near equilibrium;[16] i.e., inward and outward cotransport fluxes have similar magnitudes. Therefore, no significant net sodium movements are catalyzed under physiological conditions. This is so because membrane potential in enucleated erythrocytes is unusually dependent on chloride permeability. Thus, the electrochemical outward potassium gradient supplies the energy to catalyze high outward sodium movements. The importance of such outward sodium movements is illustrated by the fact that in sodium-loaded erythrocytes the [Na^+,K^+,Cl^-] cotransport system helps the Na^+,K^+ pump in extruding the excess in cell Na^+ content.[16] However, such ''second pump'' function cannot be directly extrapolated to other nonepithelial cells, with membrane potential dependent on potassium permeability and with small electrochemical chloride gradients.

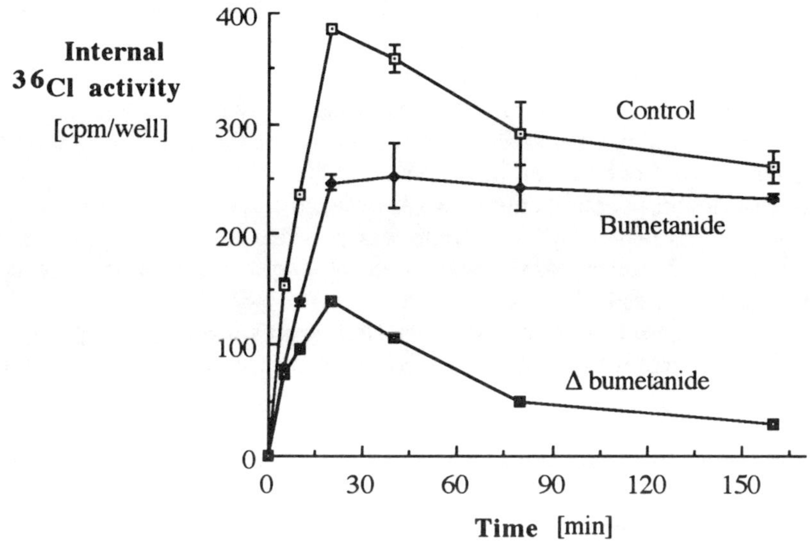

FIGURE 2. $^{36}Cl^-$ uptake in A10 vascular smooth muscle cells. Values are given as mean ± SD of triplicates. Assuming an internal [Na^+ + K^+ content] = 150 m*M*, steady-state basal $^{36}Cl^-$ levels (at 160 min) were 30.0 ± 8.7 m*M* (mean ± SD, n = 4). Bumetanide (20 μ*M*) induced a −17.3 ± 5.9% decrease in steady-state $^{36}Cl^-$ levels (n = 3). Initial rate of bumetanide-sensitive $^{36}Cl^-$ influx was 38 ± 14 mmol (liters of cell water h^{-1}). For technical details on ion fluxes in A10 cells, see References 22 and 23.

C. VASCULAR SMOOTH MUSCLE CELLS

Due to technical reasons, the [Na^+,K^+,Cl^-] cotransport system was very difficult to explore in vascular smooth muscle cells. Nevertheless, as early as 1982 we first reported the existence of a very active [Na^+,K^+,Cl^-] cotransport system in these cells.[17]

Intriguingly, in vascular smooth muscle the [Na^+,K^+,Cl^-] cotransport system resembles more human erythrocytes than epithelial cells. Thus, in spite of important unidirectional inward and outward fluxes, the cotransport system catalyzes a very small net sodium influx. Of course, in vascular smooth muscle cells, changes in internal sodium and potassium contents are rapidly regulated by the Na^+,K^+ pump. However, even when the Na^+,K^+ pump is blocked by ouabain, the net sodium influx via the cotransport system is very small.

As previously mentioned, a potassium to sodium stoichiometry higher than one was found in human erythrocytes[8] and in peritoneal mouse macrophages.[9] Assuming an electroneutral cotransport, this suggests the presence of relatively high chloride fluxes. In vascular smooth muscle, with small but outwardly directed electrochemical Cl^- gradient, high chloride fluxes can stimulate outward sodium movements, thus decreasing net sodium influx.

Several authors have suggested that the physiological role of the [Na^+,K^+,Cl^-] cotransport system in nonepithelial cells is the handling of cell chloride contents.[18] Figure 2 shows that bumetanide slightly decreased steady-state chloride contents, suggesting that the cotransport system can catalyze a small but significant net chloride influx. On the other hand, under physiological conditions chloride ions passively diffuse out of the cell by chloride channels, a process that tends to depolarize the cell membrane (by the loss of negatively charged ions). Then the cotransport system may help the cell to recover such chloride ion loss, a process that tends to repolarize the cell membrane.

A very important contribution to our knowledge of the [Na^+,K^+,Cl^-] cotransport system in vascular smooth muscle was provided by Owen et al.,[19-21] who showed that this transport system was stimulated by the atrial natriuretic factor (ANF) via cGMP, and that it was inhibited by cAMP.[21,22]

Several observations suggested that the cotransport system could be particularly helpful in the recovery of cell chloride loss in activated vascular smooth muscle cells:

1. In sodium loaded cells, bumetanide had a more powerful action in decreasing steady-state chloride contents (Figure 3)
2. Endothelin-1 and other vasoconstrictors stimulate cotransport activity[23]
3. Physiological increases in basal levels of cytosolic free calcium contents were able to stimulate cotransport activity (Figure 4)

III. [Na^+,K^+,Cl^-] COTRANSPORT IN PRIMARY HYPERTENSION

A. RED BLOOD CELLS

To our knowledge, the [Na^+,K^+,Cl^-] cotransport system is the membrane carrier in which the highest number of abnormalities were reported in erythrocytes from humans and rats with primary hypertension. Table 1 summarizes six cotransport abnormalities.

In spontaneously hypertensive rats, the most frequent abnormality seems to be an increased V_{max} for cotransport, which is usually detected as an increased bumetanide-sensitive Rb^+ influx.[24-28] Increased V_{max} for cotransport was also seen in 30 to 40% of essential hypertensive patients in association with increased Na^+:Li^+ countertransport and/or increased membrane sodium leak.[16,28-30]

Another cotransport abnormality frequently seen in essential hypertensive patients is a high K_m for internal sodium.[16] High K_M for cotransport was also observed in blacks, where it seems to be a predictor of salt-sensitive hypertension.[32] Moreover, Canessa et al.[33] recently reported that high sodium intake increased the K_M for cotransport, but only in hypertensive subjects.

Kinetic studies of K_M are difficult to perform in rat erythrocytes. Nevertheless, a high K_m for internal sodium has been described in spontaneously hypertensive rat (SHR) erythrocytes.[34]

Increased K_M for internal sodium was frequently found to be associated with a low V_{max}.[13] Moreover, low V_{max} for cotransport seems to be correlated with low plasma renin activity[35] and also seems to be a predictor of salt-sensitive hypertension.[32]

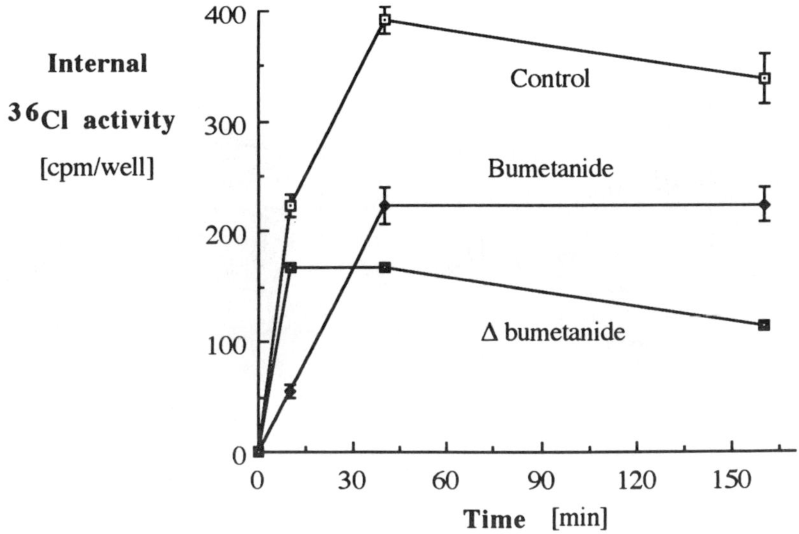

FIGURE 3. $^{36}Cl^-$ uptake in sodium loaded A10 vascular smooth muscle cells. A 74% stationary increase in internal sodium content was obtained by incubating the cells with 2 m*M* ouabain. Bumetanide induced a much more important decrease in steady-state $^{36}Cl^-$ levels ($-42.5 \pm 9.0\%$; mean ± SD, n = 5) than in basal conditions (compare with Figure 2). The initial rate of bumetanide-sensitive $^{36}Cl^-$ influx was also stimulated up to 114 ± 14 mmol (liters of cell water h^{-1}).

The results suggest that high K_m and/or low V_{max} for cotransport can be markers of low renin, salt-sensitive hypertension. One possible link explaining such correlations can be the endogenous ''bumetanide-like'' factor, a plasmatic cotransport inhibitor which seems to be secreted in the circulation in response to excess sodium intake.[36]

B. EPITHELIAL CELLS

Increased erythrocyte cotransport was proposed to be a marker of increased transepithelial NaCl movements. Evidence supporting such hypothesis was found in kidney vesicles from the Milan strain of spontaneously hypertensive rat (MHS)[37] and in the choroid plexus of the Okamoto strain of spontaneously hypertensive rats (SHR).[38]

In MHS, increased renal sodium reabsorption seems to be the primary abnormality leading to the onset of high blood pressure.[39] Moreover, high erythrocyte cotransport activity was correlated with high bumetanide-sensitive Rb^+ influx in membranes vesicles from renal outer medulla.[37]

The above results suggested that increased erythrocyte cotransport could be a genetic marker for increased sodium reabsorption in the thick ascending limb of Henle. However, care needs to be taken with such kind of direct extrapolations because in kidney vesicles from MHS, increased cotransport was due to a decreased K_m for external K^+ (Rb^+) and not to an increased V_{max} as in RBC[37] and in SHR

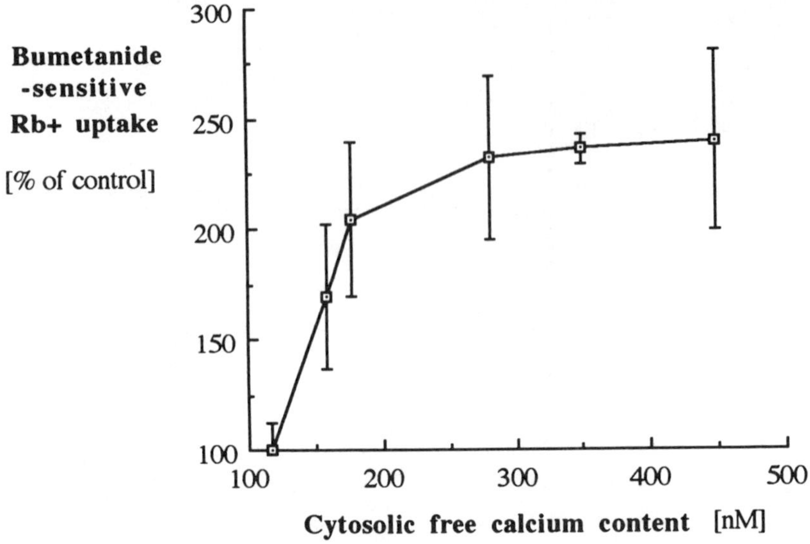

FIGURE 4. Stimulation of [Na^+,K^+,Cl^-]-cotransport system in A10 vascular smooth muscle cells by internal calcium. Physiological increases in basal levels of cytosolic free calcium contents provoked marked cotransport stimulation. Cytosolic free calcium content was measured by using the fura-2 spectrofluorimetry method. [Na^+,K^+,Cl^-]-cotransport activity was equated to the bumetanide-sensitive Rb^+ uptake. For technical details, see References 22 and 23.

and Sabra salt-sensitive hypertensive rats (SBH), sodium reabsorption in the thick ascending limb of Henle is normal[37,40,41] in spite of an increased erythrocyte cotransport.[24-27]

In SHR, high erythrocyte cotransport was correlated with high bumetanide-sensitive Rb^+ influx in isolated epithelial cells from the choroid plexus.[38] Electronic microscopy revealed intense secretory activity in the choroid plexus of the SHR, and partial loss of both the brush border in apical membranes and the invaginations of basolateral membranes. These observations suggested that a decreased surface of the secretory cell membrane tended to be compensated for by high secretory activity, thus maintaining cerebrospinal fluid (CSF) formation. Therefore, the increased cotransport activity was a secondary compensatory phenomena. In SHR-SP (stroke prone), the morphological changes were more pronounced than in SHR and cotransport fluxes were not hyperactivated, suggesting exhaustion of the compensatory phenomena.

With respect to the increased K_M of cotransport for internal sodium, it is important to note that this abnormality may also increase net NaCl entry into epithelial cells, thus enhancing transepithelial sodium movements.

C. VASCULAR SMOOTH MUSCLE CELLS

[Na^+,K^+,Cl^-] cotransport fluxes have been studied in cultured vascular smooth muscle cells from SHR, but the obtained results were controversial. Thus, high

TABLE 1
Erythrocyte [Na^+,K^+,Cl^-] Cotransport Abnormalities in Primary Hypertension

Transport abnormality	Pathological significance	Ref.
High V_{max}	Genetic increase in renal sodium reabsorption	24–31, 37–39
High K_{Na}/low V_{max}	Low-renin, salt-sensitive hypertension	16, 32, 33, 35
Low K_{Na}	?	28
High K_K	?	44
Low K_K	?	37, 44

Note: K_{Na} = K_m for internal sodium; K_K = K_m for external potassium.

and low cotransport activity were reported by Tokushige et al.[42] and by O'Donnell and Owen,[43] respectively. However, increased cotransport has been found only in calcium-deficient medium, and not in more physiological media (1 m*M* calcium[42]). Moreover, Tokushige et al. have measured $^{22}Na^+$ washout,[42] whereas O'Donnell and Owen measured bumetanide-sensitive $^{86}Rb^+$ uptake.[43]

Generally speaking, erythrocytes are classically used for ion transport studies because, among others, initial rates of ion fluxes can be precisely measured under steady-state conditions. From this point of view, erythrocyte fluxes can be directly compared with measurements of bumetanide sensitive $^{86}Rb^+$ uptake in cultured cells and not with $^{22}Na^+$ washout experiments.

Intriguingly, bumetanide sensitive rubidium uptake is high in erythrocytes of SHR[25-27] and low in cultured vascular smooth muscle cells of SHR.[43] Although both cells exhibit abnormal cotransport fluxes, the link between both cotransport abnormalities is unclear.

Decreased maximal [^{3}H] bumetanide binding suggested that low cotransport in vascular cells of SHR was due to a decreased number of available cotransport sites.[43]

Low cotransport activity can be an hypertensinogenic factor in vascular smooth muscle. Thus, low cotransport activity decreases net chloride influx, and can slightly depolarize the cell membrane (by the loss of negatively charged ions), thus increasing the opening probability of voltage-dependent calcium channels. Then, low cotransport activity can be translated into increased membrane excitability of vascular smooth muscle.

IV. SUMMARY AND CONCLUSIONS

In 1980, an abnormal [Na^+,K^+,Cl^-] cotransport system was first reported in erythrocytes from essential hypertensive patients.[4] At that time the cotransport system was poorly known, and no conclusion could be easily reached about the role of this transport system in essential hypertension. Indeed, years of research were needed to characterize this membrane carrier, perhaps the more complex of the already known ion transport proteins (under physiological conditions it moves six translocating substrates). Moreover, the cotransport system is the membrane carrier with the highest number of abnormalities (six) described in subsets of essential hypertensive patients and strains of spontaneously hypertensive rats.

In erythrocytes from spontaneously hypertensive rats, the most frequent abnormality seems to be an increased V_{max} for cotransport. Increased V_{max} for cotransport was also seen in 30 to 40% of essential hypertensive patients, in association with increased Na^+:Li^+ countertransport and/or increased membrane sodium leak.

Increased erythrocyte cotransport was proposed to be a marker of increased transepithelial NaCl movements. Evidence supporting such hypothesis was found in kidney vesicles from the Milan strain of spontaneously hypertensive rat (MHS) and in the choroid plexus of the Okamoto strain of SHR. However, in SHR and SBH, sodium reabsorption in the thick ascending limb of Henle is normal, in spite of an increased erythrocyte cotransport.

Another cotransport abnormality frequently seen in essential hypertensive patients is a high K_M for internal sodium. High K_M for cotransport was also observed in blacks, where it seems to be a predictor of salt-sensitive hypertension. Moreover, high sodium intake was found to increase the K_M for cotransport, but only in the hypertensive subjects.

Increased K_M for internal sodium was frequently found to be associated with a low V_{max}. Moreover, low V_{max} for cotransport seems to be correlated with low plasma renin activity and seems also to be a predictor of salt-sensitive hypertension.

Low bumetanide-sensitive $^{86}Rb^+$ uptake was found in cultured vascular smooth muscle from SHR. Maximal [^{3}H] bumetanide binding was also reported to be low in vascular cells of SHR, suggesting a decreased number of available cotransport sites.

In vascular smooth muscle, low cotransport activity decreases net chloride influx. This may slightly depolarize the cell membrane (by the loss of negatively charged ions), thus increasing the opening probability of voltage-dependent calcium channels. Then, low cotransport activity can be an hypertensinogenic factor for vascular smooth muscle.

REFERENCES

1. **Postnov, Y. V. and Orlov, S. N.,** Ion transport across plasma membrane in primary hypertension, *Physiol. Rev.*, 1985; 65: 904–945.
2. **Garay, R. P.,** Typology of Na^+ transport abnormalities in erythrocytes from essential hypertensive patients. A first step towards the diagnosis and specific treatment of different forms of primary hypertension, *Cardiovasc. Drugs Ther.*, 1990; 4: 373–378.
3. **Weder, A. B.,** Red-cell lithium-sodium countertransport and renal lithium clearance in hypertension, *N. Engl. J. Med.*, 1986; 314: 198–201.

4. **Garay, R. P., Dagher, G., Pernollet, M. G., Devynck, M. A., and Meyer, P.,** Inherited defect in a Na^+,K^+ cotransport system in erythrocytes from essential hypertensive patients, *Nature,* 1980; 284: 281–283.
5. **Lauf, P. K., McManus, T. J., Haas, M., Forbush, B., Duhm, J., Flatman, P. W., Saier, M. H., and Russell, J. M.,** Physiology and biophysics of chloride and cation cotransport across cell membranes, *Fed. Proc.,* 1987; 46: 2377–2395.
6. **Chipperfield, A.,** The [Na, K, Cl] cotransport system, *Clin. Sci.,* 1986; 71: 465–476.
7. **Greger, R.,** Ion transport mechanisms in the thick ascending limb of Henle's loop of mammalian nephron, *Physiol. Rev.,* 1985; 65: 760–797.
8. **Canessa, M., Brugnara, C., Cusi, D., and Tosteson, D. C.,** Modes of operation and variable stoichiometry of the furosemide-sensitive Na and K fluxes in human red cells, *J. Gen. Physiol.,* 1986; 87: 113–142.
9. **Diez, J., Braquet, P., Verna, R., Nazaret, C., and Garay, R.,** The effect of cyclic AMP on Na^+ and K^+ transport systems in mouse macrophages, *Experientia,* 1985; 41: 666–667.
10. **Altamirano, A. A., and Russell, J. M.,** Coupled Na/K/Cl cotransport efflux. Reverse unidirectional fluxes in squid giant axon, *J. Gen. Physiol.,* 1987; 89: 669–686.
11. **Palfrey, H. C. and Rao, M. C.,** Na/K/Cl co-transport and its regulation. *J. Exp. Biol.,* 1983; 106: 43–54.
12. **Liedtke, A.,** Alpha-adrenergic regulation of Na-Cl cotransport in human airway epithelium, *Am. J. Physiol.,* 1989; 257: L125–L129.
13. **Alper, S. L., Beam, K. G., and Greengard, P.,** Hormonal control of Na^+-K^+-Cl^- cotransport in turkey erythrocytes, *J. Biol. Chem.,* 1980; 255: 4864–4871.
14. **Garay, R. P.,** Inhibition of Na/K cotransport system by cyclic AMP and intracellular calcium in human red cells, *Biochim. Biophys. Acta,* 1982; 688: 786–792.
15. **Clausen, T.,** Adrenergic control of Na^+-K^+ homeostasis, *Acta Med. Scand. Suppl.,* 1983; 672: 111–115.
16. **Garay, R. P., Nazaret, C., Hannaert, P., and Price, M.,** Abnormal Na^+,K^+ cotransport function in a group of patients with essential hypertension, *Eur. J. Clin. Invest.,* 1983; 13: 311–320.
17. **Tuck M., Garay R. P., Russo-Marie F., and Meyer P.,** Na^+,K^+ cotransport system in vascular smooth muscle cells, *Am. Fed. Clin. Res. Meet.,* Washington, DC, 1982.
18. **Canessa, M., Brugnara, C., and Escobales, N.,** The Li^+-Na^+ exchange and Na^+-K^+-Cl^- cotransport system in essential hypertension, *Hypertension,* 1987; 10(Suppl. 11): 4–10.
19. **Owen, N. E.,** Regulation of Na/K/Cl cotransport in vascular smooth muscle cells, *Biochem. Biophys. Res. Commun.,* 1984; 125: 500–508.
20. **O'Donnell, M. E. and Owen, N. E.,** Atrial natriuretic factor stimulates Na/K/Cl cotransport in vascular smooth muscle cells, *Proc. Natl. Acad. Sci.,* 1986; 83: 6132–6136.
21. **Owen, N. E., Bush, E. N., Holleman, W., and O'Donnell, M. E.,** Effect of atrial natriuretic factor on Na/K/Cl cotransport in vascular smooth muscle cells, *Hypertension,* 1987; 10(Suppl. 1): 128–130.
22. **Tuck, M., Hannaert, P., Jeanclos, E., Russo-Marie, F., and Garay, R. P.,** Inhibitory action of norepinephrine on sodium transport in vascular smooth muscle in culture, *Pfluegers' Arch. Eur. J. Physiol.,* 1989; 413: 493–497.
23. **Rosati, C., Jeanclos, E., Cavalier, S., Chabrier, P. E., Hannaert, P., Braquet, P., and Garay, R. P.,** Stimulatory actions of endothelin-1 on membrane Na^+ transport system in vascular smooth muscle cells in culture, *Am. Hypertension,* 1990; 3: 711–713.
24. **DeMendonça, M., Knorr, A., Grichois, M. L., Benlshay, D., Garay, R. P., and Meyer, P.,** Erythrocytic sodium ion transport systems in primary and secondary hypertension of the rat, *Kidney Int.,* 1982; 21(Suppl. 11): 69–75.
25. **Duhm, J., Gobel, B. O., and Beck, F. X.,** Sodium and potassium ion transport accelerations in erythrocytes of DOC, DOC-salt, one-clip, two kidney and spontaneously hypertensive rats: role of hypokalemia and cell volume, *Hypertension,* 1983; 5: 642–652.

26. **Saitta, M., Hannaert, P., Rosati, C., Meyer, P., and Garay, R.,** A kinetic analysis of inward Na^+,K^+ cotransport in erythrocytes from spontaneously hypertensive rats, *J. Hypertension,* 1987; 5(Suppl. 5): S285–S286.
27. **Orlov, S. N., Postnov, I. Y., Pokudin, N. I., Kukharenko, Y., and Postnov, Y. V.,** Na^+-H^+ exchange and other ion-transport systems in erythrocytes of essential hypertensives and spontaneously hypertensive rats: a comparative analysis, *J. Hypertension,* 1989; 7: 781–788.
28. **Ferrari, P., Torielli, L., Cirillo, M., Salardi, S., and Bianchi, G.,** Sodium transport kinetics in erythrocytes and inside-out vesicles from Milan rats, *J. Hypertension,* in press.
29. **Adragna, N., Canessa, M., Solomon, H., Slater, E., and Tosteson, D. C.,** Red-cell lithium-sodium countertransport and sodium-potassium cotransport in patients with essential hypertension, *Hypertension,* 1982; 4: 795–804.
30. **Garay, R. P. and Nazaret, C.,** Na^+ leak in erythrocytes from essential hypertensive patients, *Clin. Sci.,* 1985; 69: 613–624.
31. **Garay, R. P.,** Red blood cell Na^+ content is poorly related to essential hypertension and to membrane Na^+ transport abnormalities, *Hypertension,* 1990; 15: 234–235.
32. **Canessa, M., Laski, C., and Falkner, B.,** Red blood cell Na^+ transport as a predictor of blood pressure response to Na^+ load in young blacks and whites, *Hypertension,* 1990; 16: 508–514.
33. **Canessa, M., Redgrave, J., Laski, C., and Williams, G. H.,** Does sodium intake modify red cell Na^+ transporters in normal and hypertensive subjects?, *Am. J. Hypertension,* 1989; 2: 515–523.
34. **Rosati, C., Meyer, P., and Garay, R.,** Sodium transport kinetics in erythrocytes from spontaneously hypertensive rats, *Hypertension,* 1988; 11: 41–48.
35. **Tuck, M. L., Gross, C., Maxwell, M. H., Brickman, A. S., Krasnoshtein, G., and Mayes, D.,** Erythrocyte Na^+,K^+ cotransport and Na^+,K^+ pump in black and Caucasian hypertensive patients, *Hypertension,* 1984; 6: 536–544.
36. **Dagher, G., Brossard, M., Féray, J. C., and Garay, R.,** Modulation of erythrocyte Na transport pathway(s) by excess Na intake, *Life Sci.,* 1985; 37: 243–253.
37. **Ferrandi, M., Salardi, S., Parenti, P., Ferrari, P., Bianchi, G., Braw, R., and Karlish, S. J. D.,** $Na^+/K^+/Cl^-$-cotransporter mediated Rb^+ fluxes in membrane vesicles from kidneys of normotensive and hypertensive rats, *Biochim. Biophys. Acta,* 1990; 1021: 13–20.
38. **Rosati, C., Ruchoux, M. M., Gruber, K., and Garay, R. P.,** Na^+,K^+,Cl^- cotransport system in primary hypertension: studies in red cells and in the choroid plexus of spontaneously hypertensive rats, in *Cellular Aspects of Hypertension,* Bruschi, G. and Borghetti, A., Eds. Springer-Verlag, Berlin, 1991: 257–262.
39. **Bianchi, G., Niutta, E., Ferrari, P., Salvati, P., Salardi, S., Cusi, D., Colombo, R., Cesana, B., Tripodi, G., Pati, P., and Alberghini, E.,** A possible primary role for the kidney in essential hypertension, *Am. J. Hypertension,* 1989; 2(Suppl. 2): 2S–6S.
40. **Bencsath, P., Farman, N., Vandewalle, A., and Bonvalet, J. P.,** Renal tubular reabsorption of sodium in WKR and SHR, in *New Trends in Arterial Hypertension,* Worcel, M., Ed., Elsevier/North Holland, Amsterdam, 1981: 213–224.
41. **Yagil, Y., Mekler, J., Wald, H., Popovtzer, M. M., and Ben-Ishay, D.,** Sodium handling by the Sabra hypertension prone (SBH) and resistant (SBN) rats, *Pfluegers' Arch.,* 1986; 407: 547–551.
42. **Tokushige, A., Kino, M., Tamura, H., Hopp, L., Searle, B. M., and Aviv, A.,** Bumetanide-sensitive sodium-22 transport in vascular smooth muscle cell of the spontaneously hypertensive rat, *Hypertension,* 1986; 8: 379–385.
43. **O'Donnell, M. E. and Owen, N. E.,** Reduced Na-K-Cl cotransport in vascular smooth muscle from spontaneously hypertensive rats, *Am. J. Physiol.,* 1988; 255: C169–C180.
44. **Price, M., Hannaert, P., Dagher, G., and Garay, R. P.,** The interaction of internal Na^+ and external K^+ with the erythrocyte Na^+,K^+ cotransport system in essential hypertension, *Hypertension,* 1984; 6: 352–359.
45. **Korbmacher, C., Helbig, H., Stahl, F., Coromo, M., Haller, H., Lindschau, C., Quass, P., and Wiederholt, M.,** Continuous membrane voltage recordings in A10 vascular smooth muscle cells: effect of AVP, *Am. J. Physiol.,* 1989; 257: C323–C332.

Chapter 4

KINETIC ABNORMALITIES OF THE Na^+,K^+ PUMP IN ESSENTIAL HYPERTENSION

Javier Díez and Arantxa Arrázola

TABLE OF CONTENTS

I. Introduction 59

II. General Aspects of the Na^+,K^+ Pump 59
- A. Molecular Structure 60
  - 1. The Subunits and Their Function 60
  - 2. Functional Unit 60
  - 3. Na^+,K^+-ATPase Isoforms 61
- B. Enzymatic and Functional Aspects 61
  - 1. Transport Modes of the Na^+,K^+ Pump 61
    - a. Na_i:K_o Exchange 61
    - b. K_i:Na_o Exchange 62
    - c. Na_i:Na_o Exchange 62
    - d. Na_i Efflux 63
    - e. K_i:K_o Exchange 63
  - 2. Substrate Specificity and Affinities 63
- C. Regulation 63
- D. Kinetic Studies 64

III. Kinetic Abnormalities of the Na^+,K^+ Pump in Essential Hypertension 64
- A. Is the Na^+,K^+ Pump Really Altered in Essential Hypertension? 64
  - 1. Na^+,K^+ Pump Is Not Altered in Hypertension 64
  - 2. Na^+,K^+ Pump Is Altered in Hypertension 65
- B. Increased V_{max} 65
  - 1. Decreased Affinity of the Na^+,K^+ Pump for Internal Na^+ 66
  - 2. Increased Na^+ "Leak" 66
- C. Decreased V_{max} 66
  - 1. Decreased Density of Functional Na^+,K^+ Pumps 66
  - 2. Decreased Turnover Number 66

0-8493-5474-9/94/$0.00+$.50

D. The Genetic Factor 66
1. Family Studies 67
2. Race Studies 67
3. Genes and Na^+,K^+-ATPase Structure 68
E. The Nongenetic Factor 68
1. Lipid Environment 68
2. Circulating Ouabain-Like Substances 69
F. Studies in Animals 70
G. Summary 71

IV. Pathophysiological, Clinical, and Pharmacological Aspects of the Kinetic Abnormalities of the Na^+,K^+ Pump in Essential Hypertension 72
A. Pathophysiological Implications 72
1. Hemodynamic Effects of Altered Na^+,K^+ Pump Activity *In Vivo* 73
2. Effects of Diminished Na^+,K^+ Pump Activity *In Vitro* 73
3. Molecular Mechanisms by which Diminished Na^+,K^+ Pump Activity Increases Vascular Tone 73
B. Clinical and Pharmacological Aspects 74

V. Assumptions in the Interpretation of the Kinetic Abnormalities of the Na^+,K^+ Pump in Essential Hypertension: Critical Analysis 76
A. Experimental Procedures Do Not Alter Na^+,K^+ Pump Activity 76
B. Statistical Design of the Studies Is Adequate 76
C. Differences between Populations Are Causally Associated With Hypertension Per Se 77
D. *In Vitro* Abnormalities Reflect *In Vivo* Disturbances 77
E. Changes in Blood Cells Are Markers for Changes in Cells Related to Blood Pressure 78

VI. Conclusions 79

References 80

I. INTRODUCTION

Tobian and Binion[1] reported increased arterial wall Na^+ content in human hypertension 37 years ago. When Losse and co-workers[2] reported in 1960 that erythrocyte Na^+ content was also increased in human hypertension, attention shifted from the vascular wall cation content to the membrane events which regulate the transmembrane Na^+ gradient. Because the Na^+,K^+ pump maintains Na^+ and K^+ gradients across the cell membrane by an electrogenic and active transport, the operation of the Na^+,K^+ pump was investigated in hypertension.

The Na^+,K^+ pump has been extensively investigated in blood cells from essential hypertensive patients. However, most studies were done measuring the activity of the Na^+,K^+ pump at a constant internal and external cation concentration. The results obtained by using this simple approach varied from laboratory to laboratory and were unable to provide a coherent understanding of the activity of the Na^+,K^+ pump in hypertension.[3] Transport kinetics is very complicated because of the numerous substrates and effectors acting in the different compartments. Indeed, one can conceive a profound effect on a transport system leading to low, normal, or high transport activity depending on the experimental condition. For instance, changes in cell Na^+ content are translated in high, normal, or low Na^+,K^+ pump activity depending on the use of Na^+ loaded, fresh, or Na^+ depleted cells, respectively.[4] The activity of the Na^+,K^+ pump is therefore a very complicated function of several variables and, in particular, of cell Na^+ content.[4] Thus, the modification of internal Na^+ content allows a kinetic approach to the study of the Na^+,K^+ pump.

This chapter focuses on kinetic abnormalities of the Na^+,K^+ pump in essential hypertension. It does not review studies of the Na^+,K^+ pump in animals with hereditary or experimentally induced hypertension. Therefore, studies of the pump in animal tissues and cell are discussed or cited only in the context of general observation in cells from human hypertensives. On the other hand, most investigations have used blood cells, normally erythrocytes, to identify and gain insight into abnormalities of the Na^+,K^+ pump in essential hypertension. Therefore, although blood cells are not closely representative of other cells involved in the pathophysiology of hypertension, such as the vascular smooth muscle cell and the renal tubular epithelium, abnormalities of the Na^+,K^+ pump described in those cells are reviewed here.

II. GENERAL ASPECTS OF THE Na^+,K^+ PUMP

The sodium- and potassium-activated ATPase, or the Na^+,K^+ pump (Na^+,K^+-ATPase), maintains a low intracellular concentration of Na^+ and a high intracellular concentration of K^+ in all animal cells. These concentration gradients are necessary for a variety of physiological functions, including regulation of cell volume, maintenance of osmotic pressure, Na^+ coupled transport of certain organic and inorganic molecules, and electrical excitability of nerve and muscle.[5] The Na^+,K^+-ATPase effects the coupled transports of three Na^+ ions out of the cell and two K^+ ions into the cell. The energy required for this active transport is derived from the hydrolysis of one molecule of adenosine triphosphate (ATP).[6,7]

A. MOLECULAR STRUCTURE

1. The Subunits and Their Function

The Na^+,K^+-ATPases that have been isolated from a wide range of sources are strikingly similar. In all cases the Na^+,K^+-ATPase consists of two noncovalently linked polypeptides, a catalytic α subunit, with a molecular weight of ~100,000 and a smaller glycosylated β subunit with a molecular weight of ~55,000.[8,9] A small peptide with a molecular weight of ~10,000, termed the γ subunit, has also been identified in purified preparations of the enzyme.[10,11]

Most functions of the Na^+,K^+-ATPase have been localized to the α subunit. The α subunit contains the binding sites for Na^+,K^+,ATP and ouabain (specific inhibitor); it is phosphorylated by ATP and undergoes ligand-dependent conformational changes accompanying the binding, occlusion, and translocation of ions.[9] The exact functions of the β and γ subunits remain unknown. The γ subunit does not appear to be essential for ATPase activity,[12] but recent evidence suggests that the β subunit has an important role in Na^+,K^+-ATPase function. In ouabain-resistant HeLa cells, both α and β subunits are amplified, suggesting that both subunits are required for the acquisition of ouabain resistance.[13,14] Reduction of the β subunit with 2-mercapthoethanol completely inhibits ATPase activity, suggesting that a change in the structure of the β subunit can lead to a loss in activity of the enzyme.[15] Moreover, the high degree of homology between β subunits from several diverse species[14,16-18] supports the view that the β subunit is important for Na^+,K^+-ATPase structure and function.

The complete amino acid sequences for the Na^+,K^+-ATPase subunits have been determined.[16,19] These studies have provided an important advance in the understanding of the structure of the Na^+,K^+-ATPase. Figure 1 shows a general model for Na^+,K^+-ATPase.

2. Functional Unit

Although much information is known about the structure of the α and β subunits, relatively little is known concerning the subunit interactions of the Na^+,K^+-ATPase. The exact subunit structure of the enzyme and the minimum functional unit for the active transport of cations have not yet been determined.

Although there is general agreement for 1:1 α/β ratio, there is much less agreement about whether the αβ unit alone represents the active form of the enzyme.[8]

Examinations of soluble Na^+,K^+-ATPase suggest that the αβ unit has enzymatic activity. However, molecular weight determinations and evidence from cross-linking and electron microscopy support oligomeric models for Na^+,K^+-ATPase-mediated transport (for review, see Reference 20). Thus, although it seems certain that the αβ protomer has independent catalytic activity, it cannot be excluded that

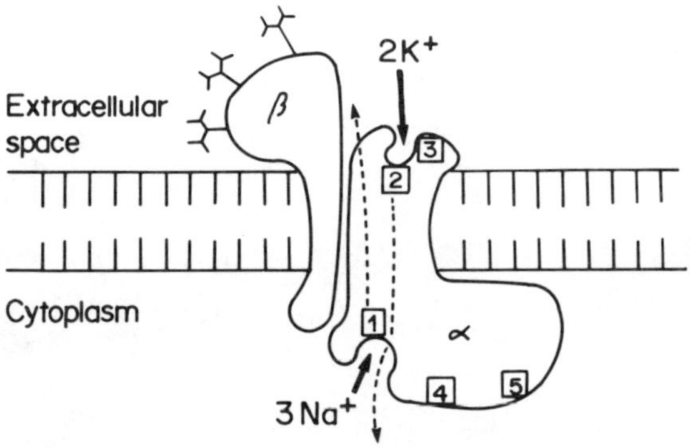

FIGURE 1. General model for Na^+,K^+-ATPase. An αβ heterodimer is represented with binding sites for Na^+ (1), K^+ (2), ouabain (3), phosphorylation (4), and ATP (5).

the transport of Na^+ and K^+ across the cellular membrane requires the formation of oligomeric complexes.

3. Na^+,K^+-ATPase Isoforms

Na^+,K^+-ATPase belongs to a multigene family.[21-23] Three α subunit (α_1, α_2, α_3) and two β subunit (β_1, β_2) isoforms have been described. Tissue-specific and developmental stage-dependent expression have been recently reviewed.[21-23] Two distinct explanations have been proposed to account for the existence of several Na^+,K^+-ATPase isoforms differentially expressed in various tissues.[24] One possible explanation for the existence of a multigene family is that it represents a selective advantage in evolution because it simplifies the problem of regulating gene expression to suit the needs of each developmental stage or each cell type of the organism. Alternatively, each isoform could be distinct from each specific functional characteristic.[24]

B. ENZYMATIC AND FUNCTIONAL ASPECTS

1. Transport Modes of the Na^+,K^+ Pump

The major physiological mode of transport mediated by the Na^+,K^+ pump is Na_i:K_o exchange, indicating that intracellular Na^+ (Na_i) is exchanged for extracellular K^+ (K_o). In addition to this normal exchange, the pump can mediate other modes of transport depending on the intra- and extracellular cation composition and on the intracellular composition of substrates, namely ATP, adenosine diphosphate (ADP), and inorganic phosphate. The existence and characterization of these other transport modes has been performed extensively in human red blood cells (RBC) and no comparably complete data exist in any other system.

a. Na_i:K_o Exchange

Early studies in human RBC established that three Na^+ ions were expelled for every two K^+ ions that were taken up,[25] then the pump should operate electrogenically. The energy source for active transport was established as ATP.[26]

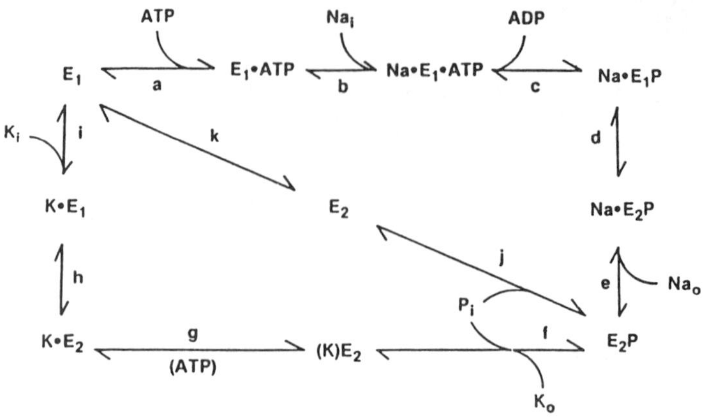

FIGURE 2. A modified version of the Post-Albers model.

The molecular mechanism of the Na^+,K^+ pump has been delineated from studies in several laboratories, notably those of Post and Alberts and their co-workers in the early 1960s.[27,28] From studies of the overall hydrolytic reaction, the partial reactions as well as side-specificity of cation requirements, it is apparent that the mechanism is characterized by a complex series of partial reaction steps. The minimal reaction sequence comprises Na_i-dependent phosphorylation and K_o-activated dephosphorylation of the enzyme linked to conformational transitions of dephospho- and phosphoforms of the enzyme. The simplified reaction mechanism depicted in Figure 2 is a modified version of the Post-Alberts model. It encompasses ion translocation modes associated with the reaction steps or sequence of steps of the Na^+,K^+ pump and is based, to a considerable extent, on results of experiments carried out with human red cells. The fundamental question as to whether the reaction pathway is ping-pong whereby the enzyme alternately binds and releases Na^+ and K^+, or is one in which both ions are bound, at least at some phase of the cycle, has been evaluated in detail by Sachs.[29] His results give strong support to the predominance of a ping-pong Na^+/K^+ exchange mechanism.

b. K_i:Na_o Exchange

This transport mode of the sodium pump is characterized by a Na_o-activated K^+ efflux from RBC that is inhibited by ouabain. This mode was first demonstrated in RBC and fulfills the thermodynamic expectation of reversibility of the entire pump cycle.[30] If the cation gradients are sufficiently steep, then the pump apparatus is driven backwards and a net synthesis of ATP from ADP and P_i is observed.

c. Na_i:Na_o Exchange

When the RBC are suspended in a K-free isotonic NaCl solution, an ouabain-sensitive isotopic Na^+ efflux can be measured that is dependent on the presence of Na_o. It was shown that the transport reaction consists of a 1:1 exchange of intra- and extracellular Na^+.[31] This flux requires intracellular ADP as well as ATP, and can be accounted for by the sequence a, b, c, d, and e in Figure 2.[32] The reaction is associated with Na^+-dependent phosphorylation of the enzyme as well as Na^+-dependent ADP-ATP exchange reactions.

d. Na_i Efflux

In the absence of alkali cations, Glynn and Karlish[33] noted a relatively slow ouabain-sensitive downhill efflux of Na^+ from RBC associated with ATP hydrolysis. The stoichiometry of this mode was approximately three Na^+ ions transport per ATP molecule hydrolyzed. Originally, the absence of an obvious countercation led these investigators to refer to this behavior as uncoupled Na^+ efflux. The association of Na_i efflux with ATP hydrolysis is similar to that of normal Na_i:K_o exchange, representing a slow turnover of the enzyme via the sequence of reactions a, b, c, d, e, j, and k in Figure 2.[32]

Several years ago, Dissing and Hoffman[34] showed that the so-called uncoupled Na^+ efflux is an electroneutral Na^+ anion-coupled efflux from red cells, at least at physiological pH.

e. K_i:K_o Exchange

Another mode of pump operation evident only in the red cells of certain species (human and goat) is ouabain-sensitive K_i:K_o exchange.[35] This mode is not associated with the hydrolysis of ATP, but is accounted for by the sequence of reversible steps denoted by f, g, h, and i in Figure 2, requiring both ATP or one of its nonhydrolyzable analogs[36] or ADP.[37]

2. Substrate Specificity and Affinities

Until recently it was thought that Na^+ alone could activate the pump at its inner surface. It is clear that the affinities of the pump for Na^+ at the cytoplasmic surface and for K^+ at the extracellular surface are not absolute. Other cations, such as Li^+, Cs^+, Rb^+, as well as K^+ were shown to compete with Na^+ at the intracellular loading site(s) and others, such as Rb^+, Cs^+, and Li^+, for K^+ at the extracellular discharge site(s).[38]

Results from experiments with inside-out vesicles (IOV) support the notion that protons can replace both Na^+ at the cytoplasmic and K^+ at the extracellular surfaces,[39] suggesting the notion of pump-mediated Na_i:H_o and H_i:K_o exchanges.

C. REGULATION

There is little evidence of physiological regulation of the sodium pump in human RBC. However, recent studies involving the cytoplasmic inhibition of the sodium pump by Ca^{2+} ions suggest the intermediacy of the regulatory protein, calnaktin, which dramatically affects the affinity with which Ca^{2+} inhibits active Na^+ pumping.[40]

In contrast, regulation of the Na^+,K^+ pump in skeletal muscle has been more extensively studied. The general properties presented below have been described in detail in a previous review.[41] The activity of this transport system is subject to acute regulation by epinephrine, norepinephrine, and insulin, all of which at physiological concentrations can induce an activation that seems mediated from specific receptors via secondary cellular messengers. In addition, the concentration of the Na^+,K^+ pump is determined by long-term regulatory factors. Muscle cell differentiation is associated with a large increase of the concentration of the enzyme. The synthesis of the Na^+,K^+ pump is markedly stimulated by thyroid hormones which together with the contractile activity (training) seem to exert a major influence on the steady-state level of Na^+,K^+ pump activity. In the intact organism, K^+ deficiency leads to a marked and reversible decrease in the concentration of the Na^+,K^+-ATPase as well as the capacity for performing active Na^+,K^+ transport.

On the other hand, alterations in the lipid composition of kidney Na^+,K^+-ATPase proteoliposomes, most notably the cholesterol content, have been shown to change its steady-state phosphoenzyme composition and kinetic behavior.[42]

D. KINETIC STUDIES

There are several approaches to study the activity of the Na^+,K^+ pump or Na^+,K^+-ATPase. Because ouabain binds specifically to this enzyme in a stoichiometry of 1:1, the maximal number of specific ouabain binding sites on the cell membrane (B_{max}) has been utilized to estimate Na^+,K^+ pump density. On the other hand, the rate of ouabain-sensitive ATP hydrolysis is used in assays of Na^+,K^+-ATPase, whereas the activity of the Na^+,K^+ pump is usually measured by ouabain-sensitive rates for Na^+ efflux and K^+ influx. Although ouabain-sensitive rate constants for Na^+ and K^+ fluxes represent innate properties of the Na^+,K^+ pump, specific kinetic analysis is necessary in order to establish the etiology of variations in Na^+,K^+ pump activity.[43] This kinetic analysis consists of the relationship between the concentrations of an ion and the rate of flux of that ion. In the case of the ouabain-sensitive Na^+ efflux, this relationship is clearly sigmoidal (Figure 3) and can be fitted by the equation:

$$V = \frac{V_{max}}{(1 + K_{Na}/Na_i)^3}$$

where V is the rate of Na^+ efflux and Na_i is the internal Na^+ concentration. This relationship is governed by two constants, the V_{max}, which is the maximal rate of Na^+ efflux, and the K_{Na}, which represents the apparent dissociation constant for internal Na^+.[44]

III. KINETIC ABNORMALITIES OF THE Na^+,K^+ PUMP IN ESSENTIAL HYPERTENSION

A. IS THE Na^+,K^+ PUMP REALLY ALTERED IN ESSENTIAL HYPERTENSION?

1. Na^+,K^+ Pump Is Not Altered in Hypertension

Certain studies have reported normal activity of the Na^+,K^+ pump in essential hypertension. In fact, some authors have described the ouabain-sensitive Na^+ efflux

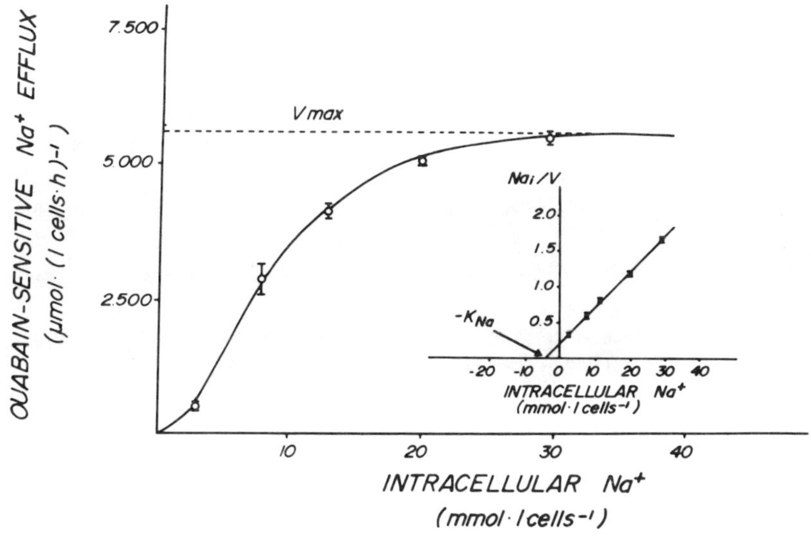

FIGURE 3. Stimulation of ouabain-sensitive Na^+ efflux by increases in erythrocyte Na^+ content. Values are given as means ± range as a measure of variability. Inset: Hanes plot (V_{max}: maximal Na^+ translocation; K_{Na}: apparent affinity of the Na^+,K^+ pump for internal Na^+).

is no different in the fresh cells of essential hypertensives than in the cells of their normotensive controls.[45,46] Alternatively, other investigators have reported that the V_{max} of sodium efflux by the pump from Na^+ loaded cells is no different in hypertensives than in normotensives.[47,48]

2. Na^+,K^+ Pump Is Altered in Hypertension

The aforementioned studies have examined relatively small groups of individuals. Furthermore, by arbitrarily defining subjects as normotensives and hypertensives, these investigations have treated the systemic blood pressure as a discontinuous variable. In reality, blood pressure levels are distributed along a continuum. Rygielski et al.[49] studied the V_{max} for Na^+,K^+-ATPase in the erythrocytes of 247 subjects that were not categorized *a priori* as hypertensives or normotensives. In this population the systolic, diastolic, and mean blood pressure levels were negatively correlated to Na^+,K^+-ATPase activity. In studies having large numbers of patients, other works have also shown that increasing levels of diastolic blood pressure are associated with diminished values for the activity of the leukocyte Na^+,K^+ pump.[50-52]

Taken together, current data suggest that hypertensives represent specific and distinct groups with a spectrum of alterations in the Na^+,K^+ pump.

B. INCREASED V_{max}

Increased Na^+,K^+ pump activity has been found in essential hypertension.[5,44,53-55] However, the character of this abnormality may be quite different with respect to its role in cellular Na^+ homeostasis.

1. Decreased Affinity of the Na^+,K^+ Pump for Internal Na^+

A decreased apparent affinity of the Na^+,K^+ pump for internal Na^+ has been reported recently by several authors in essential hypertension.[44,54,55] In all these studies the V_{max} of the Na^+,K^+ pump was increased in those patients with a decreased affinity of the pump. Because basal cell Na^+ content of hypertensives with these pump abnormalities was within the normal range, it can be suggested that the increased V_{max} of the Na^+,K^+ pump compensates the low pump affinity for internal Na^+.

2. Increased Na^+ "Leak"

Some authors have described an increased V_{max} of the Na^+,K^+ pump in hypertensives whose cells also exhibited increased Na^+ "leak".[45,53] Because basal Na^+ content is normal in these cells, it is logical to assume that the higher V_{max} also reflects an adaptive process; i.e., such cells increase their Na^+,K^+ pump activity to compensate for the increased Na^+ entry.

C. DECREASED V_{max}

Other studies have shown a diminished activity of the Na^+,K^+ pump when maximally stimulated by cellular Na^+ loading.[56-58] Again, analysis of the character of these abnormalities deserves particular consideration.

1. Decreased Density of Functional Na^+,K^+ Pumps

As shown by Ringel et al.,[56] the number of Na^+,K^+ pumps, as assessed by the ouabain binding sites, is diminished in those previously treated essential hypertensive patients who simultaneously exhibit a low V_{max} of the Na^+,K^+ pump. Such changes may be caused by secondary factors accompanying the development of hypertension, e.g., a circulating Na^+,K^+ pump inhibitor,[56] or they may be related to prolonged treatment, e.g., with diuretics.[59]

2. Decreased Turnover Number

Cells from a subpopulation of patients with essential hypertension manifest both diminished values of ouabain-sensitive rate constants for Na^+ efflux in basal conditions and diminished V_{max} after maximal stimulation by cellular Na^+ loading.[57,58] The ouabain-sensitive rate constant for Na^+ efflux reflects the density of the pump, its affinity for Na^+, and its turnover number (the frequency of a cycle of ATP hydrolysis with the transport of three Na^+ and two K^+ ions). Because neither the density of functional pumps nor the affinity of the Na^+,K^+ pump for internal Na^+ have been reported to be altered in those cells,[57,58] it is suggested that this additional abnormality of the Na^+,K^+ pump lies in a decrease of its turnover number.

D. THE GENETIC FACTOR

A number of investigators explored alterations in the cellular Na^+,K^+ pump system as genetic markers for predisposition to essential hypertension. Two major approaches were undertaken. The first was to examine Na^+,K^+ pump parameters in normotensive relatives of patients with essential hypertension; the second was to examine differences in the Na^+,K^+ pump between black and white people.

1. Family Studies

The findings related to the Na^+,K^+ pump in family members of hypertensive patients are controversial. Both inhibition and stimulation of the Na^+,K^+ pump have been reported. For example, Woods et al.,[60] using the ^{86}Rb uptake method, measured an increased erythrocyte sodium pump activity both in essential hypertensive patients and in a significant proportion of their normotensive relatives. In addition several authors[61,62] found a small, nonsignificant increase in the V_{max} of the Na^+,K^+ pump of hypertensives and their children. In contrast, other studies reported a diminished ouabain-sensitive Na^+ efflux rate constant in leukocytes from normotensives with a family history of hypertension[63] and a lower activity of Na^+,K^+-ATPase in erythrocytes from normotensive children of hypertensive subjects.[64]

These controversial data could be due in part to the absence of kinetic analyses in most of the studies described. It must be emphasized, however, that some of these variations may be environmentally determined, as Cusi et al.[65] have identified a strong correlation in erythrocyte Na^+,K^+ pump activity between husbands and wives.

2. Race Studies

Another approach to distinguishing genetic factors in the predisposition to hypertension is to examine cellular differences between blacks and whites, because it is well known that blacks in the U.S. manifest a higher frequency of essential hypertension than whites,[66-70] particularly the salt sensitivity form of the disease.[71-73]

Most studies show that blacks have reduced V_{max} for erythrocyte Na^+,K^+-ATPase activity[45,74-76] as well as decreased Na^+,K^+ pump density.[76,77] In contrast, some investigators identified no racial differences in the activity of the Na^+,K^+ pump in unloaded[78] and Na^+ loaded[46,47] erythrocytes. The failure to demonstrate racial differences in Na^+,K^+ pump activity (ouabain-sensitive Rb^+ uptake)[79] in unloaded cells was probably due to the low Rb (K^+) concentration in the assay medium, which was insufficient to sustain the activity of the Na^+,K^+ pump at basal levels. The reason for the inability to demonstrate racial differences in the V_{max} for the Na^+,K^+ pump (ouabain-sensitive Na^+ efflux)[46,47] is unclear, but it may relate to 2,5-choloromercuribenzoate (PCMBS) and nystatin which were used to load the cells.[43]

The consensus emerging from most studies suggests, however, that erythrocytes from blacks have a lower Na^+,K^+-ATPase activity than erythrocytes from whites.

The lower Na^+,K^+-ATPase activity in erythrocytes from blacks may indicate the lasting effect of a circulating factor that inhibits this enzyme. This contention is supported by findings that as a group blacks manifest several characteristics suggestive of salt sensitivity, a condition in which the levels of this factor are expected to be elevated.[80]

3. Genes and Na^+,K^+-ATPase Structure

As previously mentioned, the catalytic α subunit of Na^+,K^+-ATPase occurs as three isozymes, α_1, α_2, and α_3.[21-23,81,82] These isozymes are encoded by a multigene family and are expressed in a tissue-specific and developmentally regulated manner.[83] The α_2 subunit has a higher affinity for ouabain as compared to α_1. The α_1 and α_2 subunits appear to be tissue specific, and they differ from each other with respect to some kinetic properties.[84] RBC Na^+,K^+-ATPase has not been studied thoroughly in terms of its isozymes. Evidence has been recently provided that hypertension induces gene-specific modulation of Na^+,K^+-ATPase messenger RNA (mRNA) in vascular and cardiac tissues in the rat.[85] Recently, Herrera and Ruiz-Opazo[86] described a Pst I restriction fragment length polymorphism (RFLP) in the Na^+,K^+-ATPase α_1 gene of inbred Dahl salt-sensitive and inbred Dahl salt-resistant rats. Furthermore, Nojima et al.[87] reported a SacI RFLP in the Na^+,K^+-ATPase α_2 gene of spontaneously hypertensive rats (SHR) and normotensive rats. Given a genetic polymorphism, cosegregation analysis can show whether the gene involved causes blood pressure differences, or whether the polymorphism between strains occurs by chance.[88] Rapp and Dene[89] have recently demonstrated that blood pressure and the Na^+,K^+-ATPase α_1 gene are not causally related to substantial differences in the blood pressure of Dahl rats on a high-salt diet. Whether blood pressure and Na^+,K^+-ATPase α_2 RFLP cosegregate in SHR deserves to be tested. In any event it is possible that the α isoform of the Na^+,K^+-ATPase differs by several amino acids in hypertensives with abnormal kinetics of the Na^+,K^+ pump as compared to hypertensives with a normal pump. Therefore, it would be worthwhile to isolate and study the gene for this enzyme in these hypertensives, particularly in the subset of patients with abnormal V_{max} of the pump.

E. THE NONGENETIC FACTOR

Although differences exist in the Na^+,K^+ pump activity of blood cells between normotensives with a family history of hypertension and their counterparts without a family history of the disease, as well as between blacks and whites, it is not established whether these differences are related to variations that are indigenous to the cells or the lasting effects of circulating factors, or both. On the other hand, it is well known that the expression of genetic effects may be modified by environmental factors. More specifically, it has been demonstrated that some extracellular factors may influence the activity of the Na^+,K^+ pump in hypertension.

1. Lipid Environment

Previous studies have suggested a link between erythrocyte cation transport systems and plasma lipids.[90-92] Hespel et al.[93] showed that Na^+,K^+ pump activity was significantly correlated with both triglycerides and cholesterol. Hannaert et al.[94] investigated age, body mass index, and alcohol and tobacco consumption as possible factors for variations in erythrocyte Na^+,K^+ pump and plasma lipids. The authors showed that only alcohol consumption is significantly correlated with the Na^+,K^+ pump.[94] This observation is consistent with recent *in vitro* results obtained by Coca and Garay.[95] Ethanol concentrations similar to or higher than those occurring in the plasma of moderate drinkers are able to stimulate the Na^+,K^+ pump.

On the other hand, it has been published that treatment of hypercholesterolemic patients with lovastatin, a cholesterol lowering agent, results in significant decreases in both plasma cholesterol and RBC Na^+ content.[96] Because passive Na^+ permeability did not change as the result of lovastatin treatment, the authors suggest that if the fall in erythrocyte Na^+ content accompanying lovastatin treatment results from changes in membrane lipid composition, it is most likely the result of stimulation of RBC Na^+,K^+-ATPase.[96]

In fact, the membrane lipids are in dynamic equilibrium with plasma lipids, and hence it is possible that plasma lipid levels may influence its activity. It is known that the cholesterol content of erythrocytes is dependent on the unesterified cholesterol:phospholipid mole ratio of their milieu[97] and that changes in membrane cholesterol content affect a number of cellular functions, including carrier-mediated transport.[98] Some authors have established that high levels of membrane cholesterol in human erythrocytes inhibit the Na^+,K^+ pump and that low levels stimulate it.[99-102]

These considerations are in agreement with the contention of Bing et al.[103] that changes in cell membrane composition provide an explanation for the disturbances of ion transport systems, e.g., the Na^+,K^+ pump, in essential hypertension.

2. Circulating Ouabain-Like Substances

Several studies have suggested that the development of hypertension is associated with an inability of the kidney to adequately excrete Na^+.[104] According to this hypothesis, the increased reabsorption of Na^+ in the kidney is countered by the production of an endogenous Na^+,K^+ pump inhibitor, the natriuretic hormone,[104-106] perhaps from the hypothalamus.[107-109]

The existence of a Na^+,K^+ pump inhibitor was first postulated by de Wardener et al.[110] in 1961 to explain observations in saline-loaded dogs. Subsequent studies have presented evidence of increased amounts of pump inhibitor in hypertensive subjects,[111,112] in normotensive subjects with a positive family history for hypertension,[113] in saline-loaded subjects,[114-117] and in subjects with high dietary Na^+ intake.[118,119]

Most studies indicate that the Na^+,K^+ pump inhibitor is humoral; its effects have been observed to transfer with the plasma in plasma exchange studies.[51,120] On the other hand, serum from patients with hypertension has been shown to inhibit the Na^+,K^+ pump and increase the Na^+ content of normal leukocytes, as compared to leukocytes from matched control subjects.[51,121] Attempts to demonstrate a comparable effect of serum from hypertensive patients on Na^+ transport by erythrocytes have been unsuccessful to date, although inhibition of a preparation of Na^+,K^+-ATPase has been reported.[122] Several substances have been proposed as the Na^+,K^+ pump inhibitor. Common to all are two characteristics:[123] their production is volume controlled, and functionally, they closely resemble ouabain or digitalis. Recently, an endogenous digitalis-like factor has been isolated from human plasma with structural and functional characteristics, suggesting that it is either ouabain or an isomer of ouabain.[124-126]

The majority of the studies of the effects of salt on cells (namely RBC, but also white cells or WBC) have involved chronic (days to weeks) changes in dietary salt intake. To summarize the findings of these studies (see Weder[127] for review), it seems prudent to conclude that the evidence is suggestive (although by no means conclusive) that active membrane Na^+ transport is suppressed by a high salt intake. Whether Na^+,K^+ pump suppression results from the action of a circulating ouabain-like substance is certainly not yet proven. Although reports of decreased Na^+ efflux in RBC of salt-fed patients are compatible with the action of such a substance, one study that reported a significant suppression of ouabain-sensitive Na^+ efflux during a high-salt diet searched for and failed to find a circulating inhibitor.[128] Indeed, because one critical link in the hypothetical chain joining pump inhibition to hypertension is increased cell Na^+ concentration, observations of low to normal RBC Na^+ content after increase dietary Na^+ intake[96] seriously challenge the validity of the hypothesis.

With respect to kinetics of the Na^+,K^+ pump, some studies have shown that following a chronic Na^+ loading, the maximal velocity of the erythrocyte Na^+,K^+ pump becomes inhibited in hypertensive patients,[129] but not normotensive subjects.[48,129] The reduction in Na^+ efflux catalyzed by the Na^+,K^+ pump reported by Smith et al.[129] appears to be caused by a uniform alteration of all of the transport sites rather than complete inhibition in some of the sites as ^{3}H-ouabain binding studies indicated no change in the number of binding sites after the saline load. These experiments are consistent with the hypothesis that a saline load causes the production of a Na^+,K^+ pump inhibitor in hypertensives. However, the above observations do not address the question of whether the reduction in ouabain-sensitive Na^+ efflux is due to a humoral agent, as proposed by Gault et al.,[117] or to an alteration in the intracellular milieu, as proposed by Walter and Muller.[130] On the other hand, Masuyama et al.[131] have investigated erythrocyte membrane fluidity in essential hypertensives submitted to different salt intakes using electron spin resonance and spin labeling. The authors showed that the membrane fluidity of erythrocytes, significantly lower in hypertensives than in the normotensive subjects, was attenuated with low-salt intake, and to the contrary, was more prominent with high-salt intake in essential hypertension. Thus, generally available results could be interpreted to be consistent with at least three types of alterations: (1) a factor in the plasma that adheres to the RBC cell throughout the washing before the Na^+ efflux is measured, (2) an intracellular factor that interferes with Na^+ efflux, or (3) an alteration in the membrane structure causing decreased affinity of the Na^+,K^+ pump for Na^+.

The differential effect of volume expansion following saline loading on erythrocyte Na^+,K^+ pump activity in hypertensive as compared to normotensive subjects supports the hypothesis that an inhibitor of Na^+,K^+ pump may be of pathophysiological importance in human hypertension.

F. STUDIES IN ANIMALS

Several substrains of genetically hypertensive rats have been selected in different laboratories. However, rat erythrocytes have not been as extensively studied as human erythrocytes. This is partially due to the fact that these cells are fragile, show interstrain differences, and are relatively insensitive to ouabain. Nevertheless a Na^+,K^+ pump exists in these cells.[132] The Na^+ and K^+ fluxes catalyzed by the Na^+,K^+ pump were measured in Na^+ loaded rat erythrocytes incubated in a physiological Na^+,K^+-Ringer's medium.[133] Under these conditions, a slight but not significant increase in pump activity was observed in erythrocytes from SHR, Milan hypertensive rats, and Lyon hypertensive rats as compared to their respective controls.

Rosati et al.[134] have performed a kinetic study of the Na^+,K^+ pump in erythrocytes from SHR. Male SHR and their normotensive controls, Wistar Kyoto (WKY) rats, were studied at 2 to 26 weeks of age. In the young SHR, the V_{max} of the Na^+,K^+ pump beings to decrease with the onset of hypertension. In the adult SHR, pump activity reaches values that are almost half of those observed in WKY normotensive rats. Unfortunately, rat erythrocytes have a low apparent affinity for ouabain, and this hampered a systematic study of ouabain binding undertaken to distinguish if the decreased maximal velocity of the pump results from a decrease in the number of transport units, in the turnover number of cation translocation, or in both.

Interestingly, the development of high blood pressure in SHR was correlated with a progressive decrease in the V_{max} of the pump in erythrocytes.[134] Therefore, the authors suggest that the decreased V_{max} of the pump reflects the appearance of endogenous Na^+,K^+ pump inhibitors in plasma of adult SHR. These endogenous ouabain-like substances have been found to be increased in SHR.[135]

On the other hand, Sabra rats of the hypertensive-prone substrain have an increased maximal velocity of the erythrocyte Na^+,K^+ pump.[136] Because RBC of these rats exhibit an increased Na^+ leak and internal Na^+ content is normal, it has been suggested that the increased pump is compensating for the leak abnormality.[136]

Thus, as with the investigations of human essential hypertension, studies in rats with spontaneous hypertension have revealed abnormalities of the Na^+,K^+ pump. It is true that in such animal models of hypertension, more control can be exercised over the various genetic and environmental influences involved in the condition. Unfortunately, none can serve as an undisputed model for the human disease.

G. SUMMARY

Figure 4 represents a summary of the kinetic characteristics of the Na^+,K^+ pump, as well as its relation to Na^+ leak and etiologic factors (genetic and nongenetic factors), in two different populations of hypertensives. As compared to cells of normotensives, cells of group A exhibit increased V_{max} and decreased affinity of the pump for internal Na^+ or increased Na^+ leak. Under basal, steady-state conditions, the higher Na^+ concentration in these cells stimulates Na^+ pumps (density of functional units and/or turnover number) to accommodate for the increased Na^+ concentration. The decreased affinity of the Na^+,K^+ pump for internal Na^+ may be related to structural abnormalities of the Na^+,K^+-ATPase of genetic origin. On the other hand, changes in the lipid composition of the membrane may account for

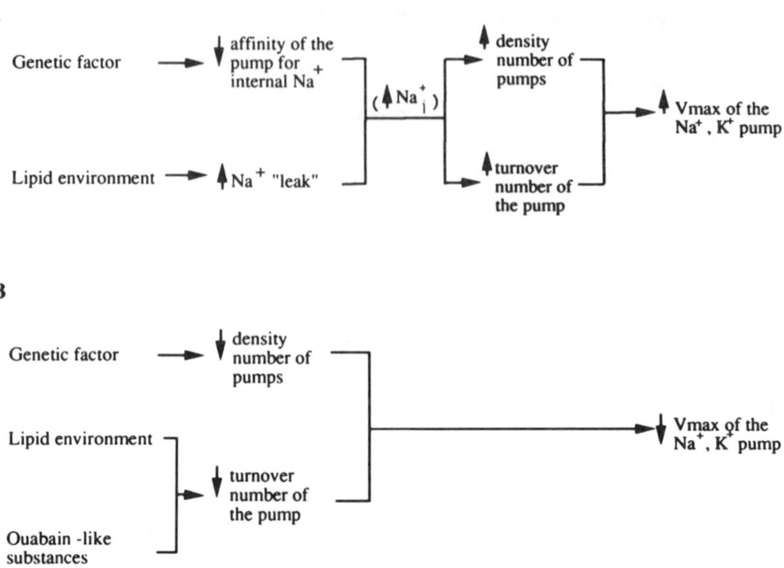

FIGURE 4. Relationships among activity of Na^+,K^+ pump, genetic factor, and nongenetic factors in various populations of hypertensives (see text for details).

the increased passive Na^+ permeability of the cell. Cells of group B have diminished V_{max} of the Na^+,K^+ pump that is associated to a decreased turnover number. A decreased synthesis of pumps during erythropoiesis probably occurs, which is genetically determined. Finally, the decrease in the turnover number may reflect the chronic influence on the pump of extracellular pump inhibitors, such as circulating ouabain-like substances, and/or of changes in the physicochemical properties of the membrane.

IV. PATHOPHYSIOLOGICAL, CLINICAL, AND PHARMACOLOGICAL ASPECTS OF THE KINETIC ABNORMALITIES OF THE Na^+,K^+ PUMP IN ESSENTIAL HYPERTENSION

A. PATHOPHYSIOLOGICAL IMPLICATIONS

Much of the current interest in the Na^+,K^+ pump activity in hypertension is due to recent suggestions that altered activity of the pump could be responsible for the increased peripheral resistance associated with hypertension. According to their pathogenic significance, kinetic abnormalities of the Na^+,K^+ pump can be divided as follows:[137]

1. Stable abnormality (diminished V_{max} of the pump). This is a defect that precedes (and is not modified by) the development (or treatment) of high

blood pressure. It is present in adult hypertensives and in some of their normotensive offspring.

2. Compensatory abnormality (increased V_{max} of the pump). This abnormality compensates other stable Na^+ transport defects, thus preventing transitory or permanent increases in cell Na^+ contents.
3. Acquired abnormality (diminished V_{max} of the pump). This is a defect that appears and develops with the increase in blood pressure. It has been observed in humans and animals following excess Na^+ intake and/or volume expansion.

Therefore, some of the mechanisms which may link a diminished activity of the Na^+,K^+ pump and changes in vascular tone will be discussed.

1. Hemodynamic Effects of Altered Na^+,K^+ Pump Activity *In Vivo*

Some indication of the *in vivo* effects of the inhibition of the Na^+,K^+ pump may be obtained from the hemodynamic responses of the cardiovascular system to the infusion of cardiac glycosides. In healthy humans and animals, cardiac glycoside infusion is followed by an acute increase in total peripheral resistance.[138-142] Whether long-term inhibition would cause sustained vasoconstriction is not clear. This is an important reservation, because chronic digitalization does not cause elevated blood pressure, even in healthy subjects,[143,144] while chronic treatment with ouabain has hypotensive action in rats.[145]

2. Effects of Diminished Na^+,K^+ Pump Activity *In Vitro*

In vitro experiments have shown that both neuronal and myogenic effects of reduced Na^+,K^+ pump activity may alter vascular tone. Exposure of innervated preparations to Na^+,K^+ pump inhibitors causes a release of transmitter noradrenaline from the vascular nerve terminals.[146] On the other hand, neural uptake of noradrenaline is at least partially dependent on neural Na^+,K^+ pump activity.[147] It has been shown recently that inhibition of the Na^+,K^+ pump by ouabain elevates the tone of resting human resistance arteries and potentiates the tone of precontracted vessels.[148] This myogenic effect of reduced Na^+,K^+ pump activity appears to be mediated by a depressant action of ouabain on the synthesis or release of endothelium-derived relaxing factor.[149,150]

3. Molecular Mechanisms by which Diminished Na^+,K^+ Pump Activity Increases Vascular Tone

The mechanism by which the inhibitors of Na^+,K^+ pump activity cause the release of noradrenaline from the nerve terminals is generally thought to be partially through Na^+,K^+ pump inhibition, with a resultant increase in intracellular Na^+ concentration of the nerve fibers. This reduces the extrusion of Ca^{2+} via a Na^+-Ca^{2+} exchange mechanism, and thus produces an increase in the intracellular free Ca^{2+} concentration.[151,152] Furthermore, release of Ca^{2+} from intracellular stores is also probably involved.[153] The mechanism by which Na^+,K^+ pump inhibition prevents the neuronal uptake of noradrenaline is still unknown.

There are several hypotheses regarding the myogenic response to Na^+,K^+ pump inhibition. First, as in nerves, the increase in intracellular Na^+ concentration resulting from Na^+,K^+ pump inhibition could cause an increase in intracellular free Ca^{2+} via Na^+-Ca^{2+} exchange. However, in contrast to cardiac muscle or aortic muscle, in more peripheral vascular smooth muscle, Na^+-Ca^{2+} exchange mechanisms play little or no role in the response to Na^+,K^+ pump inhibition.[154,155] It must be pointed out, however, that some influence of the Na^+-Ca^{2+} exchange mechanisms cannot be entirely ruled out, for under extreme conditions (where intracellular Na^+ is increased and extracellular Na^+ is reduced simultaneously) small responses of peripheral vascular smooth muscle are seen.[156,157] The second hypothesis is that depolarization which accompanies Na^+,K^+ pump inhibition may cause the response. The depolarization that accompanies the inhibition of the Na^+,K^+ pump is genetically ascribed to its electrogenicity.[158] Good evidence exists that the depolarization by Na^+,K^+ pump inhibition will potentiate the tone of activated vessels.[159] Indeed, experiments with Ca^{2+} antagonists show that these compounds eliminate the potentiating effects of Na^+,K^+ pump inhibition.[156-160] Because Ca^{2+} antagonists inhibit Ca^{2+} influx through potential-dependent channels,[161,162] the contracting effect of decreased Na^+,K^+ pump activity is most probably due to depolarization. Finally, other mechanisms for the effect of Na^+,K^+ pump inhibition on vascular tone have also been suggested. Feletou and Vanhoutte[163] have demonstrated that acetylcholine-induced hyperpolarization is sensitive to ouabain in canine coronary artery. More recent work has confirmed that hyperpolarization appears to be mediated by ATP-dependent K^+ channels.[164] It may be anticipated that ouabain would inhibit these K^+ channels and could therefore induce myogenic vasoconstrictor effects via this mechanism.[165]

In conclusion, agreement between the *in vivo* and the *in vitro* observations is that the acute inhibition of vascular Na^+,K^+ pump activity is accompanied by vasoconstriction. Neurogenic and myogenic mechanisms are involved in both cases. Agreement is also found as regards the long-term effects of the neurogenic responses, but not the myogenic mechanisms,[166] which is supported by recent observations by Nishio et al.[167] that salt-induced changes in a circulating ouabain-like substance and those in blood pressure or plasma noradrenaline showed positive correlations in essential hypertensive patients. Whether the proposed sequence of events (Figure 5) may be translated into the pathophysiology of essential hypertension remains to be established.

B. CLINICAL AND PHARMACOLOGICAL ASPECTS

We must recognize that there is still scarce information on which to draw the clinical and therapeutical characteristics of the different groups of essential hypertensives with the abnormalities of the Na^+,K^+ pump considered here. Nevertheless, some clinical findings and a particular pharmacological approach are discussed concerning those hypertensives.

Several studies have focused primarily on comparisons between relatively small numbers of hypertensives discretely categorized as patients with abnormal pump and

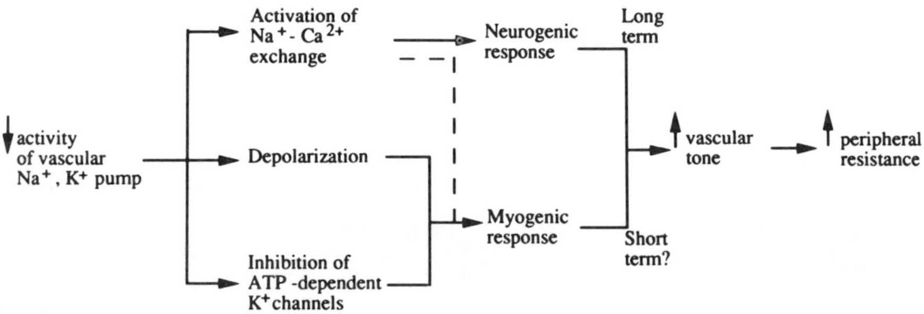

FIGURE 5. Relationships among peripheral resistance and activity of vascular Na^+,K^+ pump (see text for details).

patients with normal pump. In these studies[44,54,55] no significant differences in the clinical parameters of blood pressure (age, sex, systolic, diastolic and mean recorded blood pressure, age of first diagnosis of hypertension, number of given drugs, complications, body mass index, urinary Na^+ excretion, plasma glucose, cholesterol, triglycerides, and renin activity) were found between essential hypertensives with kinetic abnormalities of the Na^+,K^+ pump and the remaining hypertensives. However, when the relationships among the activity of the erythrocyte Na^+,K^+ pump and different clinical parameters are investigated in a large group of subjects without previous categorization as normotensives or hypertensives, two clinical observations emerge:[49] (1) male subjects demonstrated a lower pump activity than female subjects and (2) the body mass index was negatively correlated with the pump. Although sex-related differences in the erythrocyte Na^+,K^+ pump were previously demonstrated,[74] there is a lack of consensus regarding the relationship between the body mass index and the activity of the pump. Some studies suggest that such an association exists,[168,169] while others do not support this concept.[75,170-172] Relationships between the body mass index and Na^+,K^+ pump activity are likely to be established only when large numbers of subjects are investigated, as the activity of the Na^+,K^+ pump depends on multiple factors in addition to gender.

As previously mentioned, a key step in the development of essential hypertension may be the disturbance in cell ion homeostasis induced by the interaction of ouabain-like substances with the Na^+,K^+ pump. Therefore, it has been proposed that drugs that may ''protect'' the digitalis receptor site against pump inhibition are of potential interest as a new approach to the treatment of hypertension.[173]

Previous studies suggest that canrenone, an antihypertensive drug, may interfere with the above mechanism. In fact, canrenone is able to interact with the Na^+,K^+ pump *in vitro*.[173,174] This interaction is expected for a partial agonist at the digitalis receptor site. In addition, canrenone is able to partially antagonize *in vivo* the secondary effects of ouabain-like substances on cell Na^+ handling and blood pressure in rats with reduced renal mass under excess Na^+ intake.[175] These results suggest that chronic administration of canrenone to patients with essential hypertension may induce a lowering of blood pressure by antagonism with circulating ouabain-like substances at the vascular wall.

V. ASSUMPTIONS IN THE INTERPRETATION OF THE KINETIC ABNORMALITIES OF THE Na^+,K^+ PUMP IN ESSENTIAL HYPERTENSION: CRITICAL ANALYSIS

Almost every group that has reported associations of abnormalities of the Na^+,K^+ pump with hypertension has claimed that their disturbance throws light upon pathogenesis and pathophysiology. For this to be the case a certain number of assumptions must be made.

A. EXPERIMENTAL PROCEDURES DO NOT ALTER Na^+,K^+ PUMP ACTIVITY

In leukocytes, the relation between the intracellular Na^+ concentration and its efflux by means of the Na^+,K^+ pump is linear up to concentrations that are more than twice the normal values. The first order rate constant for Na^+ efflux is therefore the more satisfactory vehicle for describing the activity of the pump in these cells. In the RBC, this relation begins to break down when relatively small increases of intracellular Na^+ above the physiologic range occur as the pump approaches its maximal rate of activity.[4] In an attempt to circumvent this problem, some workers have reported the maximal velocity of Na^+ efflux by the Na^+,K^+ pump from Na^+-loaded cells. However, such experiments involve the study of cells whose composition has been manipulated until it differs greatly from the conditions that exist *in vivo*.[121] For instance, some investigators have used mercurial agents[44] and ionophores[47] to modify internal Na^+ content. These are harmful Na^+ loading methods because they alter chemical characteristics of the membrane (namely the mercurial agent PCMBS alters sulfhydryl group) and may irreversibly modify the affinity of the internal Na^+.[176] On the other hand, other investigators have developed a less harmful Na^+ loading method based on the physiological $NaHPO_4^-$ influx through the anion exchanger.[54,177] However, it is apparent that with this method the increase in intracellular Na^+ is inevitably accompanied by changes in the concentration of other intracellular ions and this also influences the pump.[121]

If a circulating inhibitor of the Na^+,K^+ pump plays a role in hypertension, observations of both increased and decreased Na^+,K^+ pump activity may be explained on the basis of different experimental conditions. For instance, with the pump partially inhibited *in vivo,* cells from hypertensive patients could manifest increased, unchanged, or decreased Na^+ pumping rates depending upon whether the inhibitor is or is not dissipated from the pump during cell preparation for the assay.[178]

B. STATISTICAL DESIGN OF THE STUDIES IS ADEQUATE

Agreement is universal that essential hypertension is associated with the decreased activity of the Na^+,K^+ pump in leukocytes; however, no unanimity exists as to whether the Na^+,K^+ pump of RBC is abnormal in patients with essential hypertension. As previously seen, a decrease in the maximal activity of the pump in essential hypertension has been reported, although this value has been said to be either normal or increased in hypertensive patients in other papers.

The analysis of the pooled data raises the question whether the inconsistent results from different centers could have been obtained purely by chance, assuming that comparable populations of control and hypertensive subjects were examined. Alternatively, it is possible that variations in the technique for measuring Na^+,K^+ pump activity marked real differences between the control and hypertensive groups, or that populations sampled by different centers were not strictly comparable.

An additional difficulty lies in the number of subjects studied. Reviewing this question in the light of recent work on intracellular Na^+, it would appear that although a number of studies do report higher intracellular Na^+ in blood cells of hypertensive patients,[179-185] almost as many negative reports have been published.[186-188] A close inspection of these reports, however, reveals that in the larger series, increases in the Na^+ content of blood cells from patients with hypertension were observed. In an overview of 20 studies involving 2822 participants Hilton[121] cites that for a study to have an 80% chance of finding a significant ($p < 0.05$) difference between normotensive and hypertensive persons, about 70 persons would have to be enrolled in each group. It is unfortunate that most studies related to the Na^+,K^+ pump do not contain an adequate number of subjects for each group.

C. DIFFERENCES BETWEEN POPULATIONS ARE CAUSALLY ASSOCIATED WITH HYPERTENSION PER SE

Even in inbred strains of rats, multiple differences are found at genetic loci throughout the genome between spontaneously hypertensive and control strains when genetic fingerprinting studies are carried out.[189] This suggests that many genetically linked factors which happen to have incorporated into the strain are not physiologically related to blood pressure. While some of the associations between ion transport processes and blood pressure may represent genetic linkage, some of the associations in humans are undoubtedly spurious and attributable to unrecognized differences between control and hypertensive groups.

On the other hand, studies of ion transport systems have overestimated the difference between normo- and hypertensive populations because of inadequate matching for confounding factors. In this regard, differences in weight, age, race, gender, diet, and lifestyle may be relevant. For instance, in 1968 Balfe and coworkers[190] described a black family with reduced erythrocyte Na^+,K^+ pump activity, and in 1983 Beutler et al.[75] demonstrated that the activity of the pump was influenced by ethnic extraction. Different groups have confirmed that the erythrocytes of black persons have a lower Na^+,K^+ pump activity than the erythrocytes of whites.[49,74,76,191] Although the lower Na^+,K^+ pump activity in blacks apparently relates to a lower pump density,[76,77,188] others have suggested that it may indicate the lasting effect of a circulating ouabain-like substance that inhibits the pump.[80] This contention is supported by findings that as a group blacks manifest several characteristics suggestive of salt sensitivity, a condition in which the levels of this factor are expected to be elevated.

D. *IN VITRO* ABNORMALITIES REFLECT *IN VIVO* DISTURBANCES

It must be assumed that disturbances of cell membrane function which can be demonstrated under laboratory conditions reflect *in vivo* abnormalities. Nevertheless, incubation media may differ radically from the body fluids in which the cell is normally bathed. Thus, humoral regulators of membrane function may be removed.[192] It seems likely, however, that processing of cells induces substantial alteration of their characteristics.[192]

Little evidence of ion transport alterations in the intact organism has been uncovered; however, one study does point to a divergence between *in vivo* and some *in vitro* studies. Boon et al.[193] investigated the distribution of administered rubidium chloride and ^{42}K in subjects with untreated hypertension. Cation influx into erythrocytes was accelerated, suggesting increased rather than reduced Na^+,K^+ pump activity as a result of inhibition by a circulating agent which some groups have reported. It was, however, possible to demonstrate the inhibition of the erythrocyte Na^+,K^+ pump by ouabain using this method.[193]

The likelihood that *in vitro* conditions do not reflect *in vivo* conditions does not, of course, explain the observed differences in hyper- and normotensive populations, because a systematic error could not create significant differences between populations unless an initial biochemical difference influenced measurements. Technical errors, however, do influence the interpretation of observed abnormalities because they may not give *in vivo* to alterations in intracellular electrolytes, postulated on the basis of *in vitro* conditions. Rather, they may indicate the potential vulnerability of cells from hypertensive patients to particular experimental conditions.

E. CHANGES IN BLOOD CELLS ARE MARKERS FOR CHANGES IN CELLS RELATED TO BLOOD PRESSURE

Remarkably little information exists to indicate how far measurements of ion handling by blood cells reflect similar changes in tissues more relevant to hypertension, e.g., the resistance vessel wall, the autonomic neuron, or the renal tubule cell.

Aalkjaer et al.[194] measured ouabain-sensitive Na^+ efflux in leukocytes and resistance vessels obtained from omental fat at operation in nonhypertensive human subjects. A significant correlation was found for ouabain-sensitive Na^+ pumping between these tissues. Thus, it is tempting to speculate on the likelihood that abnormalities of Na^+,K^+ pump activity detected in blood cells act as a marker for similar disturbances in vascular tissue.

On the other hand, erythrocyte Na^+,K^+ pump activity has been found to be inversely correlated with systolic, diastolic, and mean blood pressure levels in a large population comparing both normo- and hypertensive individuals.[49] Furthermore, the development of high blood pressure in SHR is correlated with a progressive decrease in maximal Na^+,K^+ pump activity in erythrocytes.[134] Although correlations of the RBC Na^+,K^+ pump with the systemic blood pressure do not necessarily imply a cause and effect relationship, they strongly suggest that these variables play an important role in blood pressure control.

It is certain that up to now inaccessibly has prevented the acquisition of relevant information in this field. However, recent developments have made available the

TABLE 1
Limitations to Establish the Relevance of Na^+,K^+ Pump Abnormalities in Hypertension

Experimental limitations
- Manipulation and chemicals alter physicochemical characteristics of the membrane
- Manipulation and chemicals modify intracellular composition
- Laboratory conditions do not reproduce *in vivo* situation

Statistical limitations
- The number of subjects studied is not adequate
- Differences among groups may be by chance
- Populations sampled by different authors are not comparable
- Populations studied are inadequately matched for confounding factors

Pathophysiological limitations
- There is no evidence of Na^+,K^+ pump alterations in the intact organism
- Findings on the Na^+,K^+ pump have been obtained in cells not representative of cells involved in blood pressure regulation
- Association of Na^+,K^+ pump abnormalities with hypertension do not imply a cause and effect relationship

study of ion transport in human resistance arteries obtained from small biopsies of skin and subcutaneous fat.[195,196] This experimental approach makes unnecessary the assumption that abnormalities in surrogate cells are shared by vascular cells.

In summary, although essential hypertension is associated with disturbances of Na^+,K^+ pump activity, some limitations must be resolved (Table 1) before the significance of such disturbances can be established.

VI. CONCLUSIONS

Investigation of cell Na^+ transport kinetics has confirmed the prediction of Canessa et al.[197] that the population of patients with essential hypertension is heterogeneous regarding Na^+ transport abnormality.[177] As considered in this chapter, that heterogeneity is particularly relevant as concerns the Na^+,K^+ pump. In fact, investigations using blood cells show that different patterns of abnormal kinetics of the Na^+,K^+ pump are present in patients with essential hypertension. Mechanisms responsible for the kinetic abnormalities of the Na^+,K^+ pump and their contribution to the development of essential hypertension are poorly understood. The best interpretation of the available evidence is that genetic factors are important but not exclusive determinants of Na^+,K^+ pump activity in blood cells. On the other hand, the lower Na^+,K^+ pump activity in these cells may indicate the lasting effect of a circulating substance that inhibits the pump. While the extrapolation of the findings in blood cells to vascular cells is not without its dangers, it is tempting to speculate that we may eventually find the same categories of defects in Na^+,K^+ pump activity in the blood vessels of hypertensive humans that is observed in their blood cells. Though unproved, this hypothesis remains an attractive possibility and a potent stimulus to research in the field of the Na^+,K^+ pump in hypertension. We can expect that the next several years will see the development of more adequate assays, allowing large-scale Na^+,K^+ pump abnormalities in circulating and non-circulating cells of essential hypertensive patients. This will help to characterize different pathophysiologic forms of essential hypertension, and it may help to better individualize the antihypertensive treatment.

REFERENCES

1. **Tobian, L. and Binion, J. T.,** Tissue cations and water in arterial hypertension, *Circulation,* 5, 754, 1952.
2. **Losse, H., Weymeyer, H., and Wessels, F.,** Derwasser und Elektrolyt-Ghalt von Erythrocyten bei Arterieller Hypertonie, *Klin. Wochenschr.,* 38, 393, 1960.
3. **Postnov, Y. V. and Orlov, S. N.,** Ion transport across plasma membrane in primary hypertension, *Physiol. Rev.,* 65, 904, 1985.
4. **Garay, R. P. and Garrahan, P. J.,** The interaction of sodium and potassium with the sodium pump in red cells, *J. Physiol. (London),* 231, 297, 1973.
5. **Stekhoven, F. and Bonting, S.,** Transport adenosine triphosphatases: properties and functions, *Physiol. Rev.,* 61, 1, 1981.
6. **Wallick, E., Lane, L., and Schwartz, A.,** Biochemical mechanism of the sodium pump, *Annu. Rev. Physiol.,* 41, 397, 1979.
7. **Kaplan, J.,** Ion movements through the sodium pump, *Annu. Rev. Physiol.,* 47, 535, 1985.
8. **Glynn, I. M.,** The Na^+,K^+ transporting adenosine triphosphatase, in *The Enzymes of Biological Membrane,* Vol. 3, 2nd ed., Martosoni, A., Ed., Plenum Press, New York, 1985, 35.
9. **Jorgensen, P. L.,** Mechanism of the Na^+,K^+ pump. Protein structure and conformation of the pure $(Na^+ + K^+)$-ATPase, *Biochim. Biophys. Acta,* 694, 27, 1982.
10. **Hokin, H. L., Dahl, J. L., Dupree, J. D., Dixon, J. F., Hackney, J. F., and Perdue, J. F.,** Studies on the characterization of the sodium-potassium transport of adenosine triphosphatase. X. Purification of the enzyme from rectal gland of *Squalus acanthias, J. Biol. Chem.,* 248, 2593, 1973.
11. **Forbush, B., Kaplan, J. H., and Hoffman, J. F.,** Characterization of a new photoaffinity derivative of ouabain: labeling of the large polypeptide and a proteolipid component of the Na,K-ATPase, *Biochemistry,* 17, 3667, 1978.
12. **Hardwicke, P. M. D. and Freytag, J. W.,** A proteolipid associated with Na,K-ATPase is not essential for ATPase activity, *Biochem. Biophys. Res. Commun.,* 102, 250, 1982.
13. **Schneider, J. W., Mercer, R. W., Caplan, M., Emanuel, J. R., Sweadner, K. J., Benz, E. J., Jr., and Levenson, R.,** Molecular cloning of rat brain Na,K-ATPase α-subunit cDNA, *Proc. Natl. Acad. Sci. U.S.A.,* 82, 6357, 1985.
14. **Mercer, J. W., Schneider, J. W., Savitz, A., Emanuel, J. R., Benz, E. J., Jr., and Levenson, R.,** Rat-brain Na,K-ATPase β-chain gene: primary structure, tissue specific expression, and amplification in ouabain-resistant HeLa C^+ cells, *Mol. Cell. Biol.,* 6, 3884, 1986.
15. **Kawamura, M. and Nagano, K.,** Evidence for essential disulfide bonds in the β-subunit of $(Na^+ + K^+)$-ATPase, *Biochim. Biophys. Acta,* 774, 188, 1984.
16. **Noguchi, S., Noda, M., Takahaski, H., Kawakami, K., Ohta, T., Nagano, K., Hirose, T., Inayama, S., Kawamura, M., and Numa, S.,** Primary structure of the β-subunit of *Torpedo californica* $(Na^+ + K^+)$-ATPase deduced from cDNA sequence, *FEBS Lett,* 196, 315, 1986.
17. **Kawakami, K., Nojima, H., Ohta, T., and Nagano, K.,** Molecular cloning and sequence analysis of human Na,K-ATPase β-subunit, *Nucleic Acids Res.,* 14, 2833, 1986.
18. **Schull, G. E., Lane, L. K., and Lingrel, J. B.,** Amino-acid sequence of the β-subunit of the $(Na^+ + K^+)$-ATPase deduced from a cDNA, *Nature,* 321, 429, 1986.

19. **Schull, G. E., Schwartz A., and Lingrel, J. B.,** Amino-acid sequence of the catalytic subunit of the (Na^+ + K^+)-ATPase deduced from a complementary DNA, *Nature,* 316, 691, 1985.
20. **Mercer, J. W., Schneider, J. W., and Benz, E. J., Jr.,** Na,K ATP-ase structure, in *Red Blood Cell Membranes: Structure, Function, Clinical Implications,* Agre, P. and Parker, J. G., Eds., Marcel Dekker, New York, 1989, 135.
21. **Sweadner, K. J.,** Isozymes of the Na^+/K^+-ATPase, *Biochim. Biophys. Acta,* 988, 185, 1989.
22. **Broude, N. E., Modyanov, N. N., Monastyrskaya, G. S., and Sverdlov, E. D.,** Advances in Na^+,K^+-ATPase studies: from protein to gene and back to protein, *FEBS Lett.,* 257, 1, 1989.
23. **Lingrel, J. B., Orlowski, J., Shull, M. M., and Price, E. M.,** Molecular genetics of Na,K-ATPase, *Prog. Nucleic Acids Res. Mol. Biol.,* 38, 37, 1990.
24. **Takeyasu, K., Lemas, V., and Fambrough, D. M.,** Stability of (Na^+ + K^+)-ATPase α-subunit isoforms in evolution, *Am. J. Physiol.,* 259, C619, 1990.
25. **Post, R. L. and Jolly, P. C.,** The linkage of sodium, potassium and ammonium active transport across the human erythrocyte membrane, *Biochem. Biophys. Acta,* 25, 118, 1957.
26. **Sen, A. K. and Post, R. L.,** Stoichiometry and localization of adenosine triphosphate-dependent sodium and potassium transport in the erythrocyte, *J. Biol. Chem.,* 239, 345, 1964.
27. **Alberts, R. W., Koval, G. J., and Siegel, G. J.,** Studies on the interaction of ouabain and other cardioactive steroids with Na,K-activated ATPase, *Mol. Pharmacol.,* 4, 324, 1968.
28. **Post, R. L., Kume, S., Tobin, T., Orcutt, B., and Sen, A. K.,** Flexibility of an active center in sodium-plus-potassium adenosine triphosphatase, *J. Gen. Physiol.,* 54, 304s, 1969.
29. **Sachs, J. R.,** The order of addition of sodium and release of potassium at the inside of the sodium pump of the human red cell, *J. Physiol. (London),* 381, 149, 1986.
30. **Garrahan, P. J. and Glynn, I. M.,** The incorporation of inorganic phosphate by reversal of the sodium pump, *J. Physiol. (London),* 192, 237, 1967.
31. **Garrahan, P. J. and Glynn, I. M.,** The behavior of the sodium pump in red cells in the absence of external potassium, *J. Physiol. (London),* 192, 159, 1967.
32. **Blostein, R.,** Enzymatic and functional aspects of Na^+/K^+ transport, in *The Red Blood Cell Membrane,* Raess, B. U. and Tunnicliff, G., Eds., Humana Press, Clifton, NJ, 1989, 55.
33. **Glynn, I. M. and Karlish, S. J. D.,** ATP hydrolysis associated with an uncoupled Na efflux through the sodium pump: evidence for allosteric effects of intracellular ATP and extracellular Na, *J. Physiol. (London),* 256, 465, 1967.
34. **Dissing, S. and Hoffman, J. F.,** Anion-coupled Na efflux mediated by the Na/K pump in human red blood cells, *Curr. Topics Membr. Trans.,* 19, 693, 1983.
35. **Glynn, I. M., Lew, V. L., and Lüthi, U.,** Reversal of the potassium entry mechanism in red cells, with and without reversal of the entire pump cycle, *J. Physiol. (London),* 207, 371, 1970.
36. **Simmons, T. J. B.,** The interaction of ATP-analogues possessing a blocked phosphate group with the sodium pump in human red blood cells, *J. Physiol. (London),* 244, 731, 1975.
37. **Kaplan, J. H. and Kenney, L. J.,** ADP supports ouabain-sensitive K-K exchange in human red blood cells, *Ann. N.Y. Acad. Sci.,* 402, 295, 1982.
38. **Hoffman, J. F.,** Active transport of Na^+ and K^+ by red blood cells, in *Physiology of Membrane Disorders,* 2nd ed., Andreoli, T. E., Hoffman, J. F., Fanestil, D. F., and Schulz, S. G., Eds., Plenum Press, New York, 1986, 221.
39. **Polvani, C. and Blostein, R.,** Protons as substitutes for sodium and potassium in the sodium pump reaction, *J. Biol. Chem.,* 293, 16757, 1988.
40. **Yingst, D. R.,** Modulation of the Na,K-ATPase by Ca and intracellular proteins, *Annu. Rev. Physiol.,* 50, 291, 1988.
41. **Clausen, T.,** Regulation of active Na^+,K^+ transport in skeletal muscle, *Physiol. Rev.,* 66, 542, 1986.
42. **Yoda, A. and Yoda, S.,** Two different phosphorylation dephosphorylation cycles of Na^+,K^+-ATPase proteoliposomes accompanying Na^+ transport in the absence of K^+, *J. Biol. Chem.,* 262, 110, 1987.
43. **Aviv, A. and Lasker, N.,** Proposed defects in membrane transport and intracellular ions as pathogenic factors in essential hypertension, in *Hypertension: Pathophysiology, Diagnosis, and Management,* Laragh, J. H. and Brenner, B. M., Eds., Raven Press, New York, 1990, 923.

44. **Díez, J., Hannaert, P., and Garay, R. P.,** Kinetic study of Na^+-K^+ pump in erythrocytes from essential hypertensive patients, *Am. J. Physiol.*, 252, H1, 1987.
45. **Wambach, G., Helber, A., Booner, G., and Hummerick, W.,** Natrium-Kalium-Adenosin-Triphosphatase-activitat in Erythrozyteng-Hosts von Patienten mit essentieler Hypertonie, *Klin. Wochenschr.*, 1, 349, 1979.
46. **Tuck, M. L., Gross, C., Maxwell, M. H., Brickman, A. S., Krasnoshtein, G., and Mayes, D.,** Erythrocyte Na^+,K^+ cotransport and Na^+,K^+ pump in black and Caucasian hypertensive patients, *Hypertension*, 6, 536, 1984.
47. **Tuck, M. L., Corry, D. B., Maxwell, M. H., and Stern, N.,** Kinetic analysis of erythrocyte Na^+-K^+ pump and cotransport in essential hypertension, *Hypertension*, 10, 204, 1987.
48. **Canessa, M., Redgrave, J., Laski, C., and Williams, G. H.,** Does sodium intake modify red cell Na^+ transporters in normal and hypertensive subjects?, *Am. J. Hypertension*, 2, 515, 1989.
49. **Rygielski, D., Reddi, A., Kuriyama, S., Lasker, N., and Aviv, A.,** Erythrocyte ghost Na^+,K^+-ATPase and blood pressure, *Hypertension*, 10, 259, 1987.
50. **Ambrosioni, E., Costa, F. V., Montebugnoli, L., Tartagni, F., and Magnani, V.,** Increased intralymphocytic sodium content in essential hypertension: an index of impaired Na^+ cellular metabolism, *Clin. Sci.*, 61, 181, 1981.
51. **Poston, L., Sewell, R. B., Wilkinson, S. P., Richardson, P. J., Williams, R., Clarkson, E. M., MacGregor, G. A., and de Wardener, H. E.,** Evidence for a circulating sodium transport inhibitor in essential hypertension, *Br. Med. J.*, 282, 847, 1981.
52. **Chien, Y. and Zhao, G.,** Abnormal leukocyte sodium transport in Chinese patients with essential hypertension and their normotensive offsprings, *Clin. Exp. Hypertension*, A6, 2279, 1984.
53. **Garay, R. P. and Nazaret, C.,** Na leak in erythrocytes from essential hypertensive patients, *Clin. Sci.*, 69, 613, 1985.
54. **De la Sierra, A., Coca, A., Aguilera, M. T., and Urbano, A.,** Abnormal Na^+-K^+ ATPase kinetics in a subset of essential hypertensive patients, *Eur. J. Clin. Invest.*, 18, 337, 1988.
55. **De la Sierra, A., Coca, A., Aguilera, M. T., Ingelmo, M., and Urbano-Márquez, A.,** Clinical profiles and erythrocyte Na^+ transport abnormalities of four major types of primary hypertension in Spain, *Kidney Int.*, 36, 114, 1989.
56. **Ringel, R. E., Hamlyn, J. M., Hamilton, B. P., Pinkas, G. A., Chlew, S. A., and Berman, M. A.,** Red blood cell Na^+,K^+-ATPase in men with newly diagnosed or previously treated essential hypertension, *Hypertension*, 9, 437, 1987.
57. **Postnov, Y. V., Orlov, S. N., Shevchenko, A., and Adler, A. M.,** Altered sodium permeability, calcium binding and Na^+,K^+-ATPase activity in red blood cell membrane in essential hypertension, *Pfluegers' Arch.*, 371, 263, 1977.
58. **Aderounmu, A. F. and Salako, L. A.,** Abnormal cation composition and transport in erythrocytes from hypertensive patients, *Eur. J. Clin. Invest.*, 9, 369, 1979.
59. **Zumkley, H. and Wessels, F.,** Diagnostic aspects of increased sodium concentration in red blood cell, in *Intracellular Electrolytes and Arterial Hypertension*, Zumkley, H. and Losse, H., Eds., Georg Thieme, Stuttgart, 1980, 104.
60. **Woods, K. L., Beevers, D. G., and West, M.,** Familial abnormality of erythrocyte cation transport in essential hypertension, *Br. Med. J.*, 282, 1186, 1981.
61. **Cooper, R., Miller, K., Trevisan, M., Sempos, C., Larbi, E., Ueshima, H., Le Grady, D., Ostrow, D., Stamler, J., Spalvins, A., and Canessa, M.,** Family history of hypertension and red cell cation transport in high school students, *J. Hypertension*, 1, 145, 1983.
62. **Cusi, D., Barlassina, C., Ferrandi, M., Palazzi, P., Celega, E., and Bianchi, G.,** Relationship between altered Na-K cotransport and Na-Li countertransport in the erythrocytes of essential hypertensive patients, *Clin. Sci.*, 61, 33s, 1981.
63. **Heagerty, A. M., Bing, R. F., Milner, M., Thurston, H., and Swales, J. D.,** Leukocyte membrane sodium transport in normotensive populations: dissociation of abnormalities of sodium efflux from raised blood pressure, *Lancet*, 2, 894, 1982.
64. **Svensson, A. and Sigström, L.,** Blood pressure, erythrocyte sodium and potassium concentrations and Na^+,K^+-ATPase activity in children with hypertensive mothers, *J. Hypertension*, 4, 269, 1986.

65. **Cusi, D., Tripodi, G., Alberghini, E., Niutta, E., Barlassina, C., Fossali, E., Dossi, F., and Bianchi, G.,** Heritability of sodium transport systems and hypertension, *Ann. N.Y. Acad. Sci.*, 488, 576, 1986.
66. **Cruickshank, J. K. and Beevers, D. G.,** Epidemiology of hypertension: blood pressure in blacks and whites, *Clin. Sci.*, 62, 1, 1982.
67. **Harlan, W. R., Hull, A. L., Schmouder, R. L., Landis, J. R., Larkin, F. A., and Thompson, F. E.,** High blood pressure in older Americans: the first national health and nutrition examination survey, *Hypertension,* 6, 802, 1984.
68. **Grim, C. E., Luft, F. C., Miller, J. Z., Meneely, G. R., Battarbee, H. D., Hames, C. G., and Dahl, L. K.,** Racial differences in blood pressure in Evans County, Georgia: relationship to sodium and potassium intake and plasma renin activity, *J. Chronic Dis.*, 33, 87, 1980.
69. **Boyle, E.,** Biological patterns in hypertension by race, sex, body weight and skin, *JAMA,* 213, 1637, 1973.
70. **Freis, E.,** Age, race, sex and other indices of risk in hypertension, *Am. J. Med.*, 58, 275, 1973.
71. **Dustan, H. P., Valdes, G., Bravo, E. L., and Tarazi, R. C.,** Excessive sodium retention as a characteristic of salt sensitive hypertension, *Am. J. Med. Sci.*, 292, 67, 1986.
72. **Luft, F. C., Weinberger, M. H., and Grim, C. E.,** Sodium sensitivity and resistance in normotensive human, *Am. J. Med.*, 72, 726, 1982.
73. **Weinberger, M. H., Luft, F. C., Block, R., Henry, D. P., Pratt, J. H., Weyman, A. E., Ramkin, L. I., Murray, R. H., Willis, L. R., and Grim, C. E.,** The blood pressure-raising effect of high dietary sodium intake: racial differences and the role of potassium, *J. Am. Coll. Nutr.*, 1, 139, 1982.
74. **Lasker, N., Hoop, L., Grossman, S., Bamforth, R., and Aviv, A.,** Race and sex differences in erythrocyte Na^+,K^+ and Na^+-K^+-adenosine triphosphatase, *J. Clin. Invest.*, 75, 1813, 1985.
75. **Beutler, E., Kuhl, W., and Sacks, P.,** Sodium-potassium-ATPase activity is influenced by ethnic origin and not by obesity, *N. Engl. J. Med.*, 309, 756, 1983.
76. **Izumo, H., Lear, S., Williams, M., Rosa, R., and Epstein, F. H.,** Sodium-potassium pump, ion fluxes, and cellular dehydration in sickle cell anemia, *J. Clin. Invest.*, 79, 1621, 1987.
77. **Hoop, L., Lasker, N., Grossman, S., Bamforth, R., and Aviv, A.,** [^{3}H]-ouabain binding of red blood cells in whites and blacks, *Hypertension,* 8, 1050, 1986.
78. **Woods, K. L., Beevers, D. G., and West, M. J.,** Racial differences in red cell cation transport and their relationship to essential hypertension, *Clin. Exp. Hypertension,* 3, 655, 1981.
79. **Weder, A. B., Torretti, B. A., and Julius, S.,** Racial differences in erythrocyte cation transport, *Hypertension,* 6, 115, 1984.
80. **Aviv, A. and Gardner, J.,** Racial differences in ion regulation and their possible links to hypertension in blacks, *Hypertension,* 14, 584, 1989.
81. **Sweadner, K. J.,** Two molecular forms of (Na^+,K^+)-stimulated ATP-ase in brain, *J. Biol. Chem.*, 254, 6060, 1979.
82. **Urayama, O., Shutt, H., and Sweadner, K. J.,** Identification of three isoenzyme proteins of the catalytic subunit of the Na^+,K^+-ATPase in rat brain, *J. Biol. Chem.*, 264, 8271, 1989.
83. **Herrera, V. L., Emanuel, J. R., Ruiz-Opazo, N., Levenson, R., and Nadal-Ginard, B.,** Three differentially expressed Na^+,K^+-ATPase α subunit isoforms: structural and functional implications, *J. Cell Biol.*, 105, 1855, 1987.
84. **Sweadner, K. J.,** Enzymatic properties of separated isoenzymes of the Na^+,K^+-ATPase, *J. Biol. Chem.*, 260, 11508, 1985.
85. **Herrera, V. L., Chobanian, A. V., and Ruiz-Opazo, N.,** Isoform-specific modulation of Na^+,K^+-ATPase alpha-subunit gene expression in hypertension, *Science,* 241, 221, 1988.
86. **Herrera, V. L. M. and Ruiz-Opazo, N.,** Identical Na^+,K^+-ATPase α subunit gene polymorphism in two genetic hypertensive rat strains, *Hypertension,* 12, 338, 1988.
87. **Nojima, H., Yagawa, Y., and Kawakami, K.,** The Na^+,K^+-ATPase alpha 2 subunit gene displays restriction fragment length polymorphisms between the genomes of normotensive and hypertensive rats, *J. Hypertension,* 7, 937, 1989.

88. **Rapp, J. P.,** A paradigm for identification of primary genetic causes of hypertension in rats, *Hypertension,* 5(Suppl. 1), 1198, 1983.
89. **Rapp, J. P. and Dene, H.,** Failure of alleles at the Na^+,K^+-ATPase α_1 locus to cosegregate with blood pressure in Dahl rats, *J. Hypertension,* 8, 457, 1990.
90. **Corrocher, R., Steinmayr, M., Ruzzenente, O., Brugnara, C., Bertinato, L., Mazzi, M., Furri, C., Bonfanti, D., and De Sandre, G.,** Elevation of red cell sodium-lithium countertransport in hyperlypidemias, *Life Sci.,* 36, 649, 1985.
91. **Hunt, S. C., Williams, R. R., Smith, J. B., and Ash, K. O.,** Associations of three erythrocyte cation transport systems with plasma lipids in Utah subjects, *Hypertension,* 8, 30, 1986.
92. **Hajem, S., Moreau, T., Hannaert, P., Lellouch, J., Orssaud, G., Huel, G., Claude, J. R., and Garay, R. P.,** Erythrocyte cation transport systems and plasma lipids in a general male population, *J. Hypertension,* 8, 891, 1990.
93. **Hespel, P., Lijnen, P., Fagard, R., M'Buyamba-Kabangu, J. R., Van Hoof, R., Lissens, W., Rossenew, M., and Amery, A.,** Changes in erythrocyte sodium and plasma lipids associated with physical training, *J. Hypertension,* 6, 159, 1988.
94. **Hannaert, P. A., Moreau, T., Huel, G., Orssaud, G., Lellouch, J., Claude, J. R., Sahuquillo, J., and Garay, R. P.,** Blood pressure and erythrocyte Na^+ transport systems in a French urban male population, *J. Hypertension,* 6, 905, 1988.
95. **Coca, A. and Garay, R.,** Disturbances in Na^+ transport systems induced by ethanol in human red blood cells, *Alcohol Clin. Exp. Res.,* 12, 534, 1988.
96. **Weder, A. B., Serr, C., Torretti, B. A., Basset, D. R., and Zweifler, A. J.,** Effects of lovastatin treatment on red blood cell and platelet cation transport, *Hypertension,* 17, 203, 1991.
97. **Cooper, R. A., Arner, E. C., Wiley, J. S., and Shattil, S. J.,** Modification of red cell membrane structure by cholesterol-rich lipid dispersions, *J. Clin. Invest.,* 55, 115, 1975.
98. **Spector, A. A. and Yorek, M. A.,** Membrane lipid composition and cellular function, *J. Lipid Res.,* 26, 1015, 1985.
99. **Yeagle, P. L.,** Cholesterol modulation of (Na^+,K^+)-ATPase hydrolyzing activity in the human erythrocyte, *Biochim. Biophys. Acta,* 727, 39, 1983.
100. **Kimelberg, H. K. and Papahadjopoulos, D.,** Effects of phospholipid acyl chain fluidity, phase transitions, and cholesterol on (Na^+,K^+)-adenosine triphosphatase, *J. Chem.,* 249, 1071, 1974.
101. **Claret, M., Garay, R., and Giraud, F.,** The effect of membrane cholesterol on the sodium pump in red blood cells, *J. Physiol.,* 274, 247, 1978.
102. **Gokkusu, C., Uysal, M., and Oz, H.,** Plasma and erythrocyte phospholipid levels and erythrocyte Na^+,K^+-ATPase activity in rabbits fed on cholesterol, *Med. Sci. Res.,* 15, 273, 1987.
103. **Bing, R. F., Heagerty, A. M., Thurston, H., and Swales, J. D.,** Ion transport in hypertension: are changes in the cell membrane responsible?, *Clin. Sci.,* 71, 225, 1986.
104. **de Wardener, H. E. and MacGregor, G. A.,** Dahl's hypothesis that saluretic substance may be responsible for a sustained rised arterial pressure: its possible role in essential hypertension, *Kidney Int.,* 18, 1, 1980.
105. **Haddy, F. J., Pamnani, M. B., and Clough, D. L.,** Volume over-load hypertension: a defect in the sodium-potassium pump?, *Cardiovasc. Rev. Rep.,* 1, 376, 1980.
106. **Blaustein, M. P. and Hamlyn, J. M.,** Sodium transport inhibition, cell calcium, and hypertension: the natriuretic hormone/Na^+-Ca^{++} exchange/hypertension hypothesis, *Am. J. Med.,* 5, 45, 1984.
107. **Haupert, G. T., Jr. and Sancho, J. M.,** Sodium transport inhibitor in bovine hypothalamus, *Proc. Natl. Acad. Sci. U.S.A.,* 76, 4658, 1979.
108. **Brody, M. J. and Johnson, A. K.,** Role of the anteroventral third ventricle region in fluid and electrolyte balance, blood pressure regulation and hypertension, in *Frontiers in Neuroendocrinology,* Martini, L. and Ganong, W. F., Eds., Raven Press, New York, 1980, 209.
109. **Songu-Mize, E., Bealer, S. L., and Caldwell, R. W.,** Effect of AV3V lesions on the development of DOCA-salt hypertension and vascular Na^+ pump activity, *Hypertension,* 4, 575, 1982.
110. **de Wardener, H. E., Mills, I. S., Clapham, W. F., and Hayter, C. J.,** Studies on the mechanism of the sodium diuresis which follows the administration of intravenous saline in the dog, *Clin. Sci.,* 21, 249, 1961.

111. **MacGregor, G. A., Fenton, S., Alaghband-Zadeh, J., Markandu, N. D., Roulston, J. E., and de Wardener, H. E.,** An increase in a circulating inhibitor of Na$^+$,K$^+$-dependent ATPase: a possible link between salt intake and the development of hypertension, *Clin. Sci.*, 61, 17S, 1981.
112. **Umeda, T., Naomi, S., Inoue, J., Ohno, M., Miura, F., Hamasaki, S., Iwaoka, T., and Sato, T.,** Assay of circulating sodium pump inhibitor in patients with essential hypertension and normotensive subjects, *Clin. Exp. Hypertension,* 9, 1233, 1987.
113. **Devynck, M. A., Pernollet, M. G., Rosenfeld, J. B., and Meyer, P.,** Measurement of digitalis-like compound in plasma: application in studies of essential hypertension, *Br. Med. J.*, 287, 631, 1983.
114. **Pamnani, M. B., Clough, D. L., Huot, S. J., and Haddy, F. J.,** Sodium-potassium pump activity in experimental hypertension, in *Vasodilation,* Vanhoutte, P. M. and Leusen, I., Eds., Raven Press, New York, 1981, 391.
115. **Cruber, K. A., Whitaker, J. M., and Buckalew, V. M., Jr.,** Endogenous digitalis-like substance in plasma of volume expanded dogs, *Nature,* 287, 743, 1980.
116. **Price, M. B., Pamnani, M. B., Burris, J. F., Link, W. T., Freis, E. D., and Haddy, F. J.,** Acute volume expansion in humans releases a factor which inhibits the vascular Na$^+$-K$^+$ pump, *J. Hypertension,* 2(Suppl. 3), S471, 1984.
117. **Gault, M. H., Vasder, S. C., Longerich, L. L., Fernandez, P., Prabhakaran, V., Dawe, M., and Maillet, C.,** Plasma digitalis-like factor(s) increase with salt loading, *N. Engl. J. Med.*, 309, 1459, 1983.
118. **de Wardener, H. E., MacGregor, G. A., Clarkson, E. M., Alaghband-Zadeh, J., Bitensky, L., and Chayen, J.,** Effect of sodium intake on ability of human plasma to inhibit renal Na$^+$-K$^+$ ATPase in vivo, *Lancet,* 1, 411, 1981.
119. **Morgan, T., Myers, J., and Fitzgibbon, W.,** Sodium intake, blood pressure and red cell sodium efflux, *Clin. Exp. Hypertension,* 3, 641, 1981.
120. **Pamnani, M., Huot, S., Buggy, J., Clough, D., and Haddy, F.,** Demonstration of a humoral inhibitor of the Na$^+$-K$^+$ pump in some models of experimental hypertension, *Hypertension,* 3, SII-96, 1981.
121. **Hilton, P. J.,** Factors influencing leukocyte sodium transport in hypertension, *Klin. Wochenschr.*, 63(Suppl. III), 49, 1985.
122. **Hamlyn, J. M., Ringel, R., Schaeffer, J., Levinson, P. D., Hamilton, B. P., Kowarski, A. A., and Blaustein, M. P.,** A circulating inhibitor of Na$^+$-K$^+$-dependent ATPase associated with essential hypertension, *Nature,* 300, 650, 1982.
123. **de Wardener, H. E.,** Kidney, salt intake, and Na$^+$,K$^+$-ATPase inhibitors in hypertension, *Hypertension,* 17, 830, 1991.
124. **Ludens, J. H., Clark, M. A., DuCharme, D. W., Harris, D. W., Lutzke, B. S., Mandel, F., Mathews, W. R., Sutter, D. M., and Hamlyn, J. M.,** Purification of an endogenous digitalislike factor from human plasma for structural analysis, *Hypertension,* 17, 923, 1991.
125. **Mathews, W. R., DuCharme, D. W., Hamlyn, J. M., Harris, D. W., Mandel, F., Clark, M. A., and Ludens, J. H.,** Mass spectral characterization of an endogenous digitalislike factor from human plasma, *Hypertension,* 17, 930, 1991.
126. **Bova, S., Blaustein, M. P., Ludens, J. H., Harris, D. W., DuCharme, D. W., and Hamlyn, J. M.,** Effects of an endogenous ouabainlike compound on heart and aorta, *Hypertension,* 17, 944, 1991.
127. **Weder, A. B.,** Membrane sodium transport and salt sensitivity of blood pressure, *Hypertension,* 17, 1, 1981.
128. **Weissberg, P. L., West, M. J., Kendall, M. J., Ingram, M., and Woods, K. L.,** Effect of changes in dietary sodium and potassium on blood pressure and cellular electrolyte handling in young normotensive subjects, *J. Hypertension,* 3, 475, 1985.
129. **Smith, J. B., Fineberg, N. S., Wade, M. B., and Weinberger, M. H.,** Acute sodium loading alters sodium pump in caucasian hypertensive subjects, *Hypertension,* 13, 15, 1989.
130. **Walter, V. and Muller, S.,** Evidence for a Na,K-ATPase inhibitor in erythrocytes of patients with essential hypertension, *Eur. J. Clin. Invest.*, 15, 209, 1985.

131. **Masuyama, Y., Tsuda, K., Shima, H., Ura, M., Takeda, J., Kimura, K., and Nishio, I.,** Membrane abnormality of erythrocytes is highly dependent on salt intake and renin profile in essential hypertension: an electron spin resonance study, *J. Hypertension,* 6(Suppl. 4), S266, 1988.
132. **Beaugé, L. and Ortiz, O.,** Rubidium, sodium and ouabain interaction on the influx of rubidium in rat red blood cells, *J. Physiol.,* 210, 519, 1970.
133. **De Mendonça, M., Grichois, M. L., Garay, R. P., Sassard, J., Ben Ishay, D., and Meyer, P.,** Abnormal net Na^+ and K^+ fluxes in erythrocytes of three varieties of genetically hypertensive rats, *Proc. Natl. Acad. Sci. U.S.A.,* 77, 4283, 1980.
134. **Rosati, C., Meyer, P., and Garay, R. P.,** Sodium transport kinetics in erythrocytes from spontaneously hypertensive rats, *Hypertension,* 11, 41, 1988.
135. **Wauquier, I., Pernollet, M. G., Grichois, M. L., Lacour, B., Meyer, P., and Devynck, M. A.,** Endogenous digitalislike circulating substances in spontaneously hypertensive rats, *Hypertension,* 12, 108, 1988.
136. **De Mendonça, M., Knorr, A., Grichois, M. L., Ben Ishay, D., Garay, R. P., and Meyer, P.,** Erythrocyte ion transport systems in primary and secondary hypertension of the rat, *Kidney Int.,* 21(Suppl. 11), 569, 1982.
137. **Garay, R.,** Typology of Na^+ transport abnormalities in erythrocytes from essential hypertensive patients. A first step towards the diagnosis and specific treatment of different forms of primary hypertension, *Cardiovasc. Drugs Ther.,* 4, 373, 1990.
138. **Dock, W. and Tainter, M. L.,** The circulatory changes after full therapeutic doses of digitalis, with a critical discussion of views on cardiac output, *J. Clin. Invest.,* 8, 467, 1930.
139. **Ross, J., Waldhausen, J. A., and Braunwald, E.,** Studies on digitalis. I. Direct effects on peripheral vascular resistance, *J. Clin. Invest.,* 39, 930, 1960.
140. **Harrison, L. A., Blaschke, J., Phillips, R. S., Price, W. E., Cotten, M. V., and Jacobson, E. D.,** Effects of ouabain on the splanchnic circulation, *J. Pharmacol. Exp. Ther.,* 169, 321, 1969.
141. **Treat, E., Ulano, H. B., and Jacobson, E. D.,** Effects of intra-arterial ouabain on mesenteric and carotid hemodynamics, *J. Pharmacol. Exp. Ther.,* 179, 144, 1971.
142. **DeMots, H., Rahimtoola, S. H., McAnulty, J. H., and Porte, G. A.,** Effects of ouabain on coronary and systemic vascular resistance and myocardial oxygen consumption in patients without heart failure, *Am. J. Cardiol.,* 41, 88, 1978.
143. **Haddy, F. J. and Overbeck, H. W.,** The role of humoral agents in volume expanded hypertension, *Life Sci.,* 19, 935, 1976.
144. **Guthrie, G. P.,** Effects of digoxin on responsiveness to the pressor actions of angiotensin and norepinephrine in man, *J. Clin. Endocrinol. Metab.,* 58, 76, 1984.
145. **Ayachi, S. and Brown, A. M.,** Hypotensive effects of cardiac glycosides in spontaneously hypertensive rats, *J. Pharmacol. Exp. Ther.,* 213, 520, 1980.
146. **Katsuragi, T. and Su, C.,** Release of purines and noradrenaline by ouabain and potassium chloride from vascular adrenergic nerves, *Br. J. Pharmacol.,* 58, 76, 1982.
147. **Bogdanski, D. F. and Brodie, B. B.,** The effects of inorganic ions on the storage and uptake of ^{3}H-norepinephrine by rat heart slices, *J. Pharmacol. Exp. Ther.,* 165, 181, 1969.
148. **Woolfson, R. G., Hilton, P. J., and Poston, L.,** The effect of ouabain and low sodium on the contractility of human subcutaneous resistance arteries, *Hypertension,* 15, 583, 1990.
149. **Rapoport, R. M., Schwartz, K., and Murad, F.,** Effects of sodium-potassium inhibitors and membrane depolarizing agents on sodium nitroprusside-induced relaxation and cyclic guanosine monophosphate accumulation in rat aorta, *Circ. Res.,* 57, 164, 1985.
150. **Woolfson, R. G. and Poston, L.,** Effect of ouabain in endothelium-dependent relaxation of human resistance arteries, *Hypertension,* 17, 619, 1991.
151. **Baker, P. F., Blaustein, M. P., Hodgkin, A. L., and Steinhardt, R. A.,** The influence of calcium on sodium efflux in squid axons, *J. Physiol.,* 200, 431, 1969.
152. **Nakazato, Y., Ito, S., and Ohga, A.,** Noradrenaline output induced by calcium, strontium and barium during exposure of guinea-pig vas deferens to ouabain, *Eur. J. Pharmacol.,* 68, 327, 1980.

153. **Torok, T. L., Salamon, Z., Nguyen, T. T., and Magyar, K.,** Spontaneous ^{3}H-noradrenaline release from the main pulmonary artery of the rabbit induced by sodium-pump inhibitor, *Q. J. Exp. Physiol.,* 69, 841, 1984.
154. **Mulvany, M. J.,** Effect of electrolyte transport on the response of arteriolar smooth muscle, *J. Cardiovasc. Pharmacol.,* 6(Suppl 3), S82, 1984.
155. **Vanbreemen, C., Aronson, P., and Loutzenhiser, R.,** Sodium-calcium interactions in mammalian smooth muscle, *Pharmacol. Rev.,* 30, 167, 1979.
156. **Mulvany, M. J., Aalkjaer, C., and Petersen, T. T.,** Intracellular sodium, membrane potential and contractility in rat mesenteric small arteries, *Circ. Res.,* 54, 750, 1984.
157. **Hermsmeyer, K.,** Electrogenesis of increased norepinephrine sensitivity of arterial vascular muscle in hypertension, *Circ. Res.,* 38, 362, 1976.
158. **Hendrickx, H. and Casteels, R.,** Electrogenic sodium pump in arterial smooth muscle cells, *Pfluegers' Arch.,* 346, 299, 1974.
159. **Fleming, W. W.,** The electrogenic Na^+,K^+-pump in smooth muscle: physiologic and pharmacologic significance, *Annu. Rev. Pharmacol. Toxicol.,* 20, 129, 1980.
160. **Flaim, S. F. and Dipette, D. J.,** Digoxin-norepinephrine response and calcium blocker effects in vascular smooth muscle, *Am. J. Physiol.,* 236, H613, 1979.
161. **Nyborg, N. C. B. and Mulvany, M. J.,** Effect of felodipine, new dihydropyridine vasodilator, on contractile responses to potassium, noradrenaline and calcium in mesenteric resistance vessels of the rat, *J. Cardiovasc. Pharmacol.,* 6, 499, 1984.
162. **Cauvin, C., Saida, K., and Vanbreemen, C.,** Effects of calcium antagonists on calcium fluxes in resistance vessels, *J. Cardiovasc. Pharmacol.,* 4, S287, 1982.
163. **Feletou, M. and Vanhoutte, P. M.,** Endothelium-dependent hyperpolarization of canine coronary smooth muscle, *Br. J. Pharmacol.,* 93, 515, 1988.
164. **Standen, N. B., Quayle, J. M., Davies, N. W., Brayden, J. E., Huang, Y., and Nelson, M. T.,** Hyperpolarizing vasodilators activate ATP-sensitive K^+ channels in arterial smooth muscle, *Science,* 245, 177, 1990.
165. **Taylor, S. G. and Weston, A. H.,** Endothelium-derived hyperpolarizing factor: a new endogenous inhibitor from the vascular endothelium, *TIPS,* 9, 272, 1988.
166. **Mulvany, M. J.,** Changes in sodium pump activity and vascular contraction, *J. Hypertension,* 3, 429, 1985.
167. **Nishio, I., Shima, H., Tsuda, K., Hano, T., and Masuyama, Y.,** Relationship between the sympathetic nervous system and sodium-potassium adenosine triphosphatase inhibitor in salt-sensitive patients with essential hypertension, *J. Hypertension,* 6(Suppl. 4), S216, 1988.
168. **De Luise, M., Blackburn, G. L., and Flier, J. S.,** Reduced activity of the red-cell sodium-potassium pump in human obesity, *N. Engl. J. Med.,* 303, 1017, 1980.
169. **Klimes, I., Nagulesparan, M., Unger, R. H., Aronoff, S. L., and Mott, D. M.,** Reduced Na,K-ATPase activity in intact red cells and isolated membranes from obese men, *J. Clin. Endocrinol. Metab.,* 54, 721, 1982.
170. **Simat, B. M., Mayrand, R. R., From, A. H. L., Morley, J. E., Billington, C., Fullerton, D. J., and Ahmed, K.,** Is the erythrocyte sodium pump altered in human obesity?, *J. Clin. Endocrinol. Metab.,* 56, 925, 1983.
171. **De Luise, M., Izumo, H., Grace, E. E., and Flier, J. S.,** Effect of diet upon the erythrocyte Na,K, pump, *J. Clin. Endocrinol. Metab.,* 56, 739, 1983.
172. **Martin, L. F., Dean, W. L., Flint, L. M., Jr., Suarez, C. P., Ratliffe, D. J., and Fry, D. E.,** Erythrocyte sodium-potassium-stimulated adenosine triphosphatase activity is not related to obesity, *J. Surg. Res.,* 34, 473, 1983.
173. **Garay, R. P., Díez, J., Nazaret, C., Dagher, G., and Abitbol, J. P.,** The interaction of carenone with the Na,K-pump in human red blood cells, *Naunyn-Schmiedeberg's Arch. Pharmacol.,* 329, 311, 1985.
174. **Finotti, P. and Palatini, P.,** Canrenone as a partial agonist at the digitalis receptor site of sodium-potassium activated adenosine triphosphatase, *J. Pharmacol. Exp. Ther.,* 217, 784, 1981.
175. **De Mendonça, M., Grichois, M. L., Pernollet, M. G., Thormann, B., Meyer, P., Devynck, M. A., and Garay, R. P.,** Hypotensive action of canrenone in a model of hypertension where a ouabain-like factor is present, *J. Hypertension,* 3(Suppl. 3), 573, 1985.

176. **Garrahan, P. and Rega, F.,** Cation loading of red cells, *J. Physiol.*, 193, 459, 1967.
177. **Garay, R. P.,** Kinetic aspects of red blood cell sodium transport system in essential hypertension, *Hypertension,* 10(Suppl. 1), I-11, 1987.
178. **Blaustein, M. P.,** Sodium transport and hypertension. Where are we going?, *Hypertension,* 6, 445, 1984.
179. **Cooper, R., Shamsi, N., and Katz, S.,** Increased intracellular calcium and sodium in hypertensive patients compared to normotensives, *Hypertension,* 9, 224, 1987.
180. **Ringel, R. E., Hamlyn, J. M., Schaeffer, J., Hamilton, B. P., Kowarski, A. A., Blaustein, M. P., and Berman, M. A.,** Red cell cotransport activity and sodium content in black men, *Hypertension,* 6, 724, 1984.
181. **Weissburg, P. L., Woods, K. L., and West, M. J.,** Genetic and ethnic influences on the distributions of Na^+ and K^+ in normotensive and hypertensive subjects, *J. Clin. Hypertension,* 3, 724, 1987.
182. **Forrester, T. E. and Alleyne, G. A. O.,** Sodium, potassium and rate constants for sodium efflux in leukocytes from hypertensive Jamaicans, *Br. Med. J.*, 283, 5, 1981.
183. **Aderounmu, A. F. and Salako, L. A.,** Abnormal cation composition and transport in erythrocytes from hypertensive patients, *Eur. J. Clin. Invest.*, 9, 369, 1979.
184. **Wessels, F. and Zumkley, H.,** Sodium metabolism of RBC in hypertensive patients, in *Intracellular Electrolytes and Arterial Hypertension,* Losse, H. and Zumkley, H., Eds., Georg Thieme Verlag, Stuttgart, 1980, 59.
185. **Cooper, R., Aina, O., Chaco, L., Achilihu, A. G., Shamsi, N., and Ford, E.,** Red cell sodium and potassium and hypertension among blacks, *JAMA,* 81, 365, 1989.
186. **Trevisan, M., Ostrow, D., Cooper, R., Liu, K., Sparks, S., Okonek, A., Stevens, E., Marquardt, J., and Stamler, J.,** Abnormal red blood cell ion transport and hypertension. The People's Gas Company Study, *Hypertension,* 5, 363, 1983.
187. **Smith, J. B., Wade, M. B., Feinberg, N. S., and Weinberger, M. S.,** Influence of race, sex and blood pressure on erythrocyte sodium transport in humans, *Hypertension,* 12, 251, 1988.
188. **Cannessa, M., Adragna, N., Solomon, H., Connoly, T., and Tosteson, D. C.,** Increased sodium-lithium countertransport in red cells of patients with essential hypertension, *N. Engl. J. Med.*, 382, 772, 1980.
189. **Samani, N. J., Swales, J. D., Jeffreys, A. J., Morton, D. B., Naftilan, A. J., Lindpaintner, K., Ganten, D., and Brammar, W. J.,** DNA fingerprinting of spontaneously hypertensive and Wistar-Kyoto rats: implications for hypertensive research, *J. Hypertension,* 7, 809, 1989.
190. **Balfe, J. W., Cole, C., Smith, E. K. M., Graham, J. B., and Welt, L. S.,** A hereditary sodium transport defect in the human red cell, *J. Clin. Invest.*, 47, 4, 1968.
191. **Smith, J. B., Wade, M. B., Finberg, N. S., and Weimberger, M. H.,** Influence of race, sex and blood pressure on erythrocyte sodium transport in humans, *Hypertension,* 12, 251, 1988.
192. **Swales, J. D.,** Functional disturbance of the cell membrane in hypertension, *J. Hypertension,* 8(Suppl. 7), S203, 1990.
193. **Boon, N. A., Aronson, J. K., Hallis, K. F., and Grahame-Smith, D. G.,** Cation transport abnormalities in vivo in untreated essential hypertension, *Clin. Sci.*, 70, 611, 1986.
194. **Aalkjaer, C., Heagerty, A. M., Parvin, S. D., Bell, P. R. F., Bing, R. F., and Swales, J. D.,** Cell membrane sodium transport: a correlation between human resistance vessels and leucocytes, *Lancet,* 1, 649, 1986.
195. **Aalkjaer, C., Heagerty, A. M., Petersen, K. K., Swales, J. D., and Mulvany, M. J.,** Evidence for increased media thickness, increased neuronal amine uptake, and depressed excitation-contraction coupling in isolated resistance vessels from essential hypertensives, *Circ. Res.*, 61, 181, 1987.
196. **Izzard, A. S., Cragoe, D. J., Jr., and Heagerty, A. M.,** Intracellular pH in human resistance arteries in essential hypertension, *Hypertension,* 17, 780, 1991.
197. **Canessa, M., Bize, I., and Solomon, H.,** Na^+ countertransport and cotransport in human red cells: function, dysfunction and genes in essential hypertension, *Clin. Exp. Hypertension,* 3, 783, 1981.

Chapter 5

THE Li^+/Na^+ COUNTERTRANSPORT IN HYPERTENSION

Andrea Semplicini

TABLE OF CONTENTS

I. Introduction 90

II. Kinetic Properties and Clinical Assay of Li^+/Na^+ CT 91

III. Li^+/Na^+ CT in the Population at Large 93

IV. Heritability of Li^+/Na^+ CT 96

V. Li^+/Na^+ CT and Essential Hypertension 96

VI. Li^+/Na^+ CT in Secondary Hypertension and Other Clinical Conditions 97

VII. Li^+/Na^+ CT and Associated Variables 98
- A. Li^+/Na^+ CT and Body Weight 99
- B. Li^+/Na^+ CT and Blood Lipids 99
- C. Li^+/Na^+ CT and Serum Uric Acid 100
- D. Li^+/Na^+ CT and Alcohol Consumption 100
- E. Li^+/Na^+ CT, Physical Activity, and Personality 100

VIII. Li^+/Na^+ CT and Renal Proximal Na Reabsorption 101

IX. Li^+/Na^+ CT and Antihypertensive Drug Treatment 101

X. Li^+/Na^+ CT and Peripheral Hemodynamics 101

XI. Li^+/Na^+ CT and Activity of the Renin-Angiotensin System 102

XII. Li^+/Na^+ CT, Diabetes, Reduced Glucose Tolerance, and Insulin Sensitivity 102

XIII. Li^+/Na^+ CT and Cardiovascular "Remodeling" 104

0-8493-5474-9/94/$0.00+$.50

XIV. Li^+/Na^+ and Na^+/H^+ CT 106
A. Is Li^+/Na^+ CT an Operational Mode of Na^+/H^+ CT? 106
B. Does High Li^+/Na^+ CT Reflect a Genetic Variant of Na^+/H^+ CT? 107
C. Does High Li^+/Na^+ CT Reflect Increased Na^+/H^+ CT? 107
D. Does High Li^+/Na^+ CT Reflect Abnormal Kinetic Properties of Na^+/H^+ CT? 107

XV. Summary and Conclusions 108

Acknowledgments 110

References 110

I. INTRODUCTION

Lithium, the lightest of the alkali metals, is widely present in nature but it occurs normally in the body only at trace levels. Its salts have been widely used since the early 1950s for the treatment of manic disorders to reduce the relapse and recurrence of manic-depressive episodes. Its therapeutic index is narrow (2 to 3), with therapeutic blood levels between 0.8 and 1.5 mEq/l and toxic levels above 2.5 mmol/l. Acute toxic effects include vomiting, diarrhea, ataxia, convulsions, and coma.[1] Blood levels during chronic administration should therefore be periodically monitored. This stimulated clinical studies in which it was found that during Li administration the concentration of Li in red cell water is usually only one third that in plasma.[2] Because at steady-state concentration the ratio between red cells and plasma for a passively distributed cation should be around 1.2, this observation suggested an uphill extrusion of Li.

In 1975, Haas et al.[3] was the first to report the existence of a ouabain insensitive Li^+/Na^+ exchange (or countertransport or antiport, CT) in human red cells. Their findings were independently confirmed by Duhm et al.,[4] who also underlined the existence of large interindividual differences for Li^+ distribution across the human red cell membrane.[5] The basic characteristics of this transport pathway were described by Pandey et al.,[6] Sarkadi et al.,[7] and Ehrlich and Diamond.[8]

After a few reports in manic-depressive patients, interest in the clinical measurement of Li^+/Na^+ CT in hypertension was raised by the finding by Canessa et al.[9] of an increased red cell Li^+/Na^+ CT in patients with essential hypertension and not in patients with secondary hypertension and normotensive controls. The suggestion was made that Li^+/Na^+ CT maximal velocity (V_{max}) was heritable and that an increased Li^+/Na^+ CT could be a genetic marker of susceptibility to hypertension.

These observations prompted a large number of investigations (more than 100 between 1980 and 1990 on a MEDLINE search) on Li^+/Na^+ CT in hypertension and in other related clinical conditions (diabetes mellitus, renal insufficiency, hyperlipidemia, thyroid dysfunctions, Alzheimer's disease), sometimes with conflicting results, due to methodological bias and different patients' selection.

It was first proposed that Li^+/Na^+ CT reflects Na^+/Na^+ CT. Subsequently it was independently hypothesized by Funder et al.[10] and Aronson[11] that Li^+/Na^+ CT represents a mode of functioning of the cell membrane Na^+/H^+ exchanger. Na^+/H^+ exchange is a membrane function involved in the regulation of cell volume, cell pH, in the cell response to hormones, mitogens, and growth factors, and in the renal reabsorption of Na and bicarbonate.[12] Increased Li^+/Na^+ could therefore reflect abnormal kinetic properties of the Na^+/H^+ exchanger which could account for the relationship between Li^+/Na^+ CT and hypertension. In favor of this hypothesis, strong experimental evidence was gathered in Canessa's laboratory.[13-16] However, to date the definite proof is still missing. The aim of this review is to collect the available data in the literature and our previous experience to improve the comprehension of Li^+/Na^+ CT which seems strongly correlated to the risk of developing hypertension and its major complications.

II. KINETIC PROPERTIES AND CLINICAL ASSAY OF Li^+/Na^+ CT

The red cell membrane Li^+/Na^+ CT is a heteroexchange which operates in either direction across the cell membrane. It binds either Li or Na on one side of the membrane and exchanges the transported species for either Li or Na on the opposite side at a stoichiometric ratio of 1:1.

Li^+/Na^+ CT is adenosine triphosphate (ATP) independent.[4] The energy for uphill translocation is derived from the disequilibrium of Na across the cell membrane, maintained by the Na pump.

The kinetic properties of the Li^+/Na^+ CT have been investigated. The apparent affinity (K_m) for Li is 20 times higher than that for Na on both sides of the membrane. In normotensive controls, for Li it is 0.5 m*M* inside and 1.5 m*M* outside, while that of Na is 9 and 25 m*M*, respectively.[7] Na stimulates unidirectional movement of lithium on the *trans* side and inhibits on the *cis* side. Li^+/Na^+ CT is inhibited by high external Mg concentration, phloretin, and 2,5-p-chloromercuribenzenesulforic (PCMBS),[17] it is partially inhibited by bumetanide, and is insensitive to ouabain, 4,4′-diisothiocyanatostilbene-2,2′-disulfonic acid (DIDS), furosemide, amiloride, removal of chloride and bicarbonate, and cell swelling at physiological cell pH.

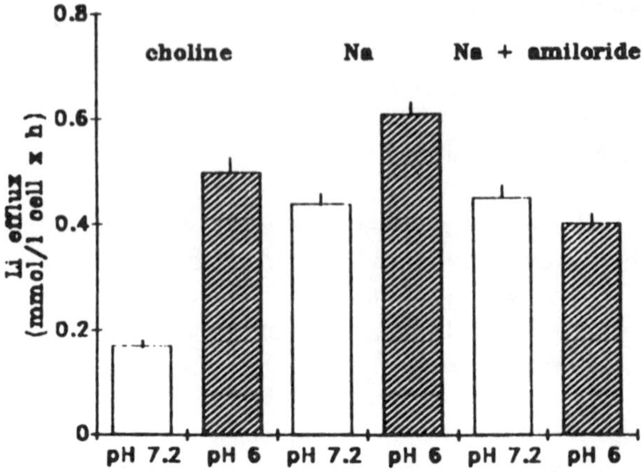

FIGURE 1. Allosteric effects of intracellular protons on Li efflux from Li loaded red cell in six normotensive controls. At physiological pH (7.2, empty bars), Li efflux was stimulated by external Na. The difference between Li efflux in Na and in choline medium is Li^+/Na^+ CT. Li efflux in Na medium was not inhibited by amiloride (1 m*M*). Red cells from the same subjects were acid loaded (cell pH 6.0) by incubation in acid medium in the presence of DIDS and methazolamide (hatched bars) and suspended in the same Na and choline media (pH 7.4) to activate Na^+/H^+ CT. Under these experimental conditions, Li efflux was stimulated to a greater extent in choline than in Na medium. Li^+/Na^+ CT was partially inhibited and Li efflux in Na medium was amiloride sensitive. This experiment thus confirms that when Na^+/H^+ CT is activated, Li^+/Na^+ CT is inhibited and amiloride sensitive.

Examination of the allosteric effects of intracellular protons on Li^+/Na^+ CT may elucidate the relationships between this exchange mode and Na^+/H^+ CT (Figure 1). In the absence of external Na, cytoplasmic acidification (from internal pH 7.2 to 6.0) stimulates unidirectional Li efflux (as uncoupled Li efflux or Li-H outward cotransport). In the presence of external Na, cytoplasmic acidification stimulates Li efflux to a smaller extent, which suggests that Li^+/Na^+ CT is partially inhibited, probably because under these experimental conditions the transporter is exchanging external Na for internal H (Na^+/H^+ CT) and not for internal Li. Under these experimental conditions Li efflux in Na medium becomes amiloride sensitive.

Detailed analysis of the kinetic properties of Li^+/Na^+ and Na^+/Li^+ exchange in human red cells are consistent with a consecutive "ping-pong" model of the transport reaction.[18] According to the model, Li and Na bind consecutively on the opposite sides of the membrane. Exchange follows binding on both sides. The rate-limiting step of the overall reaction is cation translocation, without the effect of cation binding on affinity on the other side of the membrane.

Theoretically, Li^+/Na^+ CT could be measured as Li efflux promoted by external Na (Li^+/Na^+ CT), Li influx promoted by internal Na (Na^+/Li^+ CT), Na efflux promoted by external Li, and Na influx promoted by internal Li. However, the transporter is asymmetric for Li and Na. The Na-stimulated Li flux (Li^+/Na^+ CT) is two- to threefold faster than Li stimulated Na flux (Na^+/Li^+ CT), and thus more precisely measurable. Moreover, Li is easily measured with atomic absorption spectrophotometry, it is not present normally in biological fluids, and contamination is unlikely. Extracellular Na may inhibit Li influx and its removal may be incomplete. The best method is therefore the measurement of Na-stimulated Li efflux (Li^+/Na^+ CT). To perform such measurement all other transport pathways for Li should be inhibited. These are the Na pump (with ouabain), $LiCO_3^-$ pathway (with bicarbonate free solutions), and Na-K-Cl cotransport (with furosemide).

The method for the clinical measurement of Li^+/Na^+ has been carefully standardized.[19] Briefly, the red cells are washed with Na free solution to remove extracellular Na and Li loaded by incubation in isotonic Li medium. Li loading can be achieved shortly with cold incubation in the ionophore nystatin or with 3-h incubation at 37°C. Alternatively, Li loading can be achieved with short incubation in lithium bicarbonate.[20] After loading, the red cells are washed to remove extracellular Li, bicarbonate, and nystatin, if present. Li loaded cells are divided into Na and Na-free media. The efflux of Li is measured over time. It is linear up to 1 h and the difference between efflux in the presence and in the absence of Na represents the Na-stimulated Li efflux.

Li^+/Na^+ CT was also measured as the phloretin-sensitive Li influx from Li media.[21] This method, however, cannot standardize intracellular Na concentration, which can be different from one patient to another and is very close to the apparent affinity for internal Na of the transporter (9 m*M*).

The effects of red cell age on Li^+/Na^+ CT are conflicting: Li^+/Na^+ CT has been reported to decrease[22] and to increase with red cell age due to an increase in a phloretin-insensitive component.[23]

Li^+/Na^+ CT is present in rabbit and bovine red cells, but not in dog red cells. It has been measured rarely in other cell types. Recently, however, evidence has been provided that Li^+/Na^+ CT is present in sarcolemmal vesicles from canine and bovine superior mesenteric artery.[24,25] In both preparations, it is electroneutral and phloretin- and quinidine-sensitive, as it is the red cell Li^+/Na^+ CT. Moreover, it is inhibited by ethylisopropylamiloride, one of the inhibitors of cell membrane Na^+/H^+ CT.[24,25] This body of evidence provides further proof that Li^+/Na^+ CT is mediated by the cell membrane Na^+/H^+ CT.

III. Li^+/Na^+ CT IN THE POPULATION AT LARGE

Various laboratories have investigated the distribution of Li^+/Na^+ CT in the population.[26-36] It has been shown that it is unimodally distributed but skewed to the right. Such distribution results from the superimposition of two normal distributions, one with a mean value around 0.24 mmol/l cell × h (70% of the population), the other with a mean value of 0.40 mmol/l cell × h (30% of the population).

Li^+/Na^+ CT is higher in males than in females[30-34,37-39] (Tables 1 and 2) and is correlated to body weight, body mass index,[30,38,40] and blood pressure in most,[27,30,33,38] if not all studies.[35]

Li^+/Na^+ CT is higher in whites than in blacks (Table 3) and in Chinese as compared to either Europeans or non-Chinese Asians.[41] It is ten times slower in

TABLE 1
Li^+/Na^+ CT (mol/l cell × h) in Males According to Diagnostic Category

Author	Year	Normotensives N	Normotensives M	Normotensives SD	Hypertensives N	Hypertensives M	Hypertensives SD	*p*
Canessa et al.[9]	80	17	0.24	0.06	27	0.58	0.02	<0.001
Ibsen et al.[20]	82	16	0.42	n.r.	17	0.68	n.r.	<0.005
Brugnara et al.[44]	83	31	0.20	0.06	46	0.39	0.17	<0.001
Williams et al.[38]	83	275	0.28	0.10	30	0.32	0.01	<0.05
Corrocher et al.[75]	85	40	0.21	0.09	33	0.33	0.14	<0.001
Weder[93]	86	31	0.32	0.02	14	0.38	0.03	<0.05
Semplicini et al.[94]	89	12	0.30	0.11	24	0.38	0.14	=0.06
Weighted mean			0.27			0.42		

Abbreviations: N, number of observations; M, mean; SD, standard deviation; n.r., not reported.

TABLE 2
Li^+/Na^+ CT (mmol/l cell × h) in Females According to Diagnostic Category

Author	Year	Normotensives N	Normotensives M	Normotensives SD	Hypertensives N	Hypertensives M	Hypertensives SD	*p*
Canessa et al.[9]	80	9	0.23	0.08	9	0.44	0.02	<0.001
Ibsen et al.[20]	82	10	0.34	n.r.	14	0.41	n.r.	NS
Williams et al.[38]	83	30	0.23	0.11	24	0.32	0.13	<0.01
Brugnara et al.[44]	83	27	0.18	0.10	26	0.34	0.02	<0.001
Corrocher et al.[75]	85	38	0.18	0.08	31	0.32	0.18	<0.001
Semplicini et al.[94]	89	9	0.21	0.07	17	0.32	0.19	=0.08
Weighted mean			0.21			0.34		

Abbreviations: see Table 1.

cord blood than in adulthood,[42,43] but no change occurs with aging in most, if not all studies.[44]

Li^+/Na^+ CT was investigated in many studies, which were sometimes non-representative of the general population. Moreover, Li^+/Na^+ CT was widely treated as an independent variable, with blood pressure as the dependent variable. To verify

TABLE 3
Li^+/Na^+ CT (mmol/l cell × h) According to Race, Diagnostic Category, and Family History for Hypertension

Author	Year	*White NT*			*Black NT*			
		N	M	SD	N	M	SD	*p*
Canessa et al.[140]	84	16	0.28	0.12	18	0.18	0.05	<0.005
M'Buyamba et al.[141]	84	24	0.47	0.03	22	0.24	0.02	<0.001
Weder et al.[139]	84	57	0.27	0.01	23	0.21	0.01	NS
Weinberger et al.[96]	89	21	0.21	0.10	9	0.12	0.05	<0.01
Bedford, Johnson et al.[114]	90	7	0.23	0.03	8	0.17	0.02	<0.02
Weighted mean			0.30			0.20		
		White HT			*Black HT*			
Canessa et al.[140]	84	22	0.51	0.14	18	0.18	0.02	<0.01
Weder et al.[139]	84	29	0.37	0.02	11	0.27	0.03	<0.05
Weinberger et al.[96]	89	23	0.31	0.11	9	0.23	0.12	<0.01
Bedford Johnson et al.[114]	90	6	0.23	0.02	8	0.17	0.02	<0.02
Weighted mean			0.38			0.20		
		Black NT			*Black HT*			
Canessa et al.[140]	84	18	0.18	0.05	18	0.18	0.02	NS
Weder et al.[139]	84	23	0.21	0.01	11	0.27	0.03	NS
Weinberger et al.[96]	89	9	0.12	0.05	9	0.23	0.12	<0.01
Bedford Johnson et al.[114]	90	8	0.17	0.02	11	0.17	0.03	NS
Weighted mean			0.18			0.21		
		Black NT F−			*Black NT F+*			
Woods et al.[143]	82	10	0.18	0.02	10	0.27	0.02	<0.001
Canessa et al.[140]	84	10	0.19	0.05	17	0.13	0.06	NS
Weder et al.[139]	84	12	0.20	0.03	12	0.22	0.03	NS
Bunker et al.[92]	87	19	0.25	0.12	15	0.22	0.08	NS
Weighted mean			0.21			0.20		

Abbreviations: NT, normotensives; HT, hypertensives; F−, negative family history for hypertension; F+, positive family history for hypertension; see also Table 1.

the independent effects of other potentially confounding variables on Li^+/Na^+ CT in the population, we have measured Li^+/Na^+ CT in a random sample of the general population and have confirmed that the mean value is higher in males as compared to females, and significantly and independently correlated to body mass index among males, blood pressure, and alcohol consumption. It was negatively correlated to urinary Ca excretion in females.[30]

IV. HERITABILITY OF Li^+/Na^+ CT

Large samples of kindreds have been investigated to define the mode of inheritance of Li^+/Na^+ CT, as bimodality could be either genetic or nongenetic. The coefficients of correlation for Li^+/Na^+ CT in families are larger among first-degree relatives (monozygous and dizygous twins) than between genetically unrelated individuals (spouses).[45] Because these data are consistent with a genetic component, various genetic models were tested. The most likely is a major gene with a polygenic component or an environmental factor.[28,46]

In a sib-sib pair study, Li^+/Na^+ CT was elevated in subjects with the MM blood group antigen, which is associated with increased blood pressure.[47]

V. Li^+/Na^+ CT AND ESSENTIAL HYPERTENSION

After the first report by Canessa et al.,[9] many other laboratories have confirmed the increase of the red cell Li^+/Na^+ CT V_{max} in patients with essential hypertension as compared to normotensive controls, with few exceptions (Table 4). Moreover, in patients with high V_{max}, the affinity for Na seems to be increased at the outside[31] and decreased at the inside ion-binding site.[48] On the contrary, the affinity for Li on the inside is unchanged in hypertensives as compared to normotensives.[32]

It is now well established that Li^+/Na^+ CT is not increased in all hypertensive patients, and that only a subset of 40 to 50% of them has an Li^+/Na^+ CT > 0.40 mmol/l cell $\times$ h, the upper normal limit for most laboratories. Population studies have shown that the subgroup with the highest Li^+/Na^+ CT has the largest proportion of hypertensives.[33,36] Among hypertensives, Li^+/Na^+ CT is higher in severe and drug-resistant patients than in the others.[49,50] It is also higher in hypertensive patients who do not remain normotensive with nutritional interventions, including salt and caloric restriction and therefore require drug therapy, than in the patients who remain normotensive with simple dietetic measures after ceasing administration of the drug.[51]

It is well known that sodium restriction may reduce blood pressure in salt-sensitive patients. Salt restriction, however, did not affect Li^+/Na^+ CT.[52,53]

Li^+/Na^+ CT in patients with essential hypertension shows a peculiar temperature dependence on Arrhenius plots. Li efflux in Na medium and Li^+/Na^+ CT increase with the temperature of the medium, but the increase is not linear. A change in slope (''break'') of the line is evident around 20°C in hypertensives and around 30°C in normotensives.[54]

Li^+/Na^+ CT is increased in normotensive offsprings of hypertensive parents who are prone to develop hypertension later in life (Table 5). It has been proposed, therefore, that Li^+/Na^+ CT is a potential laboratory tool to predict the risk of developing hypertension later in life. However, only the patients in whom familiar segregation analysis is able to document the existence of a recessive major gene for high Li^+/Na^+ CT have an increased probability of hypertension in a 10-year follow-up.[55] This emphasizes that increased Li^+/Na^+ CT is not only influenced by the genetic background but also by the environment.

TABLE 4
Li^+/Na^+ CT (mmol/l cell × h) in Normotensives and Essential Hypertensives

Author	Year	Normotensives N	M	SD	Hypertensives N	M	SD	*p*
Canessa et al.[9]	80	26	0.24	0.02	36	0.55	0.02	<0.001
Canali et al.[135]	81	46	0.25	0.09	15	0.33	0.11	<0.001
Cusi et al.[134]	81	12	0.25	0.03	18	0.32	0.02	<0.05
Adragna et al.[137]	82	16	0.27	0.02	22	0.53	0.36	<0.005
Clegg et al.[142]	82	38	0.28	0.09	75	0.53	0.24	<0.005
Ibsen et al.[20]	82	16	0.42	0.10	17	0.68	0.27	<0.01
Woods et al.[143]	82	9	0.17	0.02	16	0.35	0.02	<0.001
Cooper et al.[138]	83	37	0.28	0.10	18	0.36	0.15	<0.01
Fujita et al.[102]	83	35	0.33	0.02	40	0.48	0.03	<0.02
Levy et al.[54]	83	22	0.36	0.03	52	0.48	0.02	<0.001
Trevisan et al.[40]	83	64	0.29	0.08	70	0.35	0.13	<0.05
Williams et al.[38]	83	511	0.26	0.05	54	0.32	0.10	<0.001
Canessa et al.[140]	84	16	0.28	0.12	22	0.52	0.14	<0.005
Weder et al.[139]	84	57	0.27	0.01	29	0.37	0.02	<0.05
Corrocher et al.[75]	85	78	0.19	0.08	64	0.32	0.16	<0.001
Hunt et al.[144]	85	35	0.26	0.12	27	0.36	0.14	<0.01
Beuckelmann and Erdmann[145]	86	10	0.25	0.05	10	0.36	0.13	<0.05
Fallo et al.[146]	86	15	0.26	0.01	15	0.40	0.03	<0.01
Hunt et al.[73]	86	1276	0.27	0.11	143	0.34	0.14	<0.001
Morgan et al.[147]	86	367	0.40	0.01	125	0.45	0.02	<0.05
Gless et al.[63]	86	39	0.23	0.02	20	0.30	0.03	<0.025
McDonald et al.[74]	87	37	0.28	n.r.	18	0.36	n.r.	<0.05
Turner et al.[148]	87	39	0.31	0.07	104	0.44	0.15	<0.001
Weder et al.[103]	87	23	0.29	0.12	20	0.36	0.14	NS
Yap et al.[48]	89	30	0.34	0.02	50	0.36	0.03	NS
Semplicini et al.[94]	89	21	0.26	0.10	41	0.35	0.16	<0.001
Weinberger et al.[96]	89	n.r.	0.21	0.10	n.r.	0.31	0.10	<0.01
Weighted mean			0.28			0.41		

Abbreviations: see Table 1.

VI. Li^+/Na^+ CT IN SECONDARY HYPERTENSION AND OTHER CLINICAL CONDITIONS

Li^+/Na^+ CT seems to be increased only among essential hypertensives. It was evaluated in primary aldosteronism, estrogen-induced hypertension, polycystic kidney disease, renovascular hypertension, chronic glomerulonephritis, lupus erythematosus, and end stage renal disease with negative results.[9,44,54,56,57] In pigs, however, it has been shown that deoxycosterone acetate treatment may simultaneously increase blood pressure and red cell Li^+/Na^+ CT.[58]

TABLE 5
Li^+/Na^+ CT (mmol/l cell × h) in Normotensives According to Family History for Hypertension

Author	Year	Negative history			Positive history			*p*
		N	M	SD	N	M	SD	
Canessa et al.[9]	80	10	0.23	0.02	8	0.54	0.05	<0.0001
Cusi et al.[134]	81	24	0.23	0.08	24	0.23	0.09	NS
Canessa et al[17]	81	24	0.28	0.02	24	0.35	0.03	<0.001
Canali et al.[135]	81	15	0.26	0.09	43	0.36	0.12	<0.001
Woods et al.[136]	82	11	0.16	0.01	8	0.29	0.03	<0.001
Adragna et al.[137]	82	16	0.29	0.02	8	0.32	0.03	NS
Trevisan et al.[71]	83	28	0.29	0.07	12	0.23	0.09	<0.05
Cooper et al.[138]	83	26	0.30	0.13	27	0.32	0.12	NS
Levy et al.[54]	83	24	0.46	0.05	28	0.51	0.04	<0.01
Smith et al.[61]	84	63	0.24	0.01	44	0.28	0.15	<0.05
Weder et al.[139]	84	36	0.27	0.02	21	0.29	0.02	NS
Funder et al.[10]	84	9	0.35	0.12	14	0.30	0.02	NS
Weighted mean			0.27			0.33		

Abbreviations: see Table 1.

It was reported that Li^+/Na^+ CT is acutely reduced by hemodialysis and ultrafiltration in blacks with end stage renal disease, and this was attributed to the removal of a dialyzable plasma factor.[59] These data were confirmed in some,[60] but not in other studies.[57,61]

An increase of Li^+/Na^+ CT has been reported during the third trimester of normotensive and hypertensive pregnancy,[42,62,63] with oral contraceptives,[64] Alzheimer's dementia,[65] hypothyroidism,[66] and Bartter's syndrome.[67] Li^+/Na^+ CT is reduced in hyperthyroid patients,[63,66,68] normal in patients with idiopathic hypercalciuria and kidney stones,[69] and with florid psoriasis,[70] conditions which are often associated with hypertension.

VII. Li^+/Na^+ CT AND ASSOCIATED VARIABLES

It is well known that hypertension is a multifaceted clinical entity. All epidemiological studies have provided convincing evidence that the increase in pressure is not the only hallmark of the hypertensive patient. Overweight, hyperlipidemia, reduced glucose tolerance, reduced physical activity, type A behavior, smoking, and caffeine consumption are more common among hypertensives than normotensives and are additive in increasing the risk attributable to hypertension.

Soon after the first reports appeared, it became known that blood pressure is not the only variable correlated to Li^+/Na^+ CT. Actually, some of the covariables are more strongly related to Li^+/Na^+ CT than to blood pressure itself, and are discussed below.

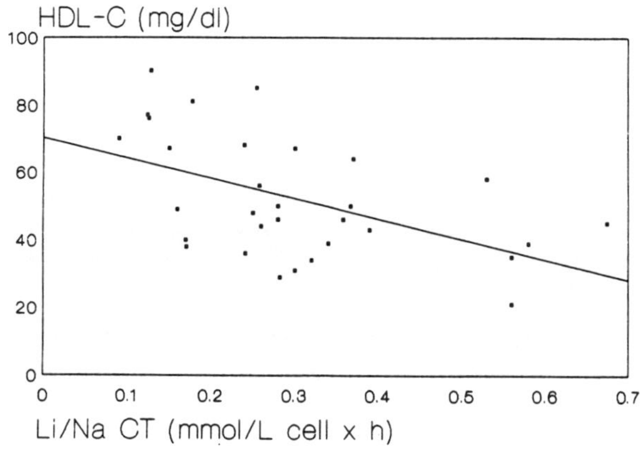

FIGURE 2. Li^+/Na^+ CT and HDL cholesterol in a group of essential hypertensives ($n = 32$, $r = -0.50$, $p < 0.01$). (From Semplicini, A. et al., *Min. Electrolyte Metab.*, 6, 207, 1992. With permission.)

A. Li^+/Na^+ CT AND BODY WEIGHT

Overweight and obese subjects have an increased Li^+/Na^+ CT as compared to lean subjects, independent of the presence of hypertension.[33,38,40,43,71-74] In view of the strong correlation between body weight and blood pressure, this underlines the importance of correcting Li^+/Na^+ CT for body weight when studying the relationship between blood pressure and Li^+/Na^+ CT. Actually, in a general population study Li^+/Na^+ CT was more strongly correlated to body weight than to blood pressure. After correction for weight, the correlation between Li^+/Na^+ CT and pressure was no longer significant, at least in males.[30]

B. Li^+/Na^+ CT AND BLOOD LIPIDS

Li^+/Na^+ CT is increased in hyperlipidemic patients as compared to subjects with normal plasma lipids in many,[73,75-77] but not all studies.[78] Li^+/Na^+ CT was positively correlated to serum total and free cholesterol,[75,76] triglycerides,[73,75,76] low-density lipoprotein (LDL) cholesterol,[48] and negatively to high-density lipoprotein (HDL) (Figure 2).[73,76] This could be due to an abnormal lipid composition of the cell membrane. It is well known that plasma lipids are in equilibrium with the cell membrane lipids and that the lipid composition of the membrane influences ion transport. Li^+/Na^+ CT was, in fact, positively correlated to the saturated and negatively to the polyunsaturated fatty acid content of the red cell membrane.[75,76] In patients with severe hyperlipidemia, extracorporeal LDL apheresis acutely reduced Li^+/Na^+ CT.[79] However, neither *in vitro* enrichment of the cell membrane with cholesteryl hemisuccinate affected Li^+/Na^+ CT[80] nor *in vivo* reduction of dietary saturated fats and supplementation with oleic[81] and linoleic acid-rich diets[82,83] modified Li^+/Na^+ CT, despite an increase in unsaturated fatty acid content of the red cell membrane. Finally, treatment with the 3-hydroxy-3-methylglutaryl coenzyme A (HMGCoA) reductase inhibitor, lovastatin, significantly reduced serum total and LDL cholesterol and increased HDL cholesterol, but did not influence Li^+/Na^+ CT.[84]

It seems, therefore, that the correlation between plasma lipids and Li^+/Na^+ CT is not strong and constant. It may be caused not by the lipid composition of the cell membrane, but by the cause of hyperlipidemia itself. It is widely known that hypertension and hyperlipidemia are often associated with overweight, reduced glucose tolerance, and diabetes. It has been proposed that the underlying mechanisms are insulin resistance and hyperinsulinemia.[85] Hyperinsulinemia stimulates sodium reabsorption in the kidney, activates the sympathetic nervous system, and favors cardiovascular remodeling (see below), and could simultaneously cause hyperlipidemia, hypertension, and activate Li^+/Na^+ CT (see below), thereby creating a correlation between these parameters.

C. Li^+/Na^+ CT AND SERUM URIC ACID

In our experience in a large group of essential hypertensives, serum uric acid is significantly correlated with Li^+/Na^+ CT ($r = 0.40$, $p < 0.01$, $n = 72$), thus confirming previous observations.[86]

The largest part of the uric acid, filtered through the glomerulus, is reabsorbed with water along the proximal tubule. It is also partly reabsorbed in the ascending limb of Henle's loop and in the collecting ducts and is secreted at the proximal tubule. Because Li^+/Na^+ CT is an operating mode of the Na^+/H^+ CT, the increased serum level of uric acid in subjects with high Li^+/Na^+ CT was attributed to an increased reabsorption of uric acid along the proximal tubule, in parallel to Na and water.[86,87] It is, however, also possible that high serum uric acid is related to the plurimetabolic syndrome (also called syndrome X)[88] characterized by obesity, hypertension, reduced glucose tolerance, hyperinsulinemia, hyperlipidemia, and hyperuricemia, a common finding in many patients with high Li^+/Na^+ CT (see below).

D. Li^+/Na^+ CT AND ALCOHOL CONSUMPTION

Chronic alcohol consumption may cause hypertension through uncertain mechanisms. It may induce alterations of Na transport in the kidney and smooth muscle cells directly or through alterations of blood lipids. A positive correlation was observed between alcohol intake and Li^+/Na^+ CT,[30,51] and *in vitro* experiments have shown that alcohol may increase Li^+/Na^+ CT.[89] Moreover, Li^+/Na^+ CT is not increased in chronic alcoholics, but it decreases with abstinence.[90]

E. Li^+/Na^+ CT, PHYSICAL ACTIVITY, AND PERSONALITY

Overfeeding and reduced physical activity are the main causes of obesity in industrialized populations. It has been shown that increased physical activity may reduce Li^+/Na^+ CT.[91] Because it corrects insulin resistance, reduces total cholesterol and blood pressure, and increases HDL cholesterol, this reemphasizes the relationships between Li^+/Na^+ CT, insulin resistance, and blood lipids.

Personality traits and red blood cell (RBC) Na transport were also related.[92] It was shown that "Type A" behavior total scores are positively correlated with Li^+/Na^+ CT among whites. High scores indicate hard-driving and time-urgent traits and reactions.

VIII. Li^+/Na^+ CT AND RENAL PROXIMAL Na REABSORPTION

Following the suggestion that Li^+/Na^+ CT is an operational mode of Na^+/H^+ CT, it appeared possible that the correlation between Li^+/Na^+ CT and hypertension could be mediated by increased proximal Na reabsorption, Na retention, plasma volume expansion, and increased cardiac output. Na^+/H^+ CT is actually responsible for the isotonic reabsorption of Na and bicarbonate in the proximal tubule. A correlation between Li^+/Na^+ CT and renal fractional reabsorption of Li, an estimate of proximal Na reabsorption, was reported by Weder,[93] but not by the author and others.[86,94-97] However, a subgroup of hypertensive patients with high Li^+/Na^+ CT has increased proximal Li reabsorption as compared to hypertensives with normal Li^+/Na^+ CT.[98] It is therefore possible that the relationship between Li^+/Na^+ CT and Li reabsorption in the kidney is not a continuous one, and that increased Li^+/Na^+ CT reflects proximal tubule Na retention only in some patients.

IX. Li^+/Na^+ CT AND ANTIHYPERTENSIVE DRUG TREATMENT

The effects of antihypertensive drugs on Li^+/Na^+ CT have been scarcely investigated.[99-101] Li^+/Na^+ CT was not affected by diuretics, but it was negatively correlated to serum potassium and increased in patients with diuretic- and laxative-induced hypokalemia.[51,63,64,76,99] This may reflect overactivity of the renin-angiotensin system in patients with high Li^+/Na^+ CT (see below), which is one of the predisposing factors to diuretic-induced hypokalemia.

Canrenone, atenolol, and captopril did not affect Li^+/Na^+ CT,[100] while the S2 inhibitor, ketanserin, *in vivo* and *in vitro* significantly increased it.[101] Finally, hypertensives with high Li^+/Na^+ CT are less sensitive to dietetic measures, such as salt and caloric restriction, and are more prone to develop hypertension when drug therapy is interrupted.[51]

X. Li^+/Na^+ CT AND PERIPHERAL HEMODYNAMICS

According to Fujita et al.[102] and Weder et al.,[36,103] Li^+/Na^+ CT is positively correlated to total peripheral resistance. On the contrary, in our experience, patients with insulin-dependent diabetes mellitus (IDDM) and some treated essential hypertensives with high Li^+/Na^+ CT (see below) have reduced peripheral resistance and increased cardiac output, consistent with sodium and water retention.[104]

XI. Li^+/Na^+ CT AND ACTIVITY OF THE RENIN-ANGIOTENSIN SYSTEM

The first description of a positive correlation between plasma renin activity and Li^+/Na^+ CT in patients with essential hypertension was provided by Brugnara et al.[44] Their findings were confirmed by others.[49,105] More recently, Redgrave et al.[106] have shown that nonmodulating essential hypertensives have increased Li^+/Na^+ CT. Nonmodulation is an ill-defined clinical entity characterized by a strong family history for hypertension, blunted vascular, renin, and adrenal response to sodium load and angiotensin II infusion, and a reduced ability to handle a sodium load, which favors salt sensitivity.

XII. Li^+/Na^+ CT, DIABETES, REDUCED GLUCOSE TOLERANCE, AND INSULIN SENSITIVITY

Clinical and epidemiological data show that hypertension and diabetes are often associated.[107] The prevalence of hypertension among patients with type 2 noninsulin-dependent diabetes mellitus (NIDDM) is increased, only in part because of obesity and overweight. NIDDM reduced glucose tolerance and hyperinsulinemia are more frequent among hypertensives than in the general population. Moreover, some hypertensives with normal glucose tolerance are insulin resistant and hyperinsulinemic.[85] Insulin resistance in patients with essential hypertension is pathway and tissue selective because it involves only glucose conversion into glycogen in skeletal muscle.[108] Hyperinsulinemia, a compensatory effect to overcome tissue resistance, may cause hypertension by salt and water retention, sympathetic nervous system activation, and effects on cation transport. However, chronic insulin infusion did not induce hypertension in dogs and the removal of insulin-producing tumors did not reduce blood pressure.[109,110] Therefore, the relationships between hypertension and hyperinsulinemia are still uncertain. It is possible that genetic predisposition is necessary for the development of hypertension in the presence of hyperinsulinemia.

In view of the association of hypertension and diabetes, a link also between diabetes, reduced glucose tolerance, and insulin resistance on one side and Li^+/Na^+ CT on the other is likely.

Trevisan et al.[111,112] measured red cell Na transport in NIDDM in two different studies. In the first study they found that Li^+/Na^+ CT was increased, but not significantly so, in NIDDM as compared to the control group.[111] More recently, in a population study they found that Li^+/Na^+ CT is increased in diabetics, mostly NIDDM, as compared to controls.[112] In patients with IDDM and hypertension but without diabetic nephropathy we have reported an increased activity of the red cell Li^+/Na^+ and Na^+/H^+ CT as compared to normotensive IDDM.[113] In a larger group we have confirmed that Li^+/Na^+ CT is increased in hypertensive IDDM compared to normotensive IDDM, but we have also shown that Li^+/Na^+ CT is increased in

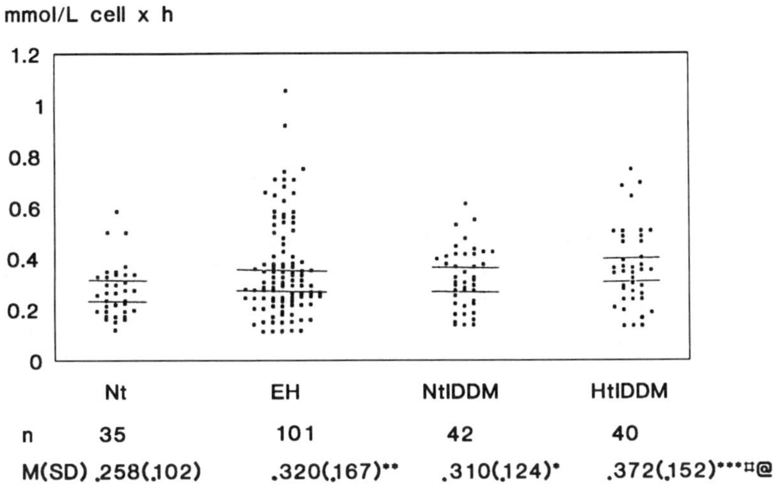

FIGURE 3. Li^+/Na^+ CT in normotensive controls (Ht), patients with essential hypertension (EH), patients with IDDM, either normotensive (NtIDDM) or hypertensive (HtIDDM). None of the patients with IDDM had overt proteinuria or diabetic nephropathy. Bars represent 95% confidence limits; * $p = 0.05$, ** $p < 0.05$, *** $p < 0.01$ vs. Ht, # $p < 0.05$ vs. NtIDDM, @ $p < 0.05$ vs. EH.

IDDM as compared to nondiabetic subjects (Figure 3). Li^+/Na^+ CT is also increased in black hypertensive diabetics as compared to nondiabetic blacks.[114] It is therefore evident that hyperinsulinemia, secondary either to insulin resistance (in NIDDM) or to exogenous administration (in IDDM), modulates Li^+/Na^+ CT even in blacks, who have reduced Li^+/Na^+ CT.

While studying patients with IDDM having good metabolic control, we were puzzled by a positive correlation between Li^+/Na^+ CT and insulin daily dose. Because insulin requirement is a rough measure of insulin sensitivity, we assessed insulin sensitivity during hyperinsulinemic euglycemic clamp in patients with IDDM and found that Li^+/Na^+ CT was significantly inversely correlated to glucose disposal ($r = -0.53$, $n = 21$, $p < 0.05$). Similar studies in patients with essential hypertension show that hypertensives with high Li^+/Na^+ CT have a 40% reduction of whole body glucose disposal during euglycemic hyperinsulinemic clamp, indicating reduced insulin sensitivity.[115]

In patients with IDDM and high Li^+/Na^+ CT, the reduced insulin sensitivity could cause poor metabolic control and favor the development of diabetic nephropathy. The patients with IDDM who develop diabetic nephropathy have higher Li^+/Na^+ CT than the patients free of this renal complication.[116,117] Other possibilities, however, exist to account for the risk of developing diabetic nephropathy in these patients. Hyperactivity of Na^+/H^+ CT in the kidney, reflected by high Li^+/Na^+ CT in the red cells, could favor cell growth, mesangial expansion, and glomerular hyperfiltration, thereby causing glomerulosclerosis.[118]

XIII. Li^+/Na^+ CT AND CARDIOVASCULAR "REMODELING"

The cardiovascular system in the hypertensive patient is remodeled to normalize wall stress. In the heart, the typical response is concentric left ventricle hypertrophy (LVH); in the resistance arteries, the wall thickness and the wall/lumen ratio are increased. It has been proposed that such "remodeling" of the cardiovascular system is not only due to hemodynamic overload, but also to growth factor stimulation and increased cellular response, favored by abnormal cation transport.[119] It is well known that cardiac hypertrophy cannot be accounted for only by increased afterload. Genetic factors may be of relevance, as normotensive offsprings of hypertensives with LVH have increased cardiac mass compared to normotensives with hypertensive parents with no LVH.[120]

Na^+/H^+ CT plays a permissive role in cellular growth.[121] After the suggestion was made that Li^+/Na^+ CT was a functioning mode of the Na^+/H^+ CT, we therefore looked for a correlation between LVH and Li^+/Na^+ CT. We compared hypertensives with Li^+/Na^+ CT higher than 0.4 mmol/l cell × h with hypertensives with normal Li^+/Na^+ CT but comparable for other clinical and demographic variables.[98] The former had greater interventricular septum and posterior and relative wall thickness than the latter on echocardiography. Moreover, the former had greater kidney volume, glomerular filtration rate, and proximal sodium reabsorption, which supports the hypothesis of common cardiac and kidney abnormalities in some hypertensive patients. An increased prevalence of LVH on electrocardiogram was also reported by Yap et al..[48] Weder et al.[36] did not observe increased left ventricular mass on echocardiogram in patients with high Li^+/Na^+ CT. However, they did report a reduced left ventricular internal diameter and increased relative wall thickness, which is an early indicator of cardiac remodeling.

We have also studied the relationships between Li^+/Na^+ CT and cardiac "remodeling" in other clinical situations. In a group of predominantly normotensive male IDDM, we observed a significant independent correlation between Li^+/Na^+ CT and interventricular septum and posterior and relative wall thickness.[104] Also, in a large family affected by dominant autosomic familial hypertrophic cardiomyopathy we observed a significant correlation between Li^+/Na^+ CT and interventricular septum thickness, relative wall thickness, and indexes of diastolic disfunction. Li^+/Na^+ CT was not greater in the affected members as compared to the nonaffected. We therefore think that Li^+/Na^+ CT exerts a permissive and aggravating role in the clinical manifestation of the disease.

Finally, to verify the role of increased Li^+/Na^+ CT on arteriolar remodeling we have also studied minimal postischemic vascular resistances in the calf. According to the concept elaborated and experimentally validated by Folkow,[122] the luminal size of resistance arteries, brought to a state of complete relaxation, is determined by its structural characteristics and distending pressure. Accordingly, minimal vascular resistance can be taken as a hemodynamic index of the integrated arteriolar wall to lumen ratio. This led to the determination of minimal vascular

TABLE 6
Clinical, Plethysmographic, and Echocardiographic Parameters in Treated Essential Hypertensives According to Basal Li^+/Na^+ CT

	Li^+/Na^+ CT		
	Below the mean	**Above the mean**	*p*
n	15	16	
Sex ratio (M/F)	8/7	9/7	
Li^+/Na^+ CT (mmol/l cell × h)	0.16 ± 0.11	0.40 ± 0.19	0.001
SBP (mmHg)	151 ± 14	165 ± 11	0.009
DBP (mmHg)	89 ± 11	97 ± 11	0.009
HR (beats min^{-1})	88 ± 11	82 ± 9	NS
BMI (kg m^{-2})	25 ± 3	27 ± 3	0.024
Calf plethysmography			
RFL (ml min^{-1} dl^{-1})	6.56 ± 3.14	7.89 ± 2.33	0.03
PFL (ml min^{-1} dl^{-1})	43.4 ± 13	36.1 ± 15	0.067
IF (ml min^{-1} dl^{-1})	36.8 ± 12.7	28.2 ± 14.1	0.04
BRL (AU)	19.6 ± 7.36	17 ± 7	0.069
MRL (AU)	2.75 ± 0.82	3.91 ± 1.66	0.02
Echocardiography			
IVST (mm)	9.8 ± 1.4	10 ± 1.5	NS
PWT (mm)	9.2 ± 1.2	9.3 ± 1.1	NS
h/r	0.40 ± 0.09	0.38 ± 0.06	NS
Mi (g m^{-2})	107 ± 21	118 ± 27	NS
ESS (10^3 dyne cm^{-2})	70 ± 20.7	66.5 ± 19.2	NS
CI (l min^{-1} m^{-2})	3.35 ± 0.97	3.94 ± 0.81	0.06
TPRI (dyne s cm^{-5})	1720 ± 834	1423 ± 464	NS

Abbreviations: SBP, systolic blood pressure; DBP, diastolic blood pressure; HR, heart rate; BMI, body mass index; RFL, rest flow; PFL, maximal postischemic flow; IF, increase in flow after prolonged ischemia; BRL, basal resistance; MRL, minimal postischemic resistance; IVST, interventricular septum thickness; PWT, posterior wall thickness; h/r, relative wall thickness; Mi, left ventricular mass index; ESS, end systolic stress; CI, cardiac index; TPRI, total peripheral resistance index. Mean ± SD.

Modified from Semplicini, A. et al., *Min. Electrolyte Metab.*, 6, 207, 1992. With permission.

resistance after prolonged ischemia as a noninvasive way of assessing the morphological status of systemic arteries in hypertensive patients. This parameter is easily obtained and the method has been recently validated. Minimal vascular resistance is increased in the untreated hypertensive patients, but can be reduced by prolonged antihypertensive treatment. A group of 31 patients with essential hypertension was actively traced after 1 to 2 years Li^+/Na^+ CT had been measured on drug washout. Of these, 22 were still on regular antihypertensive drug treatment, and the others reported a satisfactory home blood pressure control. Echocardiogram and calf plethysmography were performed and the results are reported in Table 6, according to basal Li^+/Na^+ CT. In the patients with Li^+/Na^+ CT above the mean for this series (Li^+/Na^+ CT 0.4 ± 0.19 mmol/l cell × h), blood pressure, body mass index, rest calf flow, and minimal postischemic vascular resistance were significantly greater than in the patients with Li^+/Na^+ CT below the mean (Li^+/Na^+ CT 0.16 ± 0.11 mmol/l cell × h). The postischemic increase in calf flow was significantly lower in the former than in the latter. No difference of echocardiographic parameters was observed. These data confirm that the patients with the highest Li^+/Na^+ CT are more frequently resistant to antihypertensive therapy, that an increase of Li^+/Na^+ CT may favor vascular remodeling, or that it prevents its correction by antihypertensive treatment. The association between high minimal vascular postischemic vascular resistance and increased blood pressure confirms that structural abnormalities of the resistance vessels may contribute to the development and maintenance of hypertension. High Li^+/Na^+ CT did not prevent the correction of cardiac hypertrophy with prolonged antihypertensive treatment, thus confirming that cardiac remodeling is more easily corrected than structural vascular abnormalities.[123]

XIV. Li^+/Na^+ AND Na^+/H^+ CT

A. IS Li^+/Na^+ CT AN OPERATIONAL MODE OF Na^+/H^+ CT?

First, it was shown that Li^+/Na^+ CT may perform the exchange of Na for Na across the cell membrane (Na^+/Na^+ CT). Later, it was proposed that Li^+/Na^+ CT is an operational mode of the cell membrane Na^+/H^+ CT.[10,11] Na^+/Na^+ CT does not affect cation composition of the cell and it is of no clear physiopathologic significance. On the contrary, an increased activity of the cell membrane Na^+/H^+ CT could contribute to the development of hypertension and of its complications by facilitating vascular smooth muscle cell contraction and growth, cardiac contractility and hypertrophy, and finally, salt and water retention by the kidney.[12] Na^+/H^+ CT is involved in the regulation of cell pH and cell volume, in the response to hormones, mitogens, and growth factors, and in the renal proximal reabsorption of Na and bicarbonate.

After the proposal that Li^+/Na^+ CT may represent an operational mode of Na^+/H^+ CT various attempts were conducted to confirm this hypothesis and to show heterogeneity of Na^+/H^+ CT, which may account for the variability of Li^+/Na^+ CT. Technically, the problem is made difficult by the fact that Na^+/H^+ CT is a "housekeeping" function largely diffused in all the eukaryotic cells. The transmembrane protein responsible for Na^+/H^+ CT has not been purified and there is no perfect inhibitor to be used for binding studies.

The problem was therefore approached indirectly by comparing the kinetic properties of the two transport modes and the effects of inhibitors. Striking kinetic similarities were shown in human and rabbit red cells.[16] It was demonstrated that both are asymmetrical and have a higher affinity for H and Li than for Na. Na^+/H^+ CT is only partially sensitive to amiloride while Li^+/Na^+ CT is insensitive.[15] Some amiloride sensitivity of the Li^+/Na^+ CT can, however, be elicited by proton activation (Figure 1). A similar kinetic approach was pursued in sarcolemmal vesicles from canine and bovine mesenteric arteries with similar results.[24,25] It was also shown that when one is activated the other is inhibited.

B. DOES HIGH Li^+/Na^+ CT REFLECT A GENETIC VARIANT OF Na^+/H^+ CT?

The human gene encoding the ubiquitous Na^+/H^+ CT has been cloned.[124] It has been mapped to human chromosome 1p and polymorphism has been reported.[125] Genetic linkage analysis, applied to verify whether the Na^+/H^+ CT gene is that which specifies elevated Li^+/Na^+ CT and is associated to hypertension, did not show evidence of heterogeneity or linkage in any of 14 pedigrees, with major gene segregation for elevated Li^+/Na^+ CT.[126] This cannot, however, rule out the possibility that elevated Li^+/Na^+ is caused by post-transcriptional effects on the antiporter, by alteration of the chemical gradient for Na or H or by modification of the intrinsic activity of the antiporter, for example, by phosphorylation.[127] Moreover, the possibility exists that a distinct Na^+/H^+ CT, encoded by an unlinked gene, is responsible for Li^+/Na^+ CT.

C. DOES HIGH Li^+/Na^+ CT REFLECT INCREASED Na^+/H^+ CT?

Various pieces of evidence suggest that high Li^+/Na^+ CT does not simply reflect increased maximal velocity of translocation of the Na^+/H^+ CT. In man, Li^+/Na^+ CT is more than 100 times slower than Na^+/H^+ CT, and their maximal velocities are only weakly correlated.[94] Moreover, in a large group of patients with uncomplicated IDDM in good metabolic control, Li^+/Na^+ CT was higher in the hypertensives as compared to the normotensives (0.37 ± 0.15 mmol/l cell $\times$ h, $n = 40$, vs. 0.31 ± 0.12, $n = 42$, $p < 0.05$) (Figure 3), while Na^+/H^+ CT was only minimally increased (77 ± 36 and 71 ± 29 mmol/l cell $\times$ h, respectively) (Figure 4). It appears therefore that Li does not pass through the main pathway of the transporter and prolonged exogenous administration of insulin and the resultant chronic hyperinsulinemia in IDDM can increase Na^+/H^+ CT to a greater extent than Li^+/Na^+ CT by increasing the number of transport units or the velocity of translocation. Caution should be used to extrapolate results obtained with the measurement of Li^+/Na^+ CT to Na^+/H^+ CT.

D. DOES HIGH Li^+/Na^+ CT REFLECT ABNORMAL KINETIC PROPERTIES OF Na^+/H^+ CT?

Kinetic heterogeneity of the red cell Na^+/H^+ CT has been shown in patients with essential hypertension.[128] To verify whether an increased Li^+/Na^+ CT reflects abnormal kinetic properties or an increased number of transport units of the Na^+/H^+ CT we have studied normo- and hypertensive subjects of both sexes. They were classified as "low Li^+/Na^+ CT" or "high Li^+/Na^+ CT" according to red cell Li^+/Na^+ CT below or above the mean of the study group. In comparison to the subjects with "low Li^+/Na^+ CT", the subjects with "high Li^+/Na^+ CT" were heavier, had higher blood pressure, and had significantly different kinetic properties of the red cell Na^+/H^+ CT but similar V_{max} (Table 7).

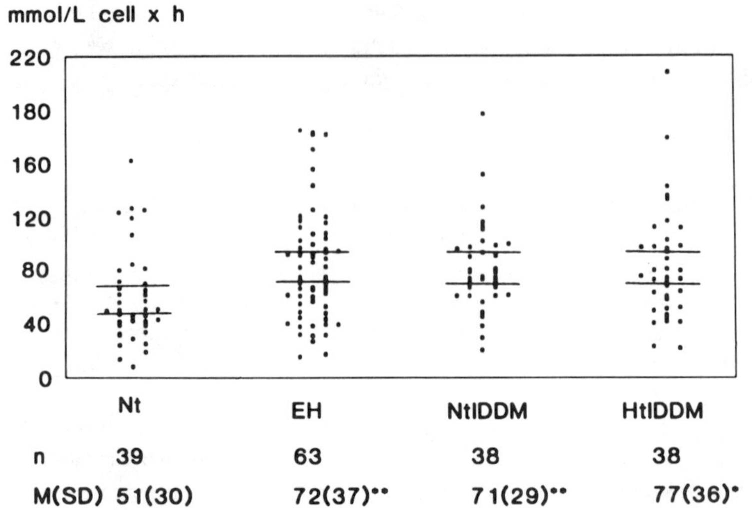

FIGURE 4. Red cell Na^+/H^+ CT in normotensive controls (Ht), in patients with essential hypertension (EH), patients with IDDM, either normotensive (NtIDDM) or hypertensive (HtIDDM). The patients are the same reported in Figure 3. Bars represent 95% confidence limits; * $p < 0.05$, ** $p < 0.01$ vs. Ht.

These data suggest that an increased Li^+/Na^+ CT is more likely to reflect abnormal kinetic properties of Na^+/H^+ CT (reduced affinity for internal H and low Hill's number) than an increased number of transport units. These kinetic abnormalities may facilitate Li movement across the membrane at physiological (7.2) cell pH.

The molecular basis for such abnormalities is uncertain. Because genetic abnormalities of the Na^+/H^+ CT in patients with high Li^+/Na^+ CT have been excluded, our working hypothesis is that the difference is in the regulation of the exchange protein, possibly caused by phosphorylation and/or intracellular Ca.

XV. SUMMARY AND CONCLUSIONS

Among the various alterations of cation transport reported in hypertension, the increase of red cell Li^+/Na^+ CT is that which has been most widely investigated and confirmed. Moreover, it raised interest in the study of cation transport in hypertension.

The pathophysiological significance of this finding is still incompletely clarified. We do not know if it is primary or secondary to other alterations of the cell metabolism. Our working hypothesis is that the increase of Li^+/Na^+ CT reflects abnormal kinetic properties of the Na^+/H^+ CT, either structural or functional (related to the phosphorylation of the transporter and to cytoplasmic calcium).

It seems unlikely that the alterations of Na^+/H^+ CT are secondary to heterogeneity of the transporter after the negative report by Lifton et al.,[126] at least with

TABLE 7
Clinical Data and Kinetic Parameters of the Red Cell Na^+/H^+ CT According to Li^+/Na^+ CT

	Li^+/Na^+ CT		
	Below the mean	**Above the mean**	*p*
n	17	16	
Sex ratio (M/F)	8/9	8/8	
BMI (kg m^{-2})	24 ± 5	28 ± 5	0.008
SBP (mmHg)	129 ± 19	163 ± 16	0.0001
DBP (mmHg)	84 ± 11	105 ± 8	0.0001
HR (beats min^{-1})	77 ± 12	77 ± 10	NS
Li^+/Na^+ CT (mmol/l cell × h)	0.24 ± 0.06	0.36 ± 0.04	0.0003
Na^+/H^+ CT			
V_{max} (mmol/l cell × h)	67 ± 32	59 ± 17	NS
K_m H (nmol/l)	283 ± 273	407 ± 219	0.03
pHi	6.8 ± 0.5	6.5 ± 0.3	0.03
Hill's n	2.67 ± 1.01	1.94 ± 0.65	0.03

Abbreviations: see Table 6.

Modified from Semplicini, A. et al., *Renal Failure,* 15, 333, 1993. With permission.

the first probe used. Other genes could be involved and this is currently under investigation.

Altered phosphorylation of the transporter, secondary to protein kinase activation or phosphatase inactivation, is another possibility. Angiotensin II, insulin, and growth factors activate Na^+/H^+ CT through direct or indirect activation of membrane protein kinases.[129]

Cytoplasmic calcium is increased in different cells of hypertensive patients, and the links between cytoplasmic calcium and Na^+/H^+ CT are strong. Calcium activates Na^+/H^+ CT[13] and Li^+/Na^+ CT,[130] while Na^+/H^+ CT on its own modulates free cytoplasmic calcium.[131,132] It is therefore likely that the high Li^+/Na^+ and Na^+/H^+ CT of many hypertensive patients reflects a genetically determined alteration of the phosphorylation state of the cell membrane and/or increased cytoplasmic calcium.

Regardless of the pathophysiological relevance of the Li^+/Na^+ CT may have for the development of hypertension, its measurement could be of clinical use. Its association with severe and drug-resistant hypertension, insulin resistance, vascular and cardiac hypertrophy, hyperlipidemia and obesity, and positive family history for hypertension and for major cardiovascular accidents suggests that high Li^+/Na^+ CT could be considered a biochemical marker for increased cardiovascular risk.[133] This possibility deserves further investigation in longitudinal studies.

ACKNOWLEDGMENTS

The continuous support, constructive criticism, and encouragement of Prof. Cesare Dal Palù, Achille C. Pessina, and Mitzy Canessa is greatly appreciated. The experimental work reported was made possible by the skillful collaboration of Drs. Giulio Ceolotto, Mauro Marzola, and Maria Grazia Mozzato.

Some of the clinical and experimental work was supported by the Italian National Research Council (CNR) targeted project "Prevention and Control of Disease Factors" (FATMA). Subproject 8 "Cardiovascular Diseases" (contract no. 91.00.218 PF 41 115.06.654).

REFERENCES

1. **Baldessarini, R. J.,** Drugs and the treatment of psychiatric disorders, in *The Pharmacological Basis of the Therapeutics,* Goodman, L. S. and Gilman, A., Eds. Macmillan, New York, 391, 1980.
2. **Mendels, J. and Frazer, A.,** Intracellular lithium concentration and clinical response. Towards a membrane theory of depression, *J. Psychiatr. Res.,* 10, 9, 1973.
3. **Haas, M., Schooler, J., and Tosteson, D. C.,** Coupling of lithium to sodium transport in human red cells, *Nature,* 258, 424, 1975.
4. **Duhm, J., Eisenried, F., Becker, B. F., and Greil, W.,** Studies on the lithium transport across the red cell membrane. I. Li uphill transport by the Na-dependent Li countertransport system of human erythrocytes, *Pfluegers' Arch. Eur. J. Physiol.,* 364, 147, 1976.
5. **Duhm, J. and Becker, B. D.,** Studies on the lithium transport across the red cell membrane. III. Factors contributing to the intraindividual variability of the in vitro Li^+ distribution across the human red cell membrane, *Pfluegers' Arch. Eur. J. Physiol.,* 368, 203, 1977.
6. **Pandey, G. N., Sarkadi, B., Haas, M., Gunn, R. B., Davis, J. M., and Tosteson, D. C.,** Lithium transport pathways in human red blood cells, *J. Gen. Physiol.,* 72, 233, 1978.
7. **Sarkadi, B., Alifimoff, J. K., Gunn, R. B., and Tosteson, D. C.,** Kinetics and stoichiometry of Na-dependent Li transport in human red cells, *J. Gen. Physiol.,* 72, 249, 1978.
8. **Ehrlich, B. E. and Diamond, J. M.,** Lithium fluxes in human erythrocytes, *Am. J. Physiol.,* 237, C102, 1979.
9. **Canessa, M., Adragna, N., Solomon, H. S., Connolly, T. M., and Tosteson, D. C.,** Increased sodium-lithium countertransport in red cells of patients with essential hypertension, *N. Engl. J. Med.,* 302, 772, 1980.
10. **Funder, J., Wieth, J. O., Jensen, H. A., and Ibsen, K. K.,** The sodium/lithium exchange mechanism in essential hypertension: is it a sodium/proton exchanger?, in *Topics in Pathophysiology of Hypertension,* Villareal, H. and Sambhi, M. P., Eds., Martinus Nijhoff, Boston, 147, 1984.
11. **Aronson, P. S.,** Red-cell sodium-lithium countertransport and essential hypertension, *N. Engl. J. Med.,* 307, 317, 1982.
12. **Mahnensmith, R. L. and Aronson, P.,** The plasma membrane sodium-hydrogen exchanger and its role in physiological and pathophysiological processes, *Circ. Res.,* 56, 773, 1985.
13. **Escobales, N. and Canessa, M.,** Ca^{2+}-activated Na^+ fluxes in human red cells: amiloride sensitivity, *J. Biol. Chem.,* 260, 11914, 1985.
14. **Canessa, M., Brugnara, C., and Escobales, N.,** The Li^+-Na^+ exchange and Na^+-K^+-Cl^- cotransport systems in essential hypertension, *Hypertension,* 10, IV4, 1987.

15. **Canessa, M., Morgan, K., and Semplicini, A.,** Genetic differences in lithium-sodium exchange and regulation of the sodium-hydrogen exchanger in essential hypertension, *J. Cardiovasc. Pharmacol.,* 12(Suppl. 3), S92, 1988.
16. **Morgan, K. and Canessa, M.,** Interactions of external and internal H^+ and Na^+ with Na^+/Na^+ and Na^+/H^+ exchange of rabbit red cells: evidence for a common pathway, *J. Membr. Biol.,* 118, 193, 1990.
17. **Canessa, M., Bize, I., Solomon, H., Adragna, N., Tosteson, D. C., Dagher, G., Garay, R., and Meyer, P.,** Na countertransport and cotransport in human red cells: function, dysfunction, and genes in essential hypertension, *Clin. Exp. Hypertension,* 3, 783, 1981.
18. **Hannaert, P. A. and Garay, R. P.,** A kinetic analysis of Na-Li countertransport in human red blood cells, *J. Gen. Physiol.,* 87, 353, 1986.
19. **Canessa, M.,** Kinetic properties of Na/H exchange and Li/Na, Na/Na, and Na/Li exchanges of human red cells, *Methods Enzymol.,* 173, 176, 1989.
20. **Ibsen, K. K., Jensen, H. A., Wieth, J. O., and Funder, J.,** Essential hypertension: sodium-lithium countertransport in erythrocytes from patients and from children having one hypertensive parent, *Hypertension,* 4, 703, 1982.
21. **Duhm, J. and Gobel, B. O.,** Sodium-lithium exchange and sodium-potassium cotransport in human erythrocytes. I. Evaluation of a simple uptake test to assess the activity of the two transport systems, *Hypertension,* 4, 468, 1982.
22. **Hentschel, W. M., Wu, L. L., Tobin, G. O., Anstall, H. B., Smith, J. B., Williams, R. R., and Ash, K. O.,** Erythrocyte cation transport activities as a function of cell age, *Clin. Chim. Acta,* 157, 33, 1986.
23. **Carr, S., Thomas, T. H., and Wilkinson, R.,** Sodium-lithium countertransport activity and its sensitivity to inhibitors with erythrocyte ageing in man, *Clin. Chim. Acta,* 178, 51, 1988.
24. **Kahn, A. M., Allen, J. C., Cragoe, E. J., Jr., Zimmer, R., and Shelat, H.,** Sodium-lithium exchange in sarcolemmal vesicles from canine superior mesenteric artery, *Circ. Res.,* 62, 478, 1988.
25. **Kahn, A. M., Allen, J. C., Cragoe, E. J., Jr., and Shelat, H.,** Sodium-lithium exchange and sodium-proton exchange are mediated by the same transport system in sarcolemmal vesicles from bovine superior mesenteric artery, *Circ. Res.,* 65, 818, 1989.
26. **Smith, J. B., Ash, K. O., Hunt, S. C., Hentschel, W. M., Sprowell, W., Dadone, M. M., and Williams, R. R.,** Three red cell sodium transport systems in hypertensive and normotensive Utah adults, *Hypertension,* 6, 159, 1984.
27. **Turner, S. T., Johnson, M., Boerwinkle, E., Richelson, E., Taswell, H. F., and Sing, C. F.,** Sodium-lithium countertransport and blood pressure in healthy blood donors, *Hypertension,* 7, 955, 1985.
28. **Boerwinkle, E., Turner, S. T., Weinshilboum, R., Johnson, M., Richelson, E., and Sing, C. F.,** Analysis of the distribution of erythrocyte sodium lithium countertransport in a sample representative of the general population, *Gen. Epidemiol.,* 3, 365, 1986.
29. **Hasstedt, S. J., Wu, L. L., Ash, K. O., Kuida, H., and Williams, R. R.,** Hypertension and sodium-lithium countertransport in Utah pedigrees: evidence for major-locus inheritance, *Am. J. Hum. Gen.,* 43, 14, 1988.
30. **Mozzato, M. G., Semplicini, A., Zamboni, S., Urbani, V., Marzola, M., Mazzucato, L., Ambrosio, G. B., and Pessina, A. C.,** Il controtrasporto Li/Na eritrocitario e le variabili ad esso correlate in un campione randomizzato di popolazione, *Cardiologia,* 34, 347, 1989.
31. **Rutherford, P. A., Thomas, T. H., and Wilkinson, R.,** Increased erythrocyte sodium-lithium countertransport activity in essential hypertension is due to an increased affinity for extracellular sodium, *Clin. Sci.,* 79, 365, 1990.
32. **Siebers, R. W. and Maling, T. J.,** Kinetics of sodium-lithium countertransport in normotensive and hypertensive subjects, *J. Cardiovasc. Pharmacol.,* 16, S59, 1990.
33. **Laurenzi, M. and Trevisan, M.,** Sodium-lithium countertransport and blood pressure: the Gubbio population study, *Hypertension,* 13, 408, 1989.

34. **Turner, S. T., Weidman, W. H., Michels, V. V., Reed, T. J., Ormson, C. L., Fuller, T., and Sing, C. F.,** Distribution of sodium-lithium countertransport and blood pressure in Caucasians five to eighty-nine years of age, *Hypertension,* 13, 378, 1989.
35. **Weder, A. B. and Schork, N. J.,** Mixture analysis of erythrocyte lithium-sodium countertransport and blood pressure, *Hypertension,* 13, 145, 1989.
36. **Weder, A. B., Schork, N. J., Krause, L., and Julius, S.,** Red blood cell lithium-sodium countertransport in the Tecumseh blood pressure study, *Hypertension,* 17, 652, 1991.
37. **Laurenzi, M. W. and Trevisan, M.,** Erythrocyte sodium-lithium countertransport levels in an entire population: findings of the Gubbio study, *J. Hypertension,* 5(Suppl. 5), S273, 1987.
38. **Williams, R. R., Hunt, S. C., Kuida, H., Smith, J. B., and Ash, K. O.,** Sodium-lithium countertransport in erythrocytes of hypertension prone families in Utah, *Am. J. Epidemiol.,* 118, 338, 1983.
39. **Trevisan, M., Ostrow, D., Cooper, R. S., Sempos, C., and Stamler, J.,** Sex and race differences in sodium-lithium countertransport and red cell sodium concentration, *Am. J. Epidemiol.,* 120, 537, 1984.
40. **Trevisan, M., Ostrow, D., Cooper, R., Liu, K., Sparks, S., Okonek, A., Stevens, E., Marquardt, J., and Stamler, J.,** Abnormal red blood cell ion transport and hypertension. The Peoples Gas Company study, *Hypertension,* 5, 363, 1983.
41. **Arumanayagam, M., MacDonald, D., and Swaminathan, R.,** Differences in erythrocyte cation (sodium) transport between Chinese and non Chinese males, *Clin. Exp. Hypertension* [*A*], 9, 719, 1987.
42. **Worley, R. J., Hentschel, W. M., Cormier, C., Nutting, S. G., Zelenkov, K., Smith, J. B., Ash, K. O., and Williams, R. R.,** Increased sodium-lithium countertransport in erythrocytes of pregnant women, *N. Engl. J. Med.,* 307, 412, 1982.
43. **Canessa, M.,** The polymorphism of red cell Na and K transport in essential hypertension: findings, controversies, and perspectives, in *Erythrocyte Membranes 3: Recent Clinical and Experimental Advances,* Kruckeberg, W. C., Eaton, J. W., Aster, J., and Brewer, G. J., Eds., Alan R. Liss, New York, 293, 1984.
44. **Brugnara, C., Corrocher, R., Foroni, L., Steinmayr, M., Bonfanti, F., and De Sandre, G.,** Lithium-sodium countertransport in erythrocytes of normal and hypertensive subjects. Relationship with age and plasma renin activity, *Hypertension,* 5, 529, 1983.
45. **Kagamimori, S., Naruse, Y., Takata, M., and Fujita, T.,** Familial aggregation of red blood cell cation transport systems in Japanese families, *Am. J. Epidemiol.,* 122, 386, 1985.
46. **Motulsky, A. G., Burke, W., Billings, P. R., and Ward, R. H.,** Hypertension and the genetics of red cell membrane abnormalities, in *Molecular Approaches to Human Polygenic Disease 130 Ciba Foundation Symposium,* John Wiley & Sons, Chichester, U.K., 150, 1987.
47. **Weder, A. B., Schork, N. J., and Julius, S.,** Linkage of MN locus and erythrocyte lithium-sodium countertransport in Tecumseh, Michigan, *Hypertension,* 17, 977, 1991.
48. **Yap, L., Arrazola, A., Soria, F., and Diez, J.,** Is there increased cardiovascular risk in essential hypertensive patients with abnormal kinetics of red blood cell sodium-lithium countertransport?, *J. Hypertension,* 7, 667, 1989.
49. **De la Sierra, A., Coca, A., Aguilera, M. T., and Urbano-Marquez, A.,** Na^+-Li^+ countertransport in essential hypertension, *J. Hypertension,* 6, 931, 1988.
50. **Mongeau, J. G., Mauran, P., Poirot, G., and Davignon, A.,** Longitudinal study of various transport abnormalities as an index of severity in children and adolescents suffering from essential hypertension, *J. Hypertension,* 8, 657, 1990.
51. **McDonald, A. M., Dyer, A. R., Liu, K., Stamler, R., Gosch, F. C., Grimm, R., Berman, R., and Stamler, J.,** Sodium, lithium-countertransport and blood pressure control by nutritional intervention in 'mild' hypertension, *J. Hypertension,* 6, 283, 1988.
52. **Cooper, R., Trevisan, M., Van Horn, L., Larbi, E., Liu, K., Nanas, S., Ueshima, H., Sempos, C., Ostrow, D., and Stamler, J.,** Effect of dietary sodium reduction on red blood cell sodium concentration and sodium-lithium countertransport, *Hypertension,* 6, 731, 1984.

53. **Canessa, M., Redgrave, J., Laski, C., and Williams, G. H.,** Does sodium intake modify red cell Na transporters in normal and hypertensive subjects, *Am. J. Hypertension,* 2, 515, 1989.
54. **Levy, R., Paran, E., Keynan, A., and Livne, A.,** Essential hypertension: improved differentiation by the temperature dependence of Li efflux in erythrocytes, *Hypertension,* 5, 821, 1983.
55. **Hunt, S. C., Stephenson, S. H., Hopkins, P. N., Hasstedt, S. J., and Williams, R. R.,** A prospective study of sodium-lithium countertransport and hypertension in Utah, *Hypertension,* 17, 1, 1991.
56. **Corry, D. B., Tuck, M. L., Brickman, A. S., Yanagawa, N., and Lee, D. B.,** Sodium transport in red blood cells from dialyzed uremic patients, *Kidney Int.,* 29, 1197, 1986.
57. **DeSanto, N. G., Trevisan, M., DeColle, S., DiMuro, M., DeChiara, F., Latte, M., Franzese, A., Iacono, R., Capasso, G., and Capodicasa, G.,** Intraerythrocytic cation metabolism in children with uremia undergoing hemodialysis, *J. Lab. Clin. Med.,* 110, 231, 1987.
58. **Weder, A. B. and Torretti, B. A.,** Erythrocyte lithium transport changes induced by deoxycorticosterone acetate treatment in pigs, *Hypertension,* 7, 541, 1985.
59. **Woods, J. W., Parker, J. C., and Watson, B. S.,** Perturbation of sodium-lithium countertransport in red cells, *N. Engl. J. Med.,* 308, 1258, 1983.
60. **Trevisan, M., DeSanto, N., Laurenzi, M., DiMuro, M., DeChiara, F., Latte, M., Franzese, A., Iacone, R., Capodicasa, G., and Giordano, C.,** Intracellular ion metabolism in erythrocytes and uraemia: the effect of different dialysis treatments, *Clin. Sci.,* 71, 545, 1986.
61. **Smith, J. B., Ash, K. O., Gregory, M. C., Sprowell, W. L., Hentschel, W. M., and Williams, R. R.,** Hemodialysis does not affect erythrocyte sodium-lithium countertransport, *Clin. Chim. Acta,* 143, 275, 1984.
62. **Corrocher, R., Bertinato, L., Brugnara, C., Guadagnini, L. M., Bassi, A., Bonfanti, F., Losi, S., and Stopelli, G.,** Placental hormones and elevation of erythrocyte sodium-lithium countertransport in pregnancy, *Clin. Exp. Hypertension,* B5, 9, 1986.
63. **Gless, K. H., Sutterlin, U., Schaz, K., Schutz, V., and Hunstein, W.,** Intracellular sodium concentration and transport in red cells in essential hypertension, hyperthyroidism, pregnancy and hypokalemia, *Clin. Physiol. Biochem.,* 4, 199, 1986.
64. **Beuckelmann, D. and Erdmann, E.,** Exogenous factors influencing the human erythrocyte sodium-lithium countertransport system, *Eur. J. Clin. Invest.,* 14, 392, 1984.
65. **Diamond, J. M., Matsuyama, S. S., Meier, K., and Jarvik, L. F.,** Elevation of erythrocyte countertransport rates in Alzheimer's dementia, *N. Engl. J. Med.,* 309, 1061, 1983.
66. **Brent, G. A., Canessa, M., and Dluhy, R. G.,** Reversible alteration of red cell lithium-sodium countertransport in patients with thyroid disease, *J. Clin. Endocrinol. Metab.,* 68, 322, 1989.
67. **Mattioli, M., Delva, P., Lechi, C., Minuz, P., Lechi, A., and Scuro, L. A.,** Increased sodium-lithium countertransport in red cells of patients with Bartter's syndrome, *J. Endocrinol. Invest.,* 7, 61, 1984.
68. **Sutterlin, U., Gless, K. H., Schaz, K., Hufner, M., Schutz, V., and Hunstein, W.,** Peripheral effects of thyroid hormones: alteration of intracellular Na-concentration, ouabain-sensitive Na-transport, and Na-Li countertransport in human red blood cells, *Klin. Wochenschr.,* 62, 598, 1984.
69. **Bianchi, G., Vezzoli, G., Cusi, D., Cova, T., Elli, A., Soldati, L., Tripodi, G., Surian, M., Ottaviano, E., Rigatti, P., and Ortolani, S.,** Abnormal red cell calcium pump in patients with idiopathic hypercalciuria, *N. Engl. J. Med.,* 319, 897, 1988.
70. **Semplicini, A., Mozzato, M. G., Rigon, E., Parolin, O., Samá, B., Padovan, S., Degan, P., Peserico, A., and Pessina, A. C.,** Red blood cell sodium and potassium fluxes in psoriatic patients, *Eur. J. Clin. Invest.,* 18, 47, 1988.
71. **Trevisan, M., Cooper, R., Ostrow, D., Sempos, C., Sparks, S., Nanas, S., Miller, W., and Stamler, J.,** Red cell cation transport: differences between black and white school children, *J. Hypertension,* 1, 245, 1983.
72. **Milunpalo, S., Saarinen, R., and Marniemi, J.,** Red-cell sodium-potassium pump and sodium-lithium countertransport in human obesity. Re-evaluation of the methods and association in a Finnish population, *Int. J. Obesity,* 9, 313, 1985.

73. **Hunt, S. C., Williams, R. R., Smith, J. B., and Ash, K.,** Associations of three erythrocyte cation transport systems with plasma lipids in Utah subjects, *Hypertension,* 8, 30, 1986.
74. **McDonald, A., Trevisan, M., Cooper, R., Stamler, R., Gosch, F., Ostrow, D., and Stamler, J.,** Epidemiological studies of sodium transport and hypertension, *Hypertension,* 10, I42, 1987.
75. **Corrocher, R., Steinmayr, M., Ruzzenente, O., Brugnara, C., Bertinato, L., Mazzi, M., Furri, C., Bonfanti, F., and De Sandre, G.,** Elevation of red cell sodium-lithium countertransport in hyperlipidemias, *Life Sci.,* 36, 649, 1985.
76. **Duhm, J. and Behr, J.,** Role of exogenous factors in alterations of red cell Na-Li exchange and Na-K cotransport in essential hypertension, primary hyperaldosteronism, and hypokaliemia, *Scand. J. Clin. Lab. Invest.,* 46, 82, 1986.
77. **Carr, S. J., Thomas, T. H., Laker, M. F., and Wilkinson, R.,** Elevated sodium-lithium countertransport: a familial marker of hyperlipidaemia and hypertension?, *J. Hypertension,* 8, 139, 1990.
78. **Hajem, S., Moreau, T., Hannaert, P., Lellouch, J., Orssaud, G., Huel, G., Claude, J. R., and Garay, R. P.,** Erythrocyte cation transport systems and plasma lipids in a general male population, *J. Hypertension,* 8, 891, 1990.
79. **Messner, H., Kleophas, W., Hein, D., Gries, A., and Kobberling, J.,** Sodium lithium countertransport is acutely influenced by heparin-induced extracorporal LDL precipitation, *Eur. J. Clin. Invest.,* 21, 215, 1991.
80. **Levy, R., Hevroni, D., Cabantchik, Z. I., and Livne, A.,** Li_i-Na_o countertransport and Li leak in erythrocytes are differentially affected by membrane enrichment with cholesteryl hemisuccinate, *Biochim. Biophys. Acta,* 854, 325, 1986.
81. **Pagnan, A., Corrocher, R., Ambrosio, G. B., Ferrari, S., Guarini, P., Piccolo, D., Opportuno, A., Bassi, A., Olivieri, O., and Baggio, G.,** Effects of an olive-oil-rich diet on erythrocyte membrane lipid composition and cation transport systems, *Clin. Sci.,* 76, 87, 1989.
82. **Murray, G. E. and Patrick, J.,** Effect of dietary fat on sodium transport and sodium-lithium countertransport in rat erythrocytes and thymocytes, *J. Nutr.,* 116, 1390, 1986.
83. **Semplicini, A., Casiglia, E., Marzola, M., Ceolotto, G., Businaro, R., Olivieri, O., Guarini, P., Corrocher, R., Martines, C., and Dal Palú, C.,** Effects of linoleic acid supplementation on blood pressure and kinetics of red cell Na transport: the Piove di Sacco Study, *J. Hypertension,* 9(Suppl. 6), S310, 1991.
84. **Weder, A. B., Serr, C., Torretti, B. A., Bassett, D. R., and Zweifler, A.,** Effects of lovastatin treatment on red blood cell and platelet cation transport, *Hypertension,* 17, 203, 1991.
85. **Ferrannini, E., Buzzigoli, G., Bonadonna, R., Giorico, M. A., Oleggini, M., Graziadei, L., Pedrinelli, R., Brandi, L., and Bevilacqua, A.,** Insulin resistance in hypertension, *N. Engl. J. Med.,* 317, 350, 1987.
86. **Strazzullo, P., Cappuccio, F. P., Trevisan, M., Iacoviello, L., Iacone, R., Barba, G., De Leo, A., Farinaro, E., and Mancini, M.,** Red blood cell sodium-lithium countertransport, blood pressure, and uric acid metabolism in untreated healthy men, *Am. J. Hypertension,* 2, 634, 1989.
87. **Strazzullo, P., Cappuccio, F. P., Barba, G., Trevisan, M., Ciacci, C., Iacone, R., and Russo, L.,** Altered renal tubular function in men with high erythrocyte sodium-lithium countertransport, *J. Hypertension,* 7(Suppl. 6), S154, 1989.
88. **Reaven, G.,** Role of insulin resistance in human disease, *Diabetes,* 37, 1595, 1988.
89. **Coca, A., Garay, R. P., and Aguilera, M. T., De la Sierra, A., Urbano-Marquez, A.,** Disturbances of transmembranous sodium transport systems induced by ethanol in human erythrocytes, *Am. J. Hypertension,* 2, 784, 1989.
90. **Gobel, B. O., Ruppert, M., Ressel, C., and Stumpe, K. O.,** Erythrocyte cation transport and blood pressure in chronic alcoholics, *J. Hypertension,* 5(Suppl. 5), S295, 1987.
91. **Adragna, N. C., Chang, J. L., Morey, M. C., and Williams, R. S.,** Effect of exercise on cation transport in human red cells, *Hypertension,* 7, 132, 1985.
92. **Bunker, C. H., Mallinger, A. G., Adams, L. L., and Kuller, L. H.,** Red blood cell sodium-lithium countertransport and cardiovascular risk factors in black and white college students, *J. Hypertension,* 5, 7, 1987.

93. **Weder, A. B.,** Red-cell lithium-sodium countertransport and renal lithium clearance in hypertension, *N. Engl. J. Med.,* 314, 198, 1986.
94. **Semplicini, A., Canessa, M., Mozzato, M. G., Ceolotto, G., Marzola, M., Buzzacarini, F., Casolino, P., and Pessina, A. C.,** Red blood cell Na^+/H^+ and Li^+/Na^+ exchange in patients with essential hypertension, *Am. J. Hypertension,* 2, 903, 1989.
95. **Strazzullo, P., Cappuccio, F. P., Trevisan, M., Iacoviello, L., Iacone, R., Jossa, F., Giorgione, N., Farinaro, E., and Mancini, M.,** Erythrocyte sodium/lithium countertransport and renal lithium clearance in a random sample of untreated middle-aged men, *Clin. Sci.,* 77, 337, 1989.
96. **Weinberger, M. H., Smith, J. B., Fineberg, N. S., and Luft, F. C.,** Red-cell sodium-lithium countertransport and fractional excretion of lithium in normal and hypertensive humans, *Hypertension,* 13, 206, 1989.
97. **Maling, T. J. and Siebers, R. W.,** Sodium-lithium countertransport is not a marker of proximal tubular sodium clearance, *J. Cardiovasc. Pharmacol.,* 16, S50, 1990.
98. **Nosadini, R., Semplicini, A., Fioretto, P., Lusiani, L., Trevisan, R., Donadon, V., Zanette, G., Nicolosi, G. L., Dall'Aglio, V., Zanuttini, D., and Viberti, G. C.,** Sodium-lithium countertransport and cardio-renal abnormalities in essential hypertension, *Hypertension,* 18, 191, 1991.
99. **Lijnen, P., Hespel, P., Fagard, R., Staessen, J., Goossens, W., Lissens, W., and Amery, A.,** Erythrocyte and leucocyte sodium and potassium transport systems during long-term diuretic administration in men, *J. Hypertension,* 6, 639, 1988.
100. **Niutta, E., Cusi, D., Colombo, R., Pellizzoni, M., Cesana, C., Barlassina, C., Soldati, L., and Bianchi, G.,** Predicting interindividual variations in antihypertensive therapy: the role of sodium transport systems and renin, *J. Hypertension,* 8(Suppl. 4), S53, 1990.
101. **Sechi, L. A., Tedde, R., Cassisa, L., Marigliano, A., Uneddu, F., Melis, A., and Pala, A.,** Effects of ketanserin on transmembrane sodium transport in erythrocytes, *J. Cardiovasc. Pharmacol.,* 15, 269, 1990.
102. **Fujita, T., Noda, H., Ando, K., and Sato, Y.,** Peripheral resistance and red cell Li-Na countertransport in borderline hypertensives, *Life Sci.,* 32, 1621, 1983.
103. **Weder, A. B., Fitzpatrick, M. A., Torretti, B. A., Hinderliter, A. L., Egan, B. M., and Julius, S.,** Red blood cell Li^+-Na^+ countertransport, Na^+-K^+ cotransport, and the hemodynamics of hypertension, *Hypertension,* 9, 459, 1987.
104. **Semplicini, A., Lusiani, L., Marzola, M., Ceolotto, G., Mozzato, M. G., Zanette, G., Donadon, V., Stefanini, M. G., Zanuttini, D., and Pessina, A. C.,** Erythrocyte Li^+/Na^+ and Na^+/H^+ exchange, cardiac anatomy and function in insulin dependent diabetes, *Eur. J. Clin. Invest.,* 22, 254, 1992.
105. **Semplicini, A., Mozzato, M. G., Rigon, E., Parolin, O., Samá, B., Degan, P., Pessina, A. C., and Dal Palú, C.,** Does essential hypertension with low Na-K cotransport and/or high Li-Na countertransport represent a clinical entity, *J. Hypertension,* 4(Suppl. 5), S219, 1986.
106. **Redgrave, J., Canessa, M., Gleason, R., Hollenberg, N. K., and Williams, G. H.,** Red blood cell Li-Na countertransport in non modulating essential hypertension, *Hypertension,* 13, II 721, 1989.
107. **Ferrari, P. and Weidmann, P.,** Insulin, insulin sensitivity and hypertension, *J. Hypertension,* 8, 491, 1990.
108. **Natali, A., Santoro, D., Palombo, C., Cerri, M., Ghione, S., and Ferrannini, E.,** Impaired insulin action on skeletal muscle metabolism in essential hypertension, *Hypertension,* 17, 170, 1991.
109. **Hall, J. E., Brands, M. W., Kivlighn, S. D., Mizelle, H. L., Hidebrandt, D. A., and Gaillard, C. A.,** Chronic hyperinsulinemia and blood pressure. Interaction with catecholamines?, *Hypertension,* 15, 519, 1990.
110. **Tsutsu, N., Nunoi, K., Kodama, T., Nomiyama, R., Iwase, M., and Fujishima, M.,** Lack of association between blood pressure and insulin in patients with insulinoma, *J. Hypertension,* 8, 479, 1990.

111. **Trevisan, M., Vaccaro, O., Laurenzi, M., De Chiara, F., Di Muro, M., Iacone, R., and Franzese, A.**, Hypertension, non-insulin-dependent diabetes, and intracellular sodium metabolism, *Hypertension,* 11, 264, 1988.
112. **Trevisan, M., Cirillo, M., and Laurenzi, M.**, Sodium lithium countertransport and glucose metabolism, *J. Hypertension,* 8(Suppl. 3), S124, 1990.
113. **Semplicini, A., Mozzato, M. G., Samá, B., Nosadini, R., Fioretto, P., Trevisan, R., Pessina, A. C., Crepaldi, G., and Dal Palú, C.**, Na/H and Li/Na exchange in red blood cells of normotensive and hypertensive patients with insulin dependent diabetes mellitus (IDDM), *Am. J. Hypertension,* 2, 174, 1989.
114. **Bedford Johnson, B. A., Sowers, J. R., Zemel, P. C., Luft, F. C., and Zemel, M. B.**, Increased sodium-lithium countertransport in black non-insulin-dependent diabetic hypertensives, *Am. J. Hypertension,* 3, 363, 1990.
115. **Doria, A., Fioretto, P., Avogaro, A., Carraro, A., Morocutti, A., Trevisan, R., Frigato, F., Crepaldi, G., Verberti, G., and Nosadini, R.**, Insulin resistance is associated with high sodium-lithium countertransport in essential hypertension, *Am. J. Physiol.,* 261, E684, 1991.
116. **Mangili, R., Bending, J. J., Scott, G., Li, L. K., Gupta, A., and Viberti, G.**, Increased sodium-lithium countertransport activity in red cells of patients with insulin-dependent diabetes and nephropathy, *N. Engl. J. Med.,* 318, 146, 1988.
117. **Krolewski, A. S., Canessa, M., Warram, J. H., Laffel, L. M., Christlieb, A. R., Knowler, W. C., and Rand, L. I.**, Predisposition to hypertension and susceptibility to renal disease in insulin-dependent diabetes mellitus, *N. Engl. J. Med.,* 318, 140, 1988.
118. **Carr, S., Mbanya, J. C., Thomas, T., Keavey, P., Taylor, R., Alberti, K. G., and Wilkinson, R.**, Increase in glomerular filtration rate in patients with insulin-dependent diabetes and elevate erythrocyte sodium-lithium countertransport, *N. Engl. J. Med.,* 322, 500, 1990.
119. **Lever, A. F.**, Slow pressor mechanisms in hypertension: a role for hypertrophy of resistance vessels?, *J. Hypertension,* 4, 515, 1986.
120. **Devereux, R. B.**, Hypertensive cardiac hypertrophy. Pathophysiologic and clinical characteristics, in *Hypertension: Pathophysiology, Diagnosis and Management,* Vol. 26, Laragh, J. H. and Brenner, B. M., Eds., Raven Press, New York, 359, 1990.
121. **Grinstein, S., Rotin, D., and Mason, M. J.**, Na/H exchange and growth factor-induced cytosolic pH changes. Role in cellular proliferation, *Biochim. Biophys. Acta,* 988, 73, 1989.
122. **Folkow, B.**, Physiological aspects of primary hypertension, *Physiol. Rev.,* 62, 347, 1982.
123. **Agabiti-Rosei, E., Muiesan, M. L., Geri, A., Romanelli, G., Beschi, M., Castellano, M., and Muiesan, G.**, Long-term antihypertensive treatment may induce normalization of left ventricular mass before complete regression of vascular structural changes: consequences for cardiac function at rest and during stress, *J. Hypertension,* 6(Suppl. 4), S94, 1988.
124. **Sardet, C., Franchi, A., and Pouyssegur, J.**, Molecular cloning, primary structure and expression of the human growth factor-activatable Na^+/H^+ antiporter, *Cell,* 56, 271, 1989.
125. **Lifton, R. P., Sardet, C., Pouyssegur, J., and Lalouel, J. M.**, Cloning of the human genomic amiloride-sensitive Na^+/H^+ antiporter gene, identification of genetic polymorphisms and localization on the genetic map of chromosome 1p, *Genomics,* 7, 131, 1990.
126. **Lifton, R. P., Hunt, S. C., Williams, R. R., Pouyssegur, J., and Lalouel, J. M.**, Exclusion of the Na-H antiporter as a candidate gene in human essential hypertension, *Hypertension,* 17, 8, 1991.
127. **Sardet, C., Counillon, L., Franchi, A., and Pouyssegur, J.**, Growth factors induced phosphorylation of the Na^+/H^+ antiporter glycoprotein of 110 kD, *Science,* 247, 723, 1990.
128. **Canessa, M., Morgan, K., Goldszer, R., Moore, T. J., and Spalvins, A.**, Kinetic abnormalities of the red blood cell sodium-proton exchange in hypertensive patients, *Hypertension,* 17, 340, 1991.
129. **Pouyssegur, J., Franchi, A., L'Allemain, G., Magnaldo, I., Paris, S., and Sardet, C.**, Genetic approach to structure, function, and regulation of the Na^+/H^+ antiporter, *Kidney Int.,* 32(Suppl. 23), S144, 1987.

130. **Agam, G., Hatzav, P., Abekasis, S., Loven, A., and Livne, A.,** Elevated intracellular Ca^{2+} affects Lii-Nao countertransport in human red blood cells, *Biochim. Biophys. Acta,* 904, 207, 1987.
131. **Semrad, C. E. and Chang, E. D.,** Calcium-mediated cyclic AMP inhibition of Na-H exchange in small intestine, *Am. J. Physiol.,* 21, C315, 1987.
132. **Siffert, W., Siffert, G., Scheid, P., and Akkerman, J. W. N.,** Na^+/H^+ exchanges modulates Ca^{++} mobilization in human platelets stimulated by ADP and the thromboxane mimetic U 46619, *J. Biol. Chem.,* 264, 719, 1990.
133. **Carr, S. J., Thomas, T. H., and Wilkinson, R.,** Erythrocyte sodium-lithium countertransport in primary and renal hypertension: relation to family history, *Eur. J. Clin. Invest.,* 19, 101, 1989.
134. **Cusi, D., Barlassina, C., Ferrandi, M., Lupi, P., Ferrari, P., and Bianchi, G.,** Familial aggregation of cation transport abnormalities and essential hypertension, *Clin. Exp. Hypertension,* 3, 871, 1981.
135. **Canali, M., Borghi, L., Sani, E., Curti, A., Montanari, A., Novarini, A., and Borghetti, A.,** Increased erythrocyte lithium-sodium countertransport in essential hypertension: its relationship to family history of hypertension, *Clin. Sci.,* 61, 13s, 1981.
136. **Woods, J. W., Falk, R. J., Pittman, A. W., Klemmer, P. J., Watson, B. S., and Namboodiri, K.,** Increased red-cell sodium-lithium countertransport in normotensive sons of hypertensive parents, *N. Engl. J. Med.,* 306, 593, 1982.
137. **Adragna, N. C., Canessa, M. L., Solomon, H., Slater, E., and Tosteson, D. C.,** Red cell lithium-sodium countertransport and sodium-potassium cotransport in patients with essential hypertension, *Hypertension,* 4, 795, 1982.
138. **Cooper, R., LeGrady, D., Nanas, S., Trevisan, M., Mansour, M., Histand, P., Ostrow, D., and Stamler, J.,** Increased sodium-lithium countertransport in college students with elevated blood pressure, *JAMA,* 249, 1030, 1983.
139. **Weder, A. B., Torretti, B. A., and Julius, S.,** Racial differences in erythrocyte cation transport, *Hypertension,* 6, 115, 1984.
140. **Canessa, M., Spalvins, A., Adragna, N., and Falkner, B.,** Red cell sodium countertransport and cotransport in normotensive and hypertensive blacks, *Hypertension,* 6, 344, 1984.
141. **M'Buyamba-Kabangu, J. R., Lijnen, P., Groeseneken, D., Staessen, J., Lissens, W., Goossens, W., Fagard, R., and Amery, A.,** Racial differences in intracellular concentration and transmembrane fluxes of sodium and potassium in erythrocytes of normal male subjects, *J. Hypertension,* 2, 647, 1984.
142. **Clegg, G., Morgan, D. B., and Davidson, C.,** The heterogeneity of essential hypertension. Relation between lithium efflux and sodium content of erythrocytes and a family history of hypertension, *Lancet,* 2, 891, 1982.
143. **Woods, J. W., Falk, R. J., Pittman, A. W., Klemmer, P. J., Watson, B. S., and Namboodiri, K.,** Increased red-cell sodium-lithium countertransport in normotensive sons of hypertensive parents, *N. Engl. J. Med.,* 306, 593, 1982.
144. **Hunt, S. C., Williams, R. R., Smith, J. B., Ash, K. O., and Kuida, H.,** The relationship of lithium-potassium cotransport and the passive lithium leak to hypertension in Utah subjects, *Clin. Exp. Hypertension* [*A*], 7, 1409, 1985.
145. **Beuckelmann, D. and Erdmann, E.,** Na^+-Li^+ countertransport and electrolyte composition in erythrocytes of patients with essential hypertension before and after antihypertensive treatment, *Klin. Wochenschr.,* 64, 1101, 1986.
146. **Fallo, F., Procidano, M., deAngelis, V., Manoni, F., Mantero, F., and Girolami, A.,** Erythrocyte Na^+-Li^+ countertransport and blood viscosity in arterial hypertension, *Res. Exp. Med. (Berlin),* 186, 71, 1986.
147. **Morgan, D. B., Stewart, A. D., and Davidson, C.,** Relations between erythrocyte lithium efflux, blood pressure and family histories of hypertension and cardiovascular disease: studies in a factory workforce and hypertension clinic, *J. Hypertension,* 4, 609, 1986.
148. **Turner, S. T., Boerwinkle, E., Johnson, M., Richelson, E., and Sing, C. F.,** Sodium-lithium countertransport in ambulatory hypertensive and normotensive patients, *Hypertension,* 9, 24, 1987.

Chapter 6

THE Na^+/H^+ ANTIPORT: ITS ROLE IN CELLULAR METABOLISM AND IN THE PATHOPHYSIOLOGY OF ESSENTIAL HYPERTENSION

Abraham Aviv

TABLE OF CONTENTS

I. Introduction ... 120

II. pH_i Regulation ... 120

III. The Na^+/H^+ Antiport ... 122

IV. The Na^+/H^+ Antiport in Essential Hypertension: Its Link With Cytosolic Ca^{2+} ... 125

V. Conclusion ... 127

References ... 128

0-8493-5474-9/94/$0.00+$.50

I. INTRODUCTION

In researching the cellular etiology of essential hypertension one must accept that there is no animal that can satisfactorily function as a model for this disease in human beings. Animal models of hypertension have served two crucial purposes, namely, they have been instrumental in elucidating a number of important mechanisms that produce elevated blood pressure and in testing antihypertensive drugs. However, essential hypertension in man is distinguished from hypertension in laboratory animals both in the diversity of its origins and the broad spectrum of its manifestations. Without passing judgment on their relevance, multiple cellular abnormalities in genetic animal models of primary hypertension, e.g., the spontaneously hypertensive rat (SHR) and the Dahl salt-sensitive rat, may have little bearing on mechanisms underlying human essential hypertension. For these reasons this chapter addresses the physiology of cytosolic pH (pH_i) regulation in general and the Na^+/H^+ antiport in particular by relying on data derived from both animals and humans. However, conclusions concerning the role of the Na^+/H^+ antiport in the pathophysiology of essential hypertension are exclusively based on observations confined to human beings. This approach has its own drawbacks because at the cellular level observations in men and women with essential hypertension primarily originate from studies in circulating cells. A leap of faith is required in assuming that abnormalities in these cells represent a generalized phenomenon that can be extrapolated to specialized tissues such as the vascular smooth muscle and the renal tubular epithelium. Nonetheless, the redeeming feature of this approach is that it provides for testable hypotheses once specialized human tissues are available to explore the pathophysiology of essential hypertension at the cellular level.

II. pH_i REGULATION

The most compelling reason for tight control of the pH_i is that life itself depends on the function of a multitude of enzymes and metabolic processes that are strongly pH dependent. Dramatic and acute shifts in the pH_i would therefore impose a profound burden on cellular homeostasis, threatening the very existence of the cell, the organ, and the organism. It is no wonder that cells have developed elaborate and overlapping defense mechanisms designed to counteract extreme fluctuations in pH_i. These mechanisms include the cellular buffering capacity (power) and several transport systems which extrude either acid or alkali.

Buffering power is broadly defined by the observed pH shift produced by a given amount of an acid or base that is added to a medium. Upon addition of an acid or alkali, a medium without buffering power demonstrates the predicted pH change, based on simple physiochemical principles. In contrast, a medium with buffering capacity (i.e., a buffer) exhibits less than the predicted pH shift resulting from the addition of an acid or base. The cellular buffering power resides in its bicarbonate regulation and in the property of a variety of cellular proteins to capture or release protons. Traditionally, the cellular buffering power has been measured

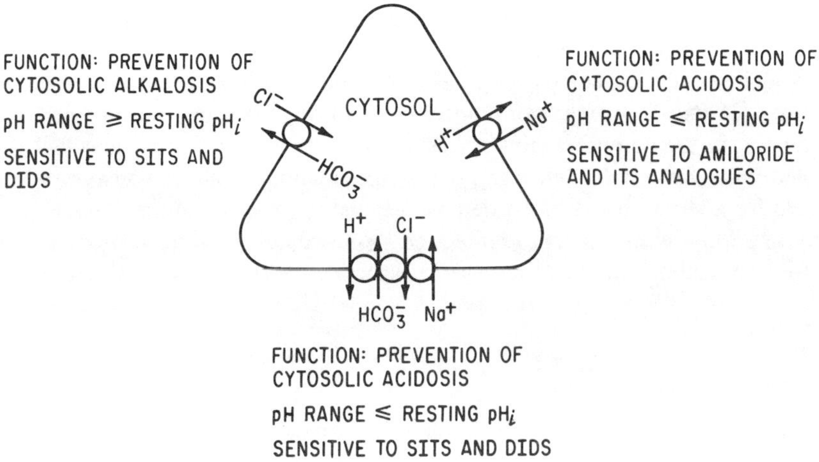

FIGURE 1. The three major alkali and acid transport systems for maintenance of pH_i.

by subjecting cells to a weak acid or base that rapidly permeates the plasma membrane and produces a detectable change in the pH_i. A striking observation arising from such measurements is that nonbicarbonate-dependent buffering power of the cell progressively increases with cytosolic acidification, whereas the bicarbonate buffering system operates more effectively around or above resting pH_i.[2-5] These cellular characteristics constitute the first line of defense against perturbations in the pH_i. The second defense mechanism resides in the capacity of cells to extrude acid or base rapidly and effectively.

Three major transport systems are engaged in acid/base transport across the plasma membrane (Figure 1):

1. The amiloride sensitive Na^+/H^+ antiport (exchanging extracellular Na^+ for intracellular H^+) that was originally considered the main acid extrusion mechanism in mammalian cells
2. The Na^+-dependent Cl^-/HCO_3^- exchange (exchanging intracellular Cl^- for extracellular HCO_3^- through coupling of the exchange of extracellular Na^+ for intracellular H^+)
3. The Na^+-independent Cl^-/HCO_3^- exchange (exchanging intracellular HCO_3^- for extracellular Cl^-)

The two Cl^-/HCO_3^- exchanges are sensitive to 4-acetamide-4′-isothiocyanatostilbene-2,2′-disulfonic acid (SITS) or to 4,4′-diisothiocyanatostilbene-2,2′-disulfonic acid (DIDS). Some cells express, in addition, an Na^+/HCO_3^- cotransport. However, information concerning this system is limited and beyond the scope of this text. The central feature of the Na^+/H^+ antiport and the two Cl^-/HCO_3^- exchanges is that they operate within specific pH_i domains and that the range of overlap of these domains determines to a certain extent the resting pH_i. Because the Na^+/H^+ antiport and the Na^+-dependent Cl^-/HCO_3^- exchange function to extrude acid, they primarily operate at pH_i lower than or close to the resting pH_i.[6-12] Their main function is to guard against cytosolic acidification. The Na^+-independent Cl^-/HCO_3^- exchange, by virtue of its alkali extrusion capacity, functions primarily near or above the resting pH_i in the defense against cytosolic alkalinization.[6-12] It is clear that when coupled with the cellular buffering power these acid and alkali transport systems provide for a strong boost to the defense against marked pH_i shifts. This is particularly important with respect to protection against cytosolic acidification, as bursts in cellular metabolic activity are usually associated with a substantial cellular acid load.

III. THE Na^+/H^+ ANTIPORT

The Na^+/H^+ antiport on the plasma membrane was originally described by Murer and co-workers[13] in brush border vesicles from rat kidney and small intestine. Subsequent studies revealed that this transport system is ubiquitous. It is very likely that more than one isoform of the Na^+/H^+ antiport exists.[14] This idea is supported by observations that in different cells and tissues the Na^+/H^+ antiport exhibits a spectrum of sensitivities to amiloride and its analogs, different activation kinetics by Na^+ and H^+, and a variety of responses to intracellular messengers. Moreover, different activities of apical and basolateral Na^+/H^+ antiports are observed in single cell types of the intestinal and renal epithelia. Perhaps the most supportive evidence for the existence of several Na^+/H^+ antiports originates from studies showing that mitochondrial inner membranes demonstrate Na^+/H^+ antiport activity oriented in a direction opposite to that of the plasmalemma Na^+/H^+ antiport (i.e., H^+ is transported into the cytosol in exchange for Na^+ entering the mitochondrial matrix).[15-17] In fact, the discovery of mitochondrial Na^+/H^+ antiport by Mitchell and Moyle[18,19] preceded by a decade the identification of the carrier in the plasma membrane.

The focus of this presentation is on the plasma membrane Na^+/H^+ antiport. The human gene for this transporter was recently cloned by Sardet et al.[20] In polarized cells, such as the renal tubular epithelium and intestinal epithelium, this antiport is likely to reside in the basolateral membrane. Substantial interest in this transporter arose when it was reported that in nominally bicarbonate free medium, the cellular response to growth factors and other agents, acting through phospholipase C (PLC) and protein kinase C (PKC), is exerted by cytosolic alkalinization through activation of the Na^+/H^+ antiport.[21,22] It was therefore proposed that cytosolic alkalinization, mediated by activation of the Na^+/H^+ antiport, is a potent signal for mitogenesis, cell growth, and other important cellular functions. More recent studies have challenged this concept by showing that in bicarbonate-containing medium the response to growth factors and other agents is not associated with alkalinization and, in fact, may be expressed by slight cytosolic acidification.[23,24] As stressed by Thomas:[25] "Intracellular pH is probably too fundamental a parameter to act as an intracellular messenger even for an event as important as

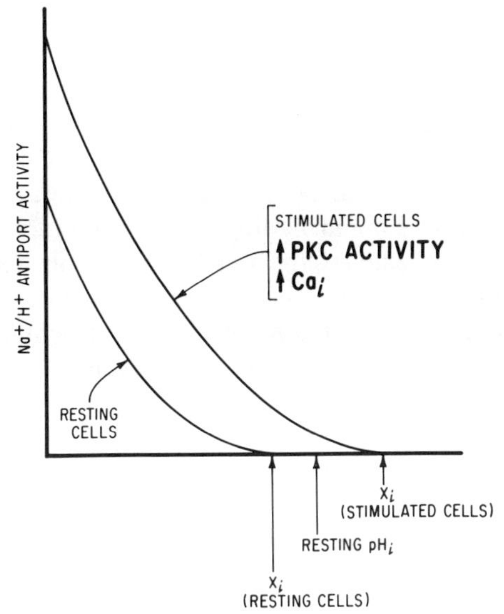

FIGURE 2. An illustration of the relationship between the Na^+/H^+ antiport activity (y axis) and the pH_i (x axis). In the resting cell the pH_i set point for activation of the Na^+/H^+ antiport (Xi) is lower than the resting pH_i. An alkaline shift in the Xi is observed in cells subjected to agonists that raise Ca_i and stimulate PKC. Note that the shift in the Xi is to a pH higher than the resting pH_i. In both resting cells and stimulated cells, the Na^+/H^+ antiport activity progressively increases as the pH_i drops below the Xi.

the initiation of growth except perhaps in acid transporting epithelia.'' This assertion should not detract from the pivotal role of the Na^+/H^+ antiport in cellular pH_i and ionic homeostasis, as the role of this acid extruder is not the promotion of cytosolic alkalosis but the prevention of cytosolic acidosis.

In addition to its involvement in mitogenesis and growth, the Na^+/H^+ antiport is an important element in numerous biological and physiological functions. These include platelet and white blood cell activation, vasoconstriction, skeletal and cardiac muscle contractions, cellular volume regulation, and Na^+ reabsorption by the renal epithelium.[26-28] Several stimuli are responsible for activation of the Na^+/H^+ antiport, of which the first and foremost is cytosolic acidification. The Na^+/H^+ antiport is usually quiescent at resting pH_i. However, acidification of the cytosol below a critical pH_i (which may vary among cells) results in triggering the transporter into action (Figure 2). This is the pH_i set point for activation of the Na^+/H^+ antiport (Xi) and it is an important parameter for characterizing this transport system. Other stimuli for the Na^+/H^+ antiport include osmotically evoked cellular volume reduction, increased PKC activity, and a rise in the cytosolic free Ca (Ca_i). The effect of Ca_i is mediated through PKC-dependent and -independent mechanisms. Agonists that act through PKC stimulate the Na^+/H^+ antiport not only by increasing the metabolic activity of the cells, and thereby promoting cytosolic acidification, but also by increasing the affinity of the transporter to the cytosolic proton. The latter effect is expressed by activation of the Na^+/H^+ antiport at pH above the resting Xi (Figure 2). This agonist-evoked alkaline shift in the Xi is mediated by direct phosphorylation of the carrier protein.[29,30]

The interest in the link between Ca_i and the Na^+/H^+ antiport stems from a number of investigations showing that a nonagonist-evoked rise in Ca_i (e.g., treatment with Ca ionophores) can activate the Na^+/H^+ antiport.[31,32] Studies in human platelets show that Ca_i is paramount for the normal operation of the Na^+/H^+ antiport.[33-35] In Ca-depleted platelets the Na^+/H^+ antiport exhibits only rudimentary activity after cytosolic acidification or treatment with thrombin. Thrombin is a universal platelet activator, the action of which is mediated through PLC, a rise in Ca_i, and the stimulation of PKC. Furthermore, an agonist- or nonagonist-mediated rise in Ca_i overrides the effect of PKC with respect to the stimulation of the Na^+/H^+ antiport, because increased Ca_i promotes an alkaline shift in the Xi even when PKC is inhibited.[33] In platelets, cyclic nucleotides (i.e., cyclic adenosine monophosphate, cAMP, and cyclic guanosine monophosphate, cGMP) diametrically oppose any agonist-evoked rise in Ca_i. This effect of cyclic nucleotides is likely to be the reason for their inhibition of agonist-evoked stimulation of Na^+/H^+ antiport in these[34] and other cells.[36,37] However, there are exceptions to this concept. For instance, Semard and Chang[38] reported that in chick enterocytes cAMP inhibits the Na^+/H^+ antiport in concert with a rise rather than a decline in Ca_i. Others showed that in the rabbit renal brush border membranes cAMP inhibits the Na^+/H^+ antiport by a mechanism that is protein kinase A (PKA) -dependent.[39]

The agonist- and Ca_i-evoked alkaline shift in the Xi appears to serve a fundamental physiological need.[33] First, the cellular response to a number of agonists (e.g., contraction of the vascular smooth muscle, cardiac and skeletal muscles, platelet aggregation, increased Na^+ reabsorption by intestinal or renal epithelia) entails increased metabolic activity and the formation of acid. Second, when the agonist-mediated response involves Ca^{2+} mobilization and enhanced Ca^{2+} influx, it promotes the activation of the Ca^{2+}-ATPase (or its physiological equivalent, the Ca^{2+} pump). This transport system exchanges Ca_i for extracellular protons, as its function is to restore the resting level of Ca_i.[40,41] Both increased metabolic function and accelerated Ca^{2+} pump activity therefore produce cytosolic acidification. One way by which the cell can extrude this acid load is to allow its pH_i to fall below the Xi. Prompt and effective proton extrusion takes place once this crucial pH_i level (i.e., the Xi) is reached. However, the trade off for this route of proton extrusion is that the pH_i must drop at least to the level of the Xi. This would be an ineffective way to maintain the resting pH_i, particularly when the cell is continuously subjected to fluctuating levels of a multitude of agonists that act through PLC, Ca_i, and PKC. An alkaline shift in the Xi, occurring in concert with a rise in Ca_i and/or activation of PKC, would resolve this problem. Such a process would promote proton extrusion without resorting to cytosolic acidification, thereby taking full advantage of the Na^+/H^+ antiport in maintaining the resting pH_i.

The resting pH_i is further guarded by the Na^+-independent Cl^-/HCO_3^- exchange, preventing the alkaline overshoot (due to the alkaline shift in the Xi) associated with agonist-evoked activation of the Na^+/H^+ antiport (Figure 1). This alkaline overshoot is routinely observed when agonist-mediated activation of the Na^+/H^+ antiport is monitored in nominally bicarbonate free medium. Another safety measure in some cells is provided by the Na^+-dependent Cl^-/HCO_3^- exchange, acting in concert with the Na^+/H^+ antiport to prevent cytosolic acidification. It is clear that the resting pH_i reflects the opposing and complementary actions of multiple systems, including acid and alkali transport systems, formation of intracellular proton, and cellular buffering power. Thus, even in nominally bicarbonate free medium, a relatively alkaline resting pH_i in one cell type compared to another does not necessarily indicate increased activity of the Na^+/H^+ antiport in the former. The resting pH_i under this condition is a steady state that represents the combined input of acid production and entry, acid extrusion via the Na^+/H^+ antiport, the cellular buffering power, and perhaps other processes.

What the aforementioned considerations suggest is that cells with increased metabolic activity should also demonstrate enhanced activity of the Na^+/H^+ antiport. This may be one of the reasons for the stimulation Na^+/H^+ antiport in kidney cells[42] and other tissues by thyroid hormone, an agent known to increase cellular oxygen consumption through the stimulation of the Na^+ pump. More importantly for the subject of this chapter, abnormalities resulting in the rise in Ca_i may also promote the stimulation of the Na^+/H^+ antiport by an alkaline shift in the Xi or by increased activity of this transport system throughout the pH_i range in which it operates. This seems to be the case in human essential hypertension.

IV. THE Na^+/H^+ ANTIPORT IN ESSENTIAL HYPERTENSION: ITS LINK WITH CYTOSOLIC Ca^{2+}

Using an optical swelling assay, Livne et al.[43] were the first to demonstrate that platelet Na^+/H^+ antiport activity was higher in patients with essential hypertension than in normotensive controls. Other studies using the same method confirmed this observation.[44-46] The optical assay method employs an ingenious concept, i.e., upon exposure to Na^+-propionate, proponic acid rapidly permeates the plasma membrane and acidifies the cytosol, leading to the activation of the Na^+/H^+ antiport and the gain of Na^+ as well as obligatory water. The resulting platelet volume expansion is used to estimate the activity of the Na^+/H^+ antiport. However, this technique can serve only for the gross estimation of Na^+/H^+ antiport activity after propionic acid-evoked acidification, as it cannot exclude the contribution to volume changes by other factors that are engaged in cellular volume control. Nonetheless, studies using this method paved the way for subsequent and direct measurements of the Na^+/H^+ antiport in platelets of essential hypertensives.

Direct monitoring of platelet pH_i with the fluorescent dye 2′,7′-bis-(2-carboxyethyl)-5(6)-carboxyfluorescein (BCECF) revealed gender, race (black vs. white), and blood pressure-related variations in the Xi.[47] In addition to an alkaline shift in the Xi of platelets from hypertensive than in normotensive white males, platelets from blacks and males showed an alkaline shift in the Xi compared with whites and females, respectively. These gender- and race-related variations in the Xi are compatible with the greater predisposition to essential hypertension of blacks and males than whites and premenopausal women. Such findings are further supported by the observation of a positive correlation between platelet Na^+/H^+ antiport activity after stimulation with thrombin and blood pressure in black females.[48] More recently, Livne et al.,[49] using BCECF to monitor platelet pH_i, confirmed the earlier observation of an alkaline shift in the Xi in hypertensive whites. They further proposed that increased activity of the Na^+/H^+ antiport in essential hypertension results from a greater number of phosphorylated Na^+/H^+ antiports rather than from an absolute increase in the density of these carriers on the plasma membrane. In support of this idea, they took advantage of the fact that phorbol esters stimulate PKC which, in turn, activates the Na^+/H^+ antiport by phosphorylation of the carrier protein. In their study, untreated platelets from essential hypertensives demonstrated a higher activity than did platelets from normotensives. However, there were no differences in Na^+/H^+ antiport activity between essential hypertensives and normotensives when their platelets were treated with a phorbol ester to maximally stimulate PKC. Livne et al. may be correct in assuming that in the resting state the higher Na^+/H^+ antiport activity in essential hypertension relates to an increased number of phosphorylated antiport units rather than a higher density of Na^+/H^+ antiport carriers. However, this conclusion is based on the yet unproven concept that a maximally stimulated PKC phosphorylates all the Na^+/H^+ antiport carriers on the platelet plasma membrane.

Increased Na^+/H^+ antiport activity has also been shown in leukocytes[50] and skeletal muscle[51] of essential hypertensives; the latter finding was inferred from the monitoring of pH_i in exercising muscle, using nuclear magnetic resonance spectroscopy. Additionally, cultured skin fibroblasts from blacks demonstrate higher Na^+/H^+ antiport activity than cells from whites,[52] complementing the findings of an alkaline shift in the Xi in platelets of this racial group. Collectively, these observations suggest that increased Na^+/H^+ antiport activity in essential hypertension and in individuals predisposed to this disease is present in several cell types and that it probably reflects a regulatory cellular process rather than an innate abnormality in the genetic makeup of this transporter. Such a concept is compatible with the findings of Lifton et al.[53] that the Na^+/H^+ antiport is an unlikely candidate gene for essential hypertension.

What then is the factor stimulating the Na^+/H^+ antiport in essential hypertension? The most likely culprit is Ca_i. In 1984 Erne et al.[54] reported that resting platelet Ca_i was positively correlated with blood pressure. Subsequent studies showed that Ca_i in resting platelets, stimulated platelets, or in both was higher in essential hypertensives than in normotensives.[55-59] Although it is clear that the mean value of platelet Ca_i is higher in essential hypertensives than in normotensives, a substantial scatter of the data is observed in most investigations. A recent study showed an age-dependent increase in resting platelet Ca_i in normotensives but not essential hypertensives.[59] Moreover, statistically significant differences in Ca_i were observed only between young essential hypertensives and normotensives. One explanation for increased Ca_i in platelets of essential hypertensives is a lower plasma membrane Ca^{2+}-ATPase activity.[60] An investigation using cultured skin fibroblasts from blacks and whites detected no racial difference in resting Ca_i.[61] However, when stimulated with human serum, fibroblasts from blacks demonstrated higher Ca_i levels than did cells from whites. This observation and the recent finding by Brickman et al.[57] that platelet Ca_i is higher in men than in women are in agreement with the higher Na^+/H^+ antiport activity in skin fibroblasts from blacks and the alkaline shift in the platelet Xi in males. Such gender- and race-related differences in the activity of the Na^+/H^+ antiport may reflect the relatively higher Ca_i levels in either fibroblasts or platelets from males and blacks than in females and whites, respectively.

It is well established that essential hypertension is marked by dyslipidemia.[62,63] Lipoproteins exert profound effects on cell function through their interactions with the plasma membrane. High levels of low-density lipoprotein (LDL) cholesterol and low levels of high-density lipoprotein (HDL) cholesterol are associated with platelet hyperactivity and increased cardiovascular risks, independent of essential hypertension.[65-68] Recent studies have demonstrated that LDL can raise the Ca_i in a variety of cells, including platelets,[67,68] and that HDL, particularly apolipoprotein E-rich HDL, can attenuate the agonist-evoked Ca_i response.[69] Such findings are compatible with the recent observation by Zentay et al.[48] that the Xi in platelets of a sample population of black females was inversely correlated with serum HDL and positively correlated with serum total cholesterol/HDL. Again, these findings point to a link between cellular Ca^{2+} homeostasis and the Na^+/H^+ antiport in that conditions which facilitate a rise in Ca_i are associated with an alkaline shift in the Xi.

The nexus between the Na^+/H^+ antiport and Ca_i regulation is central to the hypothesis that essential hypertension originates from primary abnormalities, leading to increased Ca_i and secondary cellular responses, including activation of the Na^+/H^+ antiport.[70] Implicit in this is the premise that peripheral vasoconstriction is mediated by the same mechanisms promoting the narrowing of the vascular lumen through medial hypertrophy and accelerated atherosclerosis. Both the vasoconstrictive and growth responses entail a rise in Ca_i and activation of the Na^+/H^+ antiport through PKC-dependent and PKC-independent pathways. Thus, genetic variations and environmental permutations raising the Ca_i in the vascular smooth muscle would under certain circumstances not only produce vasoconstriction, but also stimulate the growth of the vascular media and accelerate the development of atherosclerotic lesions. When such abnormalities are present in the renal tubular epithelium, they may promote augmented Na^+ reabsorption through a hyperactive Na^+/H^+ antiport and predispose to salt sensitivity. In platelets these abnormalities would underlie increased reactivity and a tendency to thromboembolic complications.

V. CONCLUSION

The polygenic nature of essential hypertension may thus originate from abnormalities of mechanisms that regulate Ca_i. A rise in Ca_i could result from variations intrinsic to the cellular processes that regulate Ca^{2+}, abnormalities in circulating factors or autacoids that modulate these processes, and intracellular signals relaying messages from receptors to specific intracellular target sites engaged in Ca_i regulation. What has emerged thus far from studies of the Na^+/H^+ antiport is that altered activity of this transport system in essential hypertension may represent the lasting imprint of elevated Ca_i and increased PKC activity.

REFERENCES

1. **Roos, A. and Boron, W. F.,** Intracellular pH, *Physiol. Rev.*, 61, 296, 1981.
2. **Vaughan-Jones, R. D. and Wu, M.-L.,** pH dependence of intrinsic H^+ buffering power in the sheep cardiac purkinje fiber, *J. Physiol.* 425, 429, 1990.
3. **Strazullo, P. and Canessa, M.,** Kinetics of human lymphocyte Na^+-H^+ exchanger, *Clin. Sci.*, 79, 531, 1990.
4. **Saleh, A. M. and Battle, D. A.,** Kinetic properties of the Na/H antiporter of lymphocytes from the spontaneously hypertensive rat: role of intracellular pH, *J. Clin. Invest.*, 85, 1734, 1990.
5. **Goldsmith, D. J. A. and Hilton, P. J.,** Relationship between intracellular proton buffering capacity and intracellular pH, *Kidney Int.*, 41, 43, 1992.
6. **Halligan, R. D., Shelat, H., and Kahn, A. M.,** Na^+-independent Cl^--HCO_3^- exchange in sarcolemmal vesicles from vascular smooth muscle, *Am. J. Physiol.*, 260(Cell Physiol. 29), C347, 1991.
7. **Vigne, P., Breittmayers, J.-P., Frelin, C., and Lazdunski, M.,** Dual control of the intracellular pH in aortic smooth muscle cells by a cAMP-sensitive HCO_3^-/Cl^- antiporter and a protein kinase C-sensitive Na^+/H^+ antiporter, *J. Biol. Chem.*, 263, 18023, 1988.
8. **Tonnessen, T. I., Sandvig, K., and Olsnes, S.,** Role of Na^+-H^+ and Cl^--HCO_3^- antiports in the regulation of cytosolic pH near neutrality, *Am. J. Physiol.*, 258(Cell Physiol. 27), C1117, 1990.
9. **Boyarsky, G., Ganz, M. B., Sterzel, R. B., and Boron, W. F.,** pH regulation in single glomerular mesangial cells. I. Acid extrusion in absence and presence of HCO_3^-, *Am. J. Physiol.*, 255(Cell Physiol. 24), C844, 1988.
10. **Boyarsky, G., Ganz, M. B., Sterzel, R. B., and Boron, W. F.,** pH regulation in single glomerular mesangial cells. II. Na^+-dependent and -independent Cl^--HCO_3^- exchangers, *Am. J. Physiol.*, 255(Cell Physiol. 24), C857, 1988.
11. **Mason, M. J., Smith, J. D., Garcia-Soto, J. D.-J., and Grinstein, S.,** Internal pH-sensitive site couples Cl^-/HCO_3^- exchange to Na^+-H^+ antiport in lymphocytes, *Am. J. Physiol.*, 256(Cell Physiol. 25), C428, 1989.
12. **Korbmacher, C., Helbig, H., Stahl, F., and Widerholt, M.,** Evidence for Na/H exchange and Cl/HCO_3^- exchange in vascular smooth muscle cells, *Pfluegers' Arch.*, 412, 29, 1988.
13. **Murer, H., Hopfer, U., and Kinne, R.,** Sodium/proton antiport in brush-border-membrane vesicles isolated from rat small intestine and kidney, *Biochem. J.*, 154, 597, 1976.
14. **Clark, J. D. and Limbird, L. E.,** Na^+-H^+ exchanger subtypes: a predictive review, *Am. J. Physiol.*, 261(Cell Physiol. 30), C945, 1991.
15. **Kapus, A., Ligeti, E., and Fonyo, A.,** Na^+/H^+ exchange in mitochondria as monitored by BCECF fluorescence, *FEBS Lett.*, 251, 49, 1989.
16. **Garlid, K. D., Shariat-Madar, Z., Nath, S., and Jezek, P.,** Reconstitution and partial purification of the Na^+-selective Na^+/H^+ antiporter of beef heart mitochondria, *J. Biol. Chem.*, 266, 6518, 1991.

17. **Brierley, G. P., Davis, M. H., and Jung, D. W.,** Intravesicular pH changes in submitochondrial particles induced by monovalent cations: relationship to the Na^+/H^+ and K^+/H^+ antiporters, *Arch. Biochem. Biophys.*, 264, 417, 1988.
18. **Mitchell, P. and Moyle, J.,** Respiration-driven proton translocation in rat liver mitochondria, *Biochem. J.*, 105, 1147, 1967.
19. **Mitchell, P. and Moyle, J.,** Translocation of some anions, cations and acids in rat liver mitochondria. *Eur. J. Biochem.* 9, 149, 1969.
20. **Sardet, C., Franchi, A., and Pouyssegur, L.,** Molecular cloning, primary structure, and expression of the human growth factor-activatable Na^+H^+ antiporter, *Cell,* 56, 271, 1989.
21. **Moolenaar, W. H., Tsien, R. Y., van der Saag, P. T., and de Laat, S. W.,** Na^+/H^+ exchange and cytoplasmic pH in the action of growth factors in human fibroblasts, *Nature,* 304, 645, 1983.
22. **Moolenaar, W. H., Tertoolen, L. G. J., and de Laat, S. W.,** Phorbol ester and diacylglycerol mimic growth factors in raising cytoplasmic pH, *Nature,* 312, 371, 1984.
23. **Ganz, M. B., Boyarsky, G., Sterzel, R. B., and Boron, W. F.,** Arginine vasopressin enhances pH_i regulation in the presence of HCO_3^- by stimulating three acid-base transport systems, *Nature,* 337, 648, 1989.
24. **Bierman, A. J., Cragoe, E. J., Jr., de Laat, S. W., and Moolenaar, W. H.,** Biocarbonate determines cytoplasmic pH and suppresses mitogen-induced alkalinization in fibroblastic cells, *J. Biol. Chem.*, 263, 15253, 1988.
25. **Thomas, R. C.,** Biocarbonate and pH_i response, *Nature,* 337, 601, 1989.
26. **Seifter, J. L. and Aronson, P. S.,** Properties and physiological roles of the plasma membrane sodium-hydrogen exchanger, *J. Clin. Invest.*, 78, 859, 1986.
27. **Hoffmann, E. K. and Simonsen, L. O.,** Membrane mechanisms in volume and pH regulation in vertebrate cells, *Physiol. Rev.*, 69, 315, 1989.
28. **Grinstein, S. and Rothstein, A.,** Mechanisms of regulation of the Na^+-H^+ exchanger, *J. Membr. Biol.*, 90, 1, 1986.
29. **Sardet, C., Counillon, L., Franchi, A., and Pouyssegur, L.,** Growth factors induce phosphorylation of the Na^+/H^+ antiporter, a glycoprotein of 110 kD, *Science,* 247, 723, 1990.
30. **Livne, A. A., Sardet, C., and Pouyssegur, J.,** The Na^+/H^+ exchanger is phosphorylated in human platelets in response to activating agents, *FEBS Lett.*, 284, 219, 1991.
31. **Hatori, N., Fine, B. P., Nakamura, A., Cragoe, E., Jr., and Aviv, A.,** Angiotensin II effect on cytosolic pH in cultured rat vascular smooth muscle cells, *J. Biol. Chem.*, 262, 5073, 1987.
32. **Little, P. J., Weissberg, P. L., Cragoe, E. J., Jr., and Bobik, A.,** Dependence of Na^+/H^+ antiport activation in cultured rat aortic smooth muscle on calmodulin, calcium, and ATP. Evidence for the involvement of calmodulin-dependent kinases, *J. Biol. Chem.*, 263, 16780, 1988.
33. **Kimura, M., Gardner, J. P., and Aviv, A.,** Agonist-evoked alkaline shift in the cytosolic pH set point for activation of Na^+/H^+ antiport in human platelets: the role of cytosolic Ca^{2+} and protein kinase C, *J. Biol. Chem.*, 265, 21068, 1990.
34. **Kimura, M., Lasker, N., and Aviv, A.,** Cyclic nucleotides attenuate thrombin-evoked alterations in parameters of platelet Na/H antiport: the role of cytosolic Ca, *J. Clin. Invest.*, in press.
35. **Kimura, M. and Aviv, A.,** Regulation of the cytosolic pH set point for activation of the Na^+-H^+ antiport in human platelets: the roles of the Na^+-Ca^{2+} exchange, the Na^+-K^+ cotransport and cellular volume, *Pfluegers' Arch.*, 422, 585, 1993.
36. **Felder, C. C., Campbell, T., Albrecht, F., and Jose, P. A.,** Dopamine inhibits Na^+-H^+ exchanger activity in renal BBMV by stimulation of adenylate cyclase, *Am. J. Physiol.*, 259(Renal Fluid Electrolyte Physiol. 28), F297, 1990.
37. **Reuss, L. and Petersen, K.-U.** Cyclic AMP inhibits Na^+/H^+ exchange at the apical membrane of necturus gallbladder epithelium, *J. Gen. Physiol.*, 85, 409, 1985.
38. **Semard, C. E. and Chang, E. B.,** Calcium-mediated cyclic AMP inhibition of Na-H exchange in small intestine, *Am. J. Physiol.*, 252(Cell Physiol. 21), C315, 1987.

39. **Weinman, E. J., Dubinsky, W. P., Steplock, D., Dinh, Q., and Shenolikar, S.,** Effect of limited trypsin digestion on the renal Na^+-H^+ exchanger and its regulation by cAMP-dependent protein kinase, *J. Membr. Biol.*, 109, 233, 1989.
40. **Carafoli, E.,** Intracellular calcium regulation, with special attention to the role of the plasma membrane calcium pump, *J. Cardiovasc. Pharmacol.*, 12(Suppl. 3), S77, 1985.
41. **Carafoli, E.,** Intracellular calcium homeostasis, *Annu. Rev. Biochem.*, 56, 395, 1987.
42. **Yonemura, K., Cheng, L., Sacktor, B., and Kinsella, J. L.,** Stimulation by thyroid hormone of Na^+-H^+ exchange activity in cultured opossum kidney cells, *Am. J. Physiol.*, 258(Renal Fluid Electrol. Physiol. 27), F333, 1990.
43. **Livne, A., Veitch, R., Grinstein, S., Balfe, J. W., Marquez-Julio, A., and Rothstein, A.,** Increased platelet Na^+/H^+ exchange rates in essential hypertension: application of a novel test, *Lancet*, 1, 533, 1987.
44. **Schmouder, R. L. and Weder, A. B.,** Platelet sodium-proton exchange is increased in essential hypertension, *J. Hypertension*, 7, 325, 1989.
45. **Roskopf, D., Morgenstern, E., Schloz, W., Osswald, U., and Siffert, W.,** Rapid determination of the elevated Na^+-H^+ exchange in platelets of patients with essential hypertension using an optical swelling assay, *J. Hypertension*, 9, 231, 1991.
46. **Weder, A. B., Schmouder, R. L., and Torretti, B. A.,** Platelet volume responses to cytoplasmic acidification in essential hypertension, *J. Hypertension*, 8, 1137, 1990.
47. **Tokudome, G., Tomonari, H., Gardner, J. P., Aladjem, M., Fine, B. P., Lasker, N., Gutkin, M., Byrd, L. H., and Aviv, A.,** Variations in the apparent pH set point for activation of platelet Na-H antiport, *Hypertension*, 16, 180, 1990.
48. **Zentay, Z., Reddi, A., Raguwanshi, M., Cho, J. H., Lasker, N., Dasmahapatra, A., and Aviv, A.,** Platelet Na/H antiport in obese and diabetic black women, *Hypertension*, 20, 549, 1992.
49. **Livne, A. A., Aharonovitz, O., and Paran, E.,** Higher Na^+-H^+ exchange rate and more alkaline intracellular pH set-point in essential hypertension: effects of protein kinase modulation in platelets, *J. Hypertension*, 9, 1013, 1991.
50. **Ng, L. L., Fennell, D. A., and Dudley, C.,** Kinetics of the human leucocyte Na^+-H^+ antiport in essential hypertension, *J. Hypertension*, 8, 533, 1990.
51. **Duddley, C. R. K., Taylor, D. J., Ng, L. L., Kemp, G. J., Ratcliffe, P. J., Radda, G. K., and Ledingham, J. G. G.,** Evidence for abnormal Na^+/H^+ antiport activity detected by phosphorus nuclear magnetic resonance spectroscopy in exercising skeletal muscle of patients with essential hypertension, *Clin. Sci.*, 79, 491, 1990.
52. **Hatori, N., Gardner, J. P., Tomonari, H., Fine, B. P., and Aviv, A.,** Differences in Na^+-H^+ antiport activity in skin fibroblasts from blacks and whites, *Hypertension*, 15, 140, 1990.
53. **Lifton, R. P., Hunt, S. C., Williams, R. R., Pouyssegur, J., and Lalouel, J.-M.,** Exclusion of the Na^+/H^+ antiporter as a candidate gene in human essential hypertension, *Hypertension*, 17, 8, 1991.
54. **Erne, P., Bolli, P., Burgisser, E., and Buhler, F. R.,** Correlation of platelet calcium with blood pressure: effect of antihypertensive therapy, *N. Engl. J. Med.*, 310, p. 1984, 1984.
55. **Lindner, A., Kenny, M., and Meacham, A. J.,** Effects of a circulating factor in patients with essential hypertension on intracellular free calcium in normal platelets, *N. Engl. J. Med.*, 316, 509, 1987.
56. **Brickman, A. S., Nyby, M. D., Von Hungen, K., Eggena, P., and Tuck, M. L.,** Calcitropic hormones, platelet calcium, and blood pressure in essential hypertension, *Hypertension*, 16, 515, 1990.
57. **Brickman, A., Nyby, M., Von Hungen, K., Eggena, P., and Tuck, M.,** Parathyroid hormone, platelet calcium, and blood pressure in normotensive subjects, *Hypertension*, 18, 176, 1991.
58. **Cooper, R. S., Shamsi, N., and Katz, S.,** Intracellular calcium and sodium in hypertensive patients, *Hypertension*, 9, 224, 1987.

59. **Duggan, J., Kilfeather, S., Sheridan, J., O'Brien, E., and O'Malley, K.,** The effects of age on platelet intracellular free calcium concentration in normotensives and hypertensives, *J. Hypertension,* 9, 845, 1991.
60. **Takaya, J., Lasker, N., Bamforth, R., Gutkin, M., Byrd, L. H., and Aviv, A.,** Kinetics of Ca^{2+}-ATPase activation in platelet membranes of essential hypertensives and normotensives, *Am. J. Physiol.,* 258(Cell Physiol. 27), C988, 1990.
61. **Nakamura, A., Gardner, J., Hatori, N., Nakamura, M., Fine, B. P., and Aviv, A.,** Differences of Ca^{2+} regulation in skin fibroblasts from blacks and whites, *J. Cell Physiol.,* 138, 367, 1989.
62. **Buhler, F. R., Tkachuk, V. A., Hahn, A. W. A., and Resink, T. J.,** Low- and high-density lipoproteins as hormonal regulators of platelet, vascular endothelial and smooth muscle cell interactions: relevance to hypertension, *J. Hypertension,* 9(Suppl. 6), S28, 1991.
63. **Reaven, G. M.,** Insulin resistance and compensatory hyperinsulinemia: role in hypertension, dyslipidemia, and coronary heart disease, *Am. Heart J.,* 121, 1283, 1991.
64. **Carvalho, A. C. A., Colman, R. W., and Lees, R. S.,** Platelet function in hyperlipoproteinemia, *N. Engl. J. Med.,* 290, 434, 1974.
65. **Aviram, M. and Brook, G.,** Platelet activation by plasma lipoproteins, *Prog. Cardiovasc. Dis.,* 30, 61, 1987.
66. **Andrews, H. E., Aitken, J. W., Hassall, D. G., Skinner, V. O., and Bruckdorfer, K. R.,** Intracellular mechanisms in the activation of human platelets by low-density lipoproteins, *Biochem. J.,* 242, 559, 1987.
67. **Block, L. H., Norr, M., Vogt, E., Locher, R., Vetter, W., Groscurth, P., Qiao, B.-Y., Pometta, D., James, R., Regenass, M., and Pletscher, A.,** Low density lipoprotein causes general cellular activation with increased phosphatidylinositol turnover and lipoprotein catabolism, *Proc. Natl. Acad. Sci. U.S.A.,* 85, 885, 1988.
68. **Norr, M., Locher, R., Vogt, E., Vetter, W., Black, L. H., Ferracin, F., Lefkovitz, H., and Pletscher, A.,** Rapid activation of human platelets by low concentrations of low-density lipoprotein via phosphatidylinositol cycle, *Eur. J. Biochem.,* 172, 753, 1988.
69. **Higashihara, M., Kinoshita, M., Tamio, T., Kume, S., and Kurokawa, K.,** The role of apo E in inhibitory effects of apoE-rich HDL on platelet function, *FEBS Lett.,* 282, 82, 1991.
70. **Aviv, A.,** Prospective review: the link between cytosolic Ca^{2+} and the Na^+-H^+ antiport: a unifying factor for essential hypertension, *J. Hypertension,* 6, 685, 1988.

Chapter 7

THE Cl^-/HCO_3^- ANION EXCHANGER IN HYPERTENSION

Javier Díez and Arantxa Arrázola

TABLE OF CONTENTS

I. Introduction 134

II. The Anion Exchanger: Basic Aspects 134
- A. The Regulation of pH_i 134
- B. Structure and Membrane Distribution 135
  - 1. Structure of the Band 3 Protein 135
    - a. Cytoplasmic Domain 136
    - b. Membrane Domain 136
    - c. Oligomeric Structure 137
  - 2. Molecular Biology of the Band 3-Related Anion Exchangers (AE) 137
- C. Transport Activity 138
  - 1. Characteristics of Band 3 Transport 138
    - a. Substrate Specificity 139
    - b. Ping-Pong Kinetics 139
    - c. Self-Inhibition 139
    - d. Proton Interactions 139
    - e. Cation Transport by Band 3 140
    - f. Inhibitors of Band 3 140
  - 2. Anion Exchanger Activity in Nonerythroid Cells 141
- D. Regulation 142

III. Potential Role of the Anion Exchanger in the Regulation of Blood Pressure 143
- A. Potential Role of Cl^-/HCO_3^- Exchange in Regulating Renal Na^+ Reabsorption 143
- B. Potential Role of Cl^-/HCO_3^- Exchange in Regulating Vascular Tone 144
- C. Potential Role of Cl^-/HCO_3^- Exchange in Regulating Growth of Vascular Smooth Muscle Cells 145

IV. Abnormalities of the Anion Exchanger in Hypertension 146
- A. Studies in Animals 146
- B. Studies in Humans 146

0-8493-5474-9/94/$0.00 + $.50

V. Conclusions 148

References 149

I. INTRODUCTION

The crucial role of bicarbonate (HCO_3^-) in pH homeostasis in the intact animal has long been recognized. Inside cells, it is often the most common anion, and outside is the second most common after chloride (Cl^-). In practice, HCO_3^--buffered solutions are difficult to handle for several reasons (usually, the difficulty is to maintain constant pCO_2). On the other hand, when it was discovered that cultured mammalian cells could regulate their intracellular pH (pH_i) perfectly well with an amiloride-sensitive sodium-proton (Na^+/H^+) exchanger, it was widely assumed that HCO_3^- would make no real difference in homeostasis. Thus, the lack of HCO_3^- in the original experiments would have exaggerated any pH_i change due to variations in the Na^+/H^+ exchanger.[1]

This was the case for studies that examined the interrelation between the Na^+/H^+ exchanger and pH_i in cells from either animals or humans with hypertension. Most studies have routinely used nominally HCO_3^--free buffers. Although this simplifies the analysis of the Na^+/H^+ exchanger, it also eliminates any influence the buffers may have in regulating cell pH.

Therefore, this chapter reviews the characteristics of several HCO_3^- transport processes that have been identified in various cell systems. In addition, the potential role of the Cl^-/HCO_3^- anion exchanger (AE) in regulating blood pressure is also considered. Finally, the history of the abnormalities of this transport system in hypertension is examined.

II. THE ANION EXCHANGER: BASIC ASPECTS

A. THE REGULATION OF pH_i

The distribution of H^+ ions across the plasma membrane of most cells is such that pH_i is much higher than that predicted if H^+ were passively distributed.[2] Therefore, all cells have mechanisms for H^+ extrusion that maintain pH_i at a value which is well above equilibrium and is compatible with the necessities of cytoplasmic reactions.

The regulation of pH_i in eukaryotic cells has received much attention recently. The main reason is that changes in pH_i have been thought to be related to the action of hormones and growth factors.[3] The role of the Na^+/H^+ antiporter in transducing

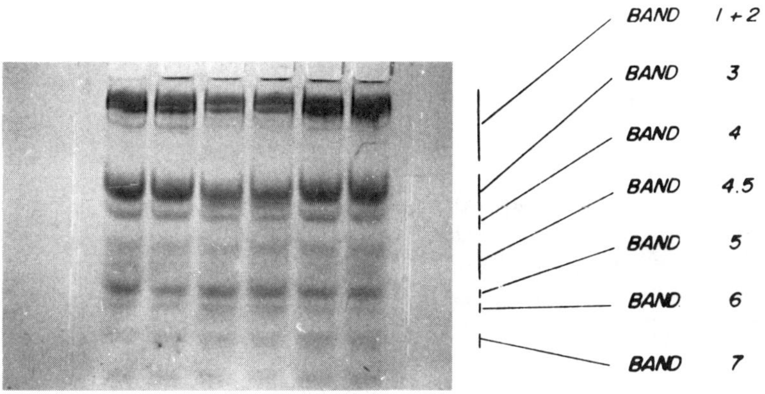

FIGURE 1. Separation of erythrocyte membrane proteins by sodium dodecyl sulfate-polyacrylamide gel electrophoresis.

hormonal messages into a pH_i signal is widely recognized.[4] Recent studies indicate, however, that the Na^+/H^+ antiporter is not the only system for pH_i regulation in eukaryotic cells and that it coexists in the plasma membrane with one or several bicarbonate transport systems. Three such systems have been identified in vertebrate cells: an Na^+-dependent Cl^-/HCO_3^- antiporter,[5-9] an Na^+-independent Cl^-/HCO_3^- antiporter [9-11] (both systems being electroneutral), and an electrogenic Na^+/HCO_3^- symporter.[7,12,13] Although bicarbonate-dependent mechanisms of pH_i regulation are still poorly understood, they seem to be of great physiological significance. Bicarbonate modifies the steady-state pH_i value in most cells and HCO_3^- transporters appear to be the principal determinants of resting pH_i in many cells in which the Na^+/H^+ antiporter is inactive at resting pH_i.[14,15]

B. STRUCTURE AND MEMBRANE DISTRIBUTION

Plasma membrane anion exchange is a nearly ubiquitous function in vertebrate cells. Anion exchange has been studied in greatest detail in the erythrocyte. Its dominant form there is the Cl^-/HCO_3^- exchange, which is mediated by the most abundant integral protein in the plasma membrane, band 3. The erythrocyte anion exchanger, band 3, is one of the most thoroughly studied plasma membrane proteins. This protein is present at $\simeq 1.2 \times 10^6$ copies per cell in mammalian erythrocytes[16] and constitutes about 25 to 30% of the total membrane protein[17] (Figure 1).

1. Structure of the Band 3 Protein

Band 3 is a transmembrane protein with a molecular weight of approximately 95 kDa.[16] This protein consists of two structurally distinct domains. Exposure of the cytoplasmic side of the red cell membranes to proteolytic enzymes under very mild conditions causes the cleavage of band 3 at a site that is located about 43 kDa from the N terminus.[18] The resultant N-terminal fragment represents a water-soluble cytoplasmic domain. The remainder of the protein, the membrane domain, has a molecular weight of 52 kDa and is hydrophobically associated with the lipid bilayer.[18,19]

a. Cytoplasmic Domain

The 43-kDa N-terminal domain is disposed to the cytoplasm, where it interacts with several cytosolic and cytoskeletal proteins.[20] Most prominent among these interactions is the association with ankyrin,[21] which forms the link between the mesh-like spectrin-actin cytoskeleton and the plasma membrane. In addition to containing the attachment site for ankyrin, the cytoplasmic domain of band 3 interacts directly with another component of the membrane skeleton, band 4.1.[23]

The cytoplasmic domain of band 3 also contains binding sites for several glycolytic enzymes and hemoglobin, and is a substrate for endogenous and exogenous tyrosine kinases.[20] This domain may play a role in red blood cell (RBC) senescence.[24,25] The binding of the N-terminal domain of human band 3 to denatured hemoglobin leads to clustering of the protein.[25] Such band 3 clusters are thought to be recognized by circulating autoantibodies, serving as a signal for the elimination of senescent erythrocytes from the bloodstream.

Lepke and Passow[26] showed that trypsin sealed inside red cell ghosts does not prevent stilbene-disulfonate-sensitive anion transport. Under the condition of these experiments, the cytoplasmic domain is proteolytically degraded. Grinstein et al.[27] subsequently demonstrated that mild proteolysis of inside-out vesicles (IOV) does not inhibit anion transport under conditions in which the cytoplasmic domain is completely removed from the membrane. Taken together, these studies are strong evidence that the cytoplasmic domain is not absolutely necessary for anion exchange. It is premature, however, to conclude that the cytoplasmic domain has absolutely no influence on anion transport, because subtle interactions between the two domains may exist which were not revealed in the above studies. A preliminary report by García et al.[28] indicates that the whole band 3 gene product induces a higher Cl^- flux in frog oocytes than does the polypeptide coded by the DNA sequence for the membrane domain alone.

b. Membrane Domain

The C-terminal 60% of band 3 is tightly, hydrophobically associated with the membrane. This membrane domain is heterogeneously glycosylated,[29] and its molecular weight is about 52 kDa. In general terms, it is probable that the membrane domain of band 3 resembles one structure in which there are several membrane-crossing α-helical segments connected by short, hydrophilic stretches. Several pieces of evidence support this assumption. The hydropathic profile of murine band 3 shows that the membrane domain is arranged in long stretches of hydrophobic residues interspersed with hydrophilic residues. All of these hydrophobic stretches are long enough to traverse the bilayer.[30] In addition, circular dichroism analysis suggests that ~90% of the membrane-associated portion of human band 3 is indeed α-helical.[31]

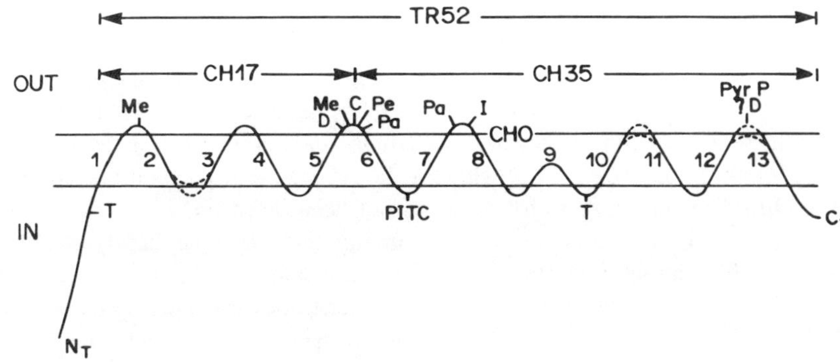

FIGURE 2. A model for the proposed transmembrane orientation of band 3. N_T: N-terminus, T, intracellular tryptic site; Me, exofacial lysine methylation; D, extracellular H_2-DIDS binding site; C, extracellular chymotryptic site; Pe, pepsin site; Pa, papain site; PITC, phenylisothiocyanate site; I, exofacial radioiodination site; CHO, proposed site for attachment of N-linked oligosaccharide; PyrP, pyridoxal phosphate site; C_T, C-terminus.

A model for the transmembrane orientation of the putative membrane-spanning region of band 3 is shown in Figure 2.[32,33] The model is based on the hydropathy profile and on proteolytic cleavage and labeling experiments which selectively modify the inside or outside of the erythrocyte membrane. Additional evidence for the model comes from the genomic structure of band 3.[30]

The membrane domain of band 3 is essential for catalyzing the 1:1, electroneutral, and reversible exchange of chloride and bicarbonate across the erythrocyte plasma membrane.[17] This domain contains the anion channel and many anion transport inhibitor binding sites: H_2-4,4′-diisothiocyanatostilbene-2,2′-disulfonic acid (H_2-DIDS), phenylisothiocyanato, phenylglyoxal, etc.[17,32]

c. *Oligomeric Structure*

Chemical crosslinking, ultracentrifugation, and a variety of spectroscopic data all indicate that band 3 is not monomeric in the native membrane.[17,34] The evidence is consistent with the idea that the protein is tetrameric, but that the tetrameter is a dimer of dimers, rather than a tetramer with fourfold rotational symmetry. Apparently, subunit interaction takes place in both the membrane and cytoplasmic domains. Although the protein is oligomeric, no evidence exists that the catalytic mechanism of transport requires concerted interactions between subunits.[35]

2. Molecular Biology of the Band 3-Related Anion Exchangers (AE)

Kopito and Lodish[30] published the cDNA sequence and deduced the amino acid sequence of AE1 (band 3) from murine anemic spleen in 1985. Since then, the postulated AE gene family[33] has taken form with two more genes. Following the isolation of the first partial AE1 cDNA clone by antibody screening, all ensuing cDNAs have been isolated by hybridization screening at high or reduced stringency.

AE1 cDNA has been cloned from mouse,[30] chicken,[36,37] human,[32,38] and rat.[39] The encoded AE1 proteins range from 848 to 929 amino acids in length. AE2 has been cloned from mouse,[40] rat,[41,42] human,[43] and rabbit.[44] The encoded AE2 proteins are 1237 and 1234 amino acids in length. AE3 cDNAs have been cloned from mouse[45] and rat[41] and encode polypeptides of 1227 amino acids in length. The human AE1 gene resides on chromosome 17,[46] whereas the AE2 gene resides on chromosome 7.[47] The chromosomal location for AE3 has not been determined.

Comparison of the sequence identity among the AE gene family members indicates that both structural domains of band 3 are conserved between individuals isoforms. Homology is highest within the membrane domains, ranging between 80 and 98%, and lowest among the cytoplasmic domains, ranging between 59 and 84%.[48] Such a high degree of sequence identity among the AE family members predicts that the proteins have similar biological activities. Recent studies in which AE2[42] and AE3[45] have been expressed in mammalian cells confirm these predictions, demonstrating that these gene products, like band 3, catalyze the electroneutral, sodium-independent Cl^-/HCO_3^- exchange. The N-terminal cytoplasmic domains of the AE proteins are not needed to mediate this exchange.[49]

The pharmacological characterization of AE2 and AE3 is just beginning. Both AE2 and AE3 are several orders of magnitude more resistant to inhibition by sulfonate stilbenes than is AE1 in the erythrocyte.[42,45] The array of other inhibitors with a range of kinetic mechanism already attempted against AE1[17] largely remains untested against AE2 and AE3 in heterologous expression systems.

Though AE mRNAs can be found in most tissues and cells, detection of the corresponding polypeptides has proven considerably more difficult. AE1 protein expression has been detected with many antibodies on the basolateral plasma membrane of the acid-secreting intercalated cells of the kidney.[50,51] AE2 protein has been convincingly localized to the choroid plexus,[42,52] the gastric parietal cell,[53] and the osteoclast.[49] AE2 protein probably mediates Na^+-independent Cl^-/HCO_3^- exchange in most cultured renal cells of tubular origin,[40,49] and perhaps in the mesangial cells as well.[49] AE3 is expressed in excitable tissues, including neurons and muscle.[48,49]

In summary, the last five years have seen the characterization of three members of the AE gene family. However, the majority of AEs in the kidney and in other epithelial and nonepithelial cells has eluded structural definition. Some of these Cl^-/base antiporters are likely new AE gene products.[49] It is possible that the different bicarbonate transport systems are all members of the same family of proteins similar to band 3 glycoprotein. In the meantime, AE sequence information and first-generation AE expression systems promise to accelerate investigation of the mechanism and regulation of Cl^-/HCO_3^- exchange and its multiple roles in cell function.[49]

C. TRANSPORT ACTIVITY

1. Characteristics of Band 3 Transport

The main function of band 3 in the RBC is to enhance the ability of the blood to carry CO_2, mediating the rapid exchange of extracellular Cl^- and intracellular

HCO_3^- ions during the RBCs' passage through the capillaries of the tissue, and the reverse exchange during their transit through the alveolar capillaries.[35,54] The kinetics of this band 3-catalyzed anion exchange has been extensively studied.

a. Substrate Specificity

In addition to Cl^- and HCO_3^-, many other anions (e.g., Br^-, SO_4^{2-}, PO_4^{2-}) are transported by way of band 3.[55-59] The rates of transport of these anions vary over a $>10^4$-fold range,[56] with Cl^- and HCO_3^- transported most rapidly. This selectivity is caused mainly by variations in the translocation rates of the anions rather than variations in the affinity of binding to transport sites. The affinity of band 3 for the different anions is nearly the same,[60-62] but the anion translocation rate is very dependent on the chemical nature of the specific anion bound to the site.[54]

b. Ping-Pong Kinetics

There is now a great deal of evidence that obligate anion exchange catalyzed by the band 3 protein proceeds by a mechanism with a single binding site, accurately described by a ping-pong kinetic scheme (Figure 3).[63,64] This mechanism involves only a single binding/transport site that has alternating access to the ions inside and outside the cell. Such a mechanism would require that the crucial transporting conformational change takes place only if an anion is bound to the transport site.[63]

c. Self-Inhibition

At Cl^- concentration up to physiological levels, anion exchange can be described by a simple ping-pong kinetic carrier scheme involving one anion binding site, but there are deviations from the Michaelis-Menten activation curve at elevated concentrations; i.e., above a certain concentration exchange flux decreases with further increasing concentration.[55,56] This phenomenon is referred to as self-inhibition. It also affects the other anions Br^-, I^-, and HCO_3^-. Dalmark[55] ascribed this phenomenon to the effect of a second, noncompetitive inhibitory anion binding site, which he referred to as a ''modifier site.''

What is the role of the modifier site in the anion transport mechanism? As discussed by Knauf[56] and Wieth and Bjerrum,[65] a close proximity between transport and modifier sites could mean that the real purpose of the modifier site is to guide the anion to its transport site.

d. Proton Interactions

Jennings[66] first showed (1976) that protons were cotransported with sulfate by measuring sulfate flux and sulfate-activated net proton transport. More recently, these studies have been expanded to measure Cl^--H^+, NO_3^--H^+, Br^--H^+ cotransport in RBC.[54,67] These experiments show that the anion-stimulated net proton fluxes are inhibited by 4,4′-dinitrostilbene-2,2′-disulfonate (DNDS), a reversible stilbene derivative. These anion-proton fluxes are small but may be an important component of net proton flux when an increased intracellular pCO_2 leads to increased internal

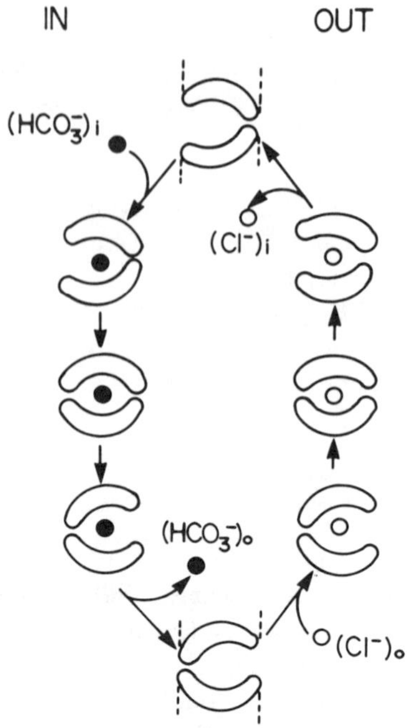

FIGURE 3. Ping-pong kinetics of band 3 Cl^-/HCO_3^- exchange.[138] The HCO_3^- and Cl^- cross the membrane in separate steps, in each case proceeding through a transition state in which the anion is probably occluded, i.e., not accessible from either side of the membrane.

H^+ and HCO_3^- concentrations, and Cl^-/HCO_3^- exchange is obligated to equilibrate HCO_3^- and Cl^- at the expense of enhancing the proton gradient.[54]

e. Cation Transport by Band 3

In physiological HCO_3^- solutions, Na^+ and Li^+ can form ion pairs $NaCO_3^-$ and $LiCO_3^-$. These anionic ion pairs are also transported by band 3.[68,69] Their transport is inhibited by stilbenes and other transported anions. Although $NaCO_3^-$ and $LICO_3^-$ are present in low concentration, their transport is not trivial because the alternative pathways for Na^+ and Li^+ have even lower turnover rates. It is estimated that in plasma $NaCO_3^-$ influx constitutes ~25 to 30% of the passive Na^+ influx.[54]

f. Inhibitors of Band 3

Most organic anions are inhibitors of band 3. Several major drugs of possible clinical important are salicylates,[70] furosemide,[71] bumetanide,[72] thiazides,[73] xipamide,[74] local anesthetics,[75] etc. For experimental use, the stilbenes, NAD-taurine, and phloretin have been the most valuable tools.[54]

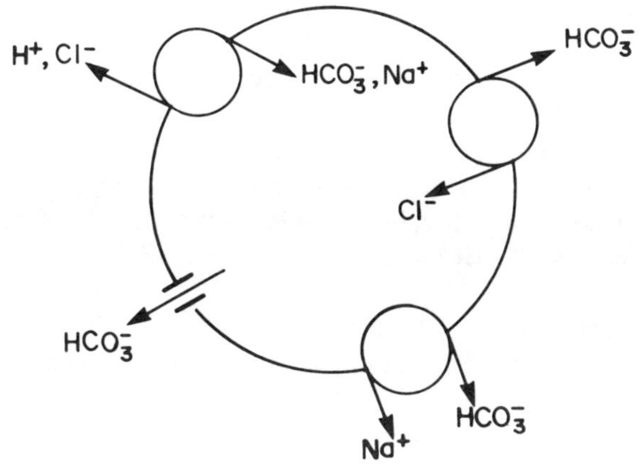

FIGURE 4. Cellular HCO_3^- transport mechanisms.

2. Anion Exchanger Activity in Nonerythroid Cells

Several major questions remain unanswered about the relationship between red cell band 3 and anion transport in general:[35] How many kinds of Cl^-/HCO_3^- exchangers are there? What are the similarities between Cl^-/HCO_3^- exchangers and other anion transport proteins? The state of understanding of these issues is yet primitive.[35]

In nonerythroid cells, Cl^-/HCO_3^- exchangers function in concert with other transport systems to regulate cell pH, cell volume, and cell Cl^-.[49] Under the conditions that prevail in most nonerythroid cells, an Na^+-independent Cl^-/HCO_3^- exchanger would act as an alkali-extruding system because the inward Cl^- gradient exceeds the inward HCO_3^- gradient[35] (Figure 4). Thus, this exchanger would be expected to be protective of cells from an alkali load.[10,11] Also functioning as acid loaders are the HCO_3^- channel and, membrane potential permitting, the electrogenic, stilbenedisulfonate-sensitive, Na^+,HCO_3^- cotransporter.[7,12,13] Countering the acid loaders are the acid extruders. One of them is another stilbenedisulfonate-inhibitable transport process: the Na^+-dependent $Cl^-HCO_3^-$ exchanger.[5-9] The function of this exchanger is to extrude acid from the cytoplasm and thereby help regulate intracellular pH, which in the steady state is known to be more alkaline than would be expected on the basis of Donnan equilibrium.[2] The protein responsible for this transport has not been identified.[35]

Renal and other epithelial cells exploit Cl^-/HCO_3^- exchange activities to regulate extracellular compartmental and systemic pH, concentration of Cl^-, and volume. They do so by restricting the expression of Cl^-/HCO_3^- exchangers to either the basolateral or the apical plasma membrane.[49] For example, good electrophysiological and kinetic evidence exists that the mammalian renal collecting duct[76] contains acid-secreting cells that have a proton pump in the apical membrane and a stilbenedisulfonate-sensitive Na^+-independent Cl^-/HCO_3^- exchanger in the basolateral membrane to redress the alkaline load imposed on the cell by the proton pump. Good evidence also exists that the basolateral membranes of gastric acid-secreting cells contain a stilbenedisulfonate-sensitive Na^+-independent Cl^-/HCO_3^- exchanger.[77]

The Cl^-/HCO_3^- exchange also plays an important role in the maintenance of intracellular Cl^- concentration above its electrochemical equilibrium concentration in many cells.[78] In addition, cell volume regulation is yet another function mediated in certain cell types by Cl^-/HCO_3^- exchange.[79]

D. REGULATION

The HCO_3^- transporters appear to be the principal determinants of resting pH_i in many cells in which the Na^+/H^+ antiporter is inactive at resting pH_i.[14,15] The acid-loading Cl^-/HCO_3^- exchangers are activated by elevated pH_i and inactivated by lowered pH_i. Each cell type displays a characteristic profile of maximal activity, hormone responsiveness, and pH_i set points at which activity is half maximal.[14,15,80,81] The pH_i set point is the major locus of rapid regulation by hormones.

Despite considerable knowledge of the ligand-activated regulation of Na^+/H^+ antiport in many cell types, there is yet little information on the action of various ligands on the regulation of the activity of the two Cl^-/HCO_3^- antiports.[82]

A large number of reports has appeared describing the stimulation of the Na^+/H^+ antiport and a rise in pH_i by serum, epidermal growth factor (EGF), platelet-derived growth factor (PDGF), vasopressin, and a number of other physiological ligands (for review, see References 3 and 83). Most of these studies were carried out in the absence of bicarbonate; however, bicarbonate-dependent processes play important roles in the regulation of cytosolic pH[2,15] and may profoundly influence the pH_i response to growth factors.[14,80] Therefore, recently, several growth factor effects on the Cl^-/HCO_3^- exchangers have been studied. In Vero cells, it has been reported that phorbol-12-myristate-13-acetate (TPA) strongly stimulates the activity of the Na^+-independent Cl^-/HCO_3^- exchange.[82] Serum has been reported to strongly activate Na^+-independent Cl^-/HCO_3^- exchange, while inhibiting Na^+-dependent Cl^-/HCO_3^- exchange. Both effects appear to be mediated by protein kinase C (PKC).[82] In addition, in mesangial cells, a single hormone, arginine-vasopressin (AVP), has been shown to activate in parallel Na^+/H^+ exchange, Na^+-dependent Cl^-/HCO_3^- exchange, and Na^+-independent Cl^-/HCO_3^- exchange.[80] The overall pattern is that of hormonal activation of multiple pH_i regulatory systems, acid loading, and base loading, so that the principal response(s) to the hormone can proceed with minimal perturbation of pH_i.[80]

The same ligand may have different effects in different cells. Thus, whereas cyclic adenosine monophosphate (cAMP) stimulates Na^+-independent Cl^-/HCO_3^- in renal cells,[84,85] an inhibition of this transporter has been shown in smooth muscle cells.[86]

Finally, in an osteoblast cell line, extracellular Ca^{2+} entry can also activate N^+-independent Cl^-/HCO_3^- exchange.[87]

III. POTENTIAL ROLE OF THE ANION EXCHANGER IN THE REGULATION OF BLOOD PRESSURE

A. POTENTIAL ROLE OF Cl^-/HCO_3^- EXCHANGE IN REGULATING RENAL Na^+ REABSORPTION

The present understanding of renal acidification is that the proximal tubule and loop of Henle utilize Na^+-coupled processes on both the apical and basolateral membranes, whereas the collecting tubule utilizes Na^+-independent transport mechanisms.[88] The net effect is that HCO_3^- absorption in the proximal, but not in the collecting tubule, is associated with Na^+ absorption.

Stilbene-sensitive transport of Cl^- in exchange for Na^+ and HCO_3^- is present in the basolateral cell membrane of the proximal tubule.[89] However, Na^+,HCO_3^- cotransporters, which coexist with Na^+-dependent Cl^-/HCO_3^- exchangers in the basolateral membrane of the proximal tubule,[90] also operate to remove Na^+ and HCO_3^- from the cell. Using the pH-sensitive dye, 2′,7′-bis(2-carboxyethyl)-5(6)-carboxyfluorescein (BCECF), Preisig and Alpern[91] have estimated that about 25% of HCO_3^- movement across the basolateral cell membrane of the rat proximal convoluted tubule is Cl^- dependent and 75% remains in the absence of Cl^-.

Friedman and Andreoli[92] reported that CO_2 stimulates NaCl reabsorption in the thick ascending limb of Henle's loop. These authors interpreted their results as the coupling of an amiloride-sensitive Na^+/H^+ exchange with a Cl^-/HCO_3^- exchange in apical plasma membranes. However, an alternative mechanism could be that Na^+ is reabsorbed through an Na^+-dependent Cl^-/HCO_3^- exchanger. On the other hand, a basolateral Na^+,HCO_3^- cotransport has been found in the rat cortical thick ascending limb,[93] and a role for this symporter in transepithelial Na^+ absorption in this segment has been suggested.[88]

In the collecting tubule, Na^+ absorption and H^+ secretion occur in separate cells. In the absence of an Na^+ entrance pathway on the apical membrane of H^+-secreting cells, it would be difficult for sufficient Na^+ to be available for the basolateral membrane HCO_3^- efflux transport mechanisms to be either Na^+-dependent or Na^+ coupled.[88]

From the above considerations we can infer that changes in the activity of the Na^+-dependent Cl^-/HCO_3^- exchanger localized in the proximal nephron could be associated to variations of Na^+ reabsorption. In this regard, it is tempting to speculate that primary hyperactivity of this AE is involved in renal Na^+ hyperreabsorption, which characterizes salt-sensitive forms of essential hypertension.[94] Accordingly, an increased capacity of the proximal tubule to reabsorb HCO_3^- has been described in chronic metabolic acidosis,[95] a condition present in patients with salt-sensitive hypertension.[96] An alternative hypothesis could be that changes in glomerular hemodynamics associated with the hypertensive process induce an adaptive increase in proximal Na^+ (and HCO_3^-) reabsorption. Interestingly, increased proximal HCO_3^- reabsorption has been reported in conditions such as glomerular hyperfiltration,[97] which is also present in essential hypertension.[98]

B. POTENTIAL ROLE OF Cl^-/HCO_3^- EXCHANGE IN REGULATING VASCULAR TONE

Although the relationship between pCO_2, pH_i, extracellular pH, and bicarbonate and vascular smooth muscle tone is still incompletely understood, the effect of these factors on a number of steps involved in the control of vascular tone has been confirmed. More specifically, it is actually accepted that several steps in smooth muscle excitation-contraction coupling are affected by pH.[99]

The importance of bicarbonate in the regulation of smooth muscle pH_i has been emphasized by Aickin[100] and Aickin and Brading,[101] based on work in the guinea pig vas deferens. More recently, a Cl^-/HCO_3^- exchange was demonstrated in rat aortic strips,[102,103] although the role in pH_i regulation was not defined. In resistance vessels, it was recently demonstrated that Na^+-dependent HCO_3^- transport[104] operates in parallel with the Na^+/H^+ exchange. The role of chloride in this transport is still undefined. In two vascular smooth muscle cell lines (A10 and A7r5) evidence has been provided for Cl^-/HCO_3^- exchange,[86,105] although these cells did not show any Na^+-dependent HCO_3^- transport. Furthermore, although Vigne et al.[86] suggested that this exchange acts as a cell-acidifying mechanism, Korbmacher et al.[105] commented that this exchange may not be pivotal for pH_i recovery from an alkaline load, and the mechanisms responsible for the recovery from an alkaline load remain largely undefined.

In the resistance vessels, Na^+-dependent HCO_3^- transport and the Na^+/H^+ exchange operate in parallel to extrude an acid load. However, the bicarbonate transport sets steady-state pH_i slightly above the detection level for any activity of the Na^+/H^+ exchange.[104] Although this suggests that bicarbonate transport plays an important role in pH_i regulation in resistance arteries, the importance of bicarbonate transport is particularly apparent during force development. In the absence of bicarbonate a fall in steady-state pH_i (0.1 to 0.2 pH units) is seen during activation with noradrenaline, suggesting that during a contraction the Na^+/H^+ exchange cannot maintain resting pH_i alone, while in the presence of bicarbonate, pH_i can be maintained at resting levels.[104,106] The vasopressin-induced contraction is also associated with a small fall in pH_i when bicarbonate transport is inhibited by omission of bicarbonate or by addition of DIDS, while in the presence of amiloride (inhibitor of Na^+/H^+ exchange) vasopressin does not cause a fall in pH_i.[107] Further, from the work with A7r3 cells it was concluded that the bicarbonate-dependent pH_i regulation dominates the Na^+/H^+ exchange-mediated pH_i regulation.[86]

If Cl^-/HCO_3^- exchange limits the rise in smooth muscle cell pH after activation of the Na^+/H^+ exchange, then a defect in regulation that leads to a decrease in Cl^-/HCO_3^- activity would allow vascular smooth muscle cell pH to rise and result in vasoconstriction. This is supported by the observation that AE inhibitors enhance contractility of vascular smooth muscle.[108] In this regard note that Cl^-/HCO_3^- exchange in vascular smooth muscle cells may be regulated by cAMP; increasing intracellular cAMP levels with β-receptor agonists inhibits Cl^-/HCO_3^- exchange.[86]

In addition to the possible relation between vascular smooth muscle cell pH and hypertension, various models have been proposed, implicating an increased rate of Na^+ influx into the cell as a cause of essential hypertension. It also has been suggested that an increase in Na^+ influx in vascular smooth muscle cells from increased rates of Na^+/H^+ exchange could raise cell Ca^{2+} levels via the Na^+/Ca^{2+} exchange.[109] The increase in cell Ca^{2+} would in turn lead to an increase in vascular tone.[110] If Cl^-/HCO_3^- exchange protects against elevated pH_i, then Na^+/H^+ exchange would not be subjected to the negative feedback of cell alkalinization. Under these circumstances, up-regulation of Cl^-/HCO_3^- exchange could accentuate the influx of cell Na^+ after activation of the Na^+/H^+ exchange by keeping pH_i low.

From this discussion, it becomes apparent that an imbalance in either direction between the rate of Cl^-/HCO_3^- exchange and the rate of Na^+/H^+ exchange could, in theory, lead to the development of hypertension. However, a definite relation between pH_i, Na^+, or Ca^{2+} and the development of hypertension is unproven at present.

C. POTENTIAL ROLE OF Cl^-/HCO_3^- EXCHANGE IN REGULATING GROWTH OF VASCULAR SMOOTH MUSCLE CELLS

The potential importance of an altered vascular structure, in the form of an increased wall (media) thickness:lumen diameter ratio, for the increased peripheral resistance in essential hypertension has often been stressed and has been unambiguously demonstrated.[111,112] The increased wall:lumen ratio could be a consequence of an increase in the vascular wall volume or growth.

In vascular smooth muscle cells in culture the vasoactive hormones angiotensin II,[113,114] noradrenaline,[115] and vasopressin[113] have all been shown to enhance proliferation and, as discussed above, these hormones also increase the pH_i of cultured vascular smooth muscle cells in a bicarbonate-free medium.

In many cell types, these hormones and other growth factors cause a rapid increase in pH_i in bicarbonate-free media. This action has been ascribed to a resetting of the Na^+/H^+ exchange,[116-119] and it has been suggested that pH_i plays an important role in mediating growth signals in cells. This hypothesis has been supported by the observation that amiloride and amiloride analogs in bicarbonate-free media prevent growth hormone-induced alkalinization and DNA synthesis.[119,120]

No study has thus far critically examined the importance of pH_i for the growth of vascular smooth muscle cells, however. Furthermore, the relationship between pH_i, Na^+/H^+ exchange activity, and the growth of vascular smooth muscle cells in the presence of bicarbonate has not been defined, making it difficult to evaluate the importance of pH_i in the growth of vascular smooth muscle cells under *in vivo* conditions.[1] In fact, Boron and co-workers[80] have shown clearly that growth factors stimulate the Na^+/H^+ exchange and Cl^-/HCO_3^- exchange mechanisms. Thus, the pH_i increase seen with growth factors in the absence of HCO_3^- is, under physiological conditions, a pH_i decrease. It is obvious that the Na^+/H^+ exchanger is unlikely to be the transmembrane signal transducer originally proposed,[118] but the Cl^-/HCO_3^- AE could be the signal transducer. This is further supported by the recent observation that phorbol esters inhibit Cl^-/HCO_3^- exchange in human leukocytes.[121] The exact role played by the inhibitory effect of phorbol esters on

Cl^-/HCO_3^- exchange in the cell proliferation response to these substances is not known at present and remains to be explored because doubt exists that the activation of the Na^+/H^+ exchange by phorbol esters is obligatory for this cell proliferative response.[122]

IV. ABNORMALITIES OF THE ANION EXCHANGER IN HYPERTENSION

A. STUDIES IN ANIMALS

Although the content of band 3 protein in membranes of spontaneously hypertensive rats (SHR) erythrocytes was 15 to 20% greater than in normotensive controls,[123] there is no evidence available that the activity of the AE is increased in red cells from SHR. With respect to other blood cells, Batlle et al.,[109] by analyzing changes in pH_i of cells incubated in the presence and absence of HCO_3^-, have excluded any abnormality in HCO_3^--dependent acid or base transport mechanisms in lymphocytes from young and adult SHR as compared to control Wistar-Kyoto (WKY) rats.

On the other hand, in experiments on aortic strips incubated in HCO_3^- buffer it was demonstrated that the rate of $^{36}Cl^-$ turnover was 1.5-fold higher in SHR than in normotensive controls.[124] A similarly altered Cl^- transport has been found by McMahon and Jones[103] in arteries from aldosterone salt-sensitive rats. Izzard and Heagerty[125] have found that at 5 weeks of age resistance arterioles from SHR were more alkaline as compared to WKY vessels, at a time when the blood pressure was rising. Although the authors argue that the increased pH_i in resistance arteries from SHR is due to enhanced Na^+/H^+ exchange,[126] their findings do not exclude a role for an abnormally high activity of the Na^+-dependent Cl^-/HCO_3^- AE. On the other hand, the observation that arteriolar pH is elevated when the media:lumen ratio is increased in hypertension-prone animals suggests that the alkaline cytoplasmic pH may be related to the processes responsible for the structural abnormalities seen in the arterioles when hypertension is established.[126] In this regard it is interesting to note that the same authors have very recently reported an abnormal HCO_3^--dependent pH regulation in mesenteric resistance arteries from rats with coarctation of the aorta 9 d postsurgery.[126] Again, the HCO_3^--dependent homeostasis appeared to be related to arterial remodeling present in these hypertensive rats.[126]

Finally, preliminary findings have shown a defective epithelial transport of Cl^- and HCO_3^- in SHR,[127] suggesting a possible abnormality of Cl^-/HCO_3^- AE in epithelial cells of this animal model of hypertension.

B. STUDIES IN HUMANS

The involvement of HCO_3^- transport under physiological conditions has been recently examined in human resistance arterioles in essential hypertension.[128] The AE inhibitor DIDS produced a fall in arteriolar pH that was identical to that in hypertensive patients and control subjects.[128] Accordingly, these authors suggest that there is no disturbance in DIDS-sensitive pH_i regulation in resistance arteries in established essential hypertension.

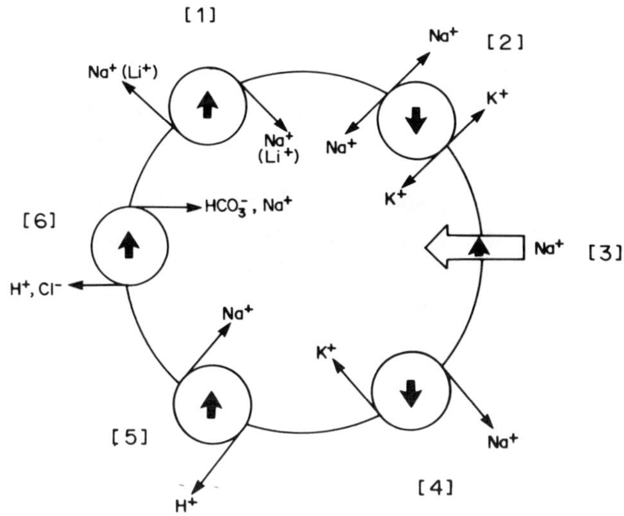

FIGURE 5. Stable Na^+ transport abnormalities that have been previously described in erythrocytes from essential hypertensive patients. (1) Increased activity of the Na^+,Li^+ countertransport; (2) diminished activity of the Na^+,K^+ cotransport; (3) increased passive entry of Na^+; (4) decreased activity of the Na^+,K^+ pump; (5) enhanced activity of the Na^+,H^+ exchange; (6) increased activity of the Na^+-dependent Cl^-/HCO_3^- AE.

One may argue, however, that *in vivo* differences in arteries from hypertensive patients compared to those from control subjects are lost as a result of removing the tissues from the body and studying them *in vitro*. At least two reasons support this notion:

1. Izzard et al.[129] recently reported significant differences in the effects of DIDS on resting pH_i in resistance arteries from rats with experimentally induced hypertension at various time points from the inception of hypertension.[129]
2. The activity of the AE in surrogate tissues such as blood cells studied in similar conditions *ex vivo* reported differences in hypertension.[130-132]

In fact, the inward Cl^- flux in erythrocytes of patients with essential hypertension has been found to be >20% that in normotensive patients.[130] On the other hand, our group has recently reported that the activity of the Na^+-dependent Cl^-/HCO_3^- AE is abnormally increased in erythrocytes from a subgroup (23%) of essential hypertensive patients.[131] When hypertensives with abnormal AE were followed over a long period of time, it was found that the increased activity of the exchange remained stable.[131] Therefore, hyperactivity of the Na^+-dependent Cl^-/HCO_3^- AE is the sixth stable Na^+ transport abnormality that may be found in RBC from essential hypertensive patients (Figure 5).

In a further study we have investigated the clinical characteristics of this subgroup of patients with increased activity of the Na^+-dependent AE. As compared to patients with normal activity of the exchanger, they were characterized by a higher frequency of family history of hypertension, lower serum high-density lipoprotein-(HDL) cholesterol levels, diminished Na^+ excretion, and higher plasma aldosterone concentrations.[132] Thus, seen from a clinical point of view patients with increased activity of the Na^+-dependent Cl^-/HCO_3^- AE apparently represent a particular subset of essential hypertensives.

On the other hand, the presence of such an abnormality may permit the specific treatment of these patients. In fact, it has been reported that xipamide, a diuretic drug with well-known antihypertensive properties, inhibits *in vitro* the Na^+-dependent Cl^-/HCO_3^- AE in human RBC.[74] Moreover, it has been suggested that the inhibition of the AE could be involved in the diuretic and/or antihypertensive action of the drug.[133] We can therefore hypothesize that xipamide represents the drug of choice for the treatment of hypertensives with increased activity of the Na^+-dependent Cl^-/HCO_3^- AE.

Little information is also available concerning the activity of the Na^+-independent Cl^-/HCO_3^- AE in cells from essential hypertensives. In a preliminary investigation we observed that the activity of this exchanger is abnormally increased in red cells from both normotensive men with a family history of hypertension and men with essential hypertension.[134] This observation would suggest that the abnormality of this AE mechanism is genetically linked to the development of hypertension.

V. CONCLUSIONS

Over the last 10 to 20 years a vast literature dealing with the relation between hypertension and abnormalities in transport and intracellular concentrations of a variety of ions including Na^+, H^+, and Ca^{2+} (see review in Reference 130) has appeared. Most of these studies have been conducted with blood cells and one of the interpretation problems, particularly in essential hypertension but also in experimental forms of hypertension, has been the relatively limited information available on the role of the various transport pathways in tissues such as vascular smooth muscle, kidney, and nerve which are more relevant for hypertension. Thus, even if it is assumed that the ion transport abnormalities detected in blood cells reflect a global abnormality, the functional consequences in terms of, for example, muscle tone and muscle growth are difficult to predict. The situation is therefore that multitudes of ion transport abnormalities have been described, but it has been difficult to organize the observations into a pathophysiological context based on experimental data.

On the other hand, we have described recently that the activity of the Na^+-independent Cl^-/HCO_3^- AE is increased in RBC of patients with essential hypertension as compared to normotensive controls.[135] Interestingly, the activity of this transport system was inversely correlated with pH_i, and directly correlated with blood pressure.[135] Thus, it appears that this AE mechanism could serve as a marker for alterations in pH_i-dependent control of vascular tone in hypertension. Again, a potential consideration arises when considering antihypertensive treatment of patients with this abnormality. In fact, the antihypertensive drug cicletanine has been shown to inhibit the Na^+-independent Cl^-/HCO_3^- AE both in erythrocytes and in vascular smooth muscle cells.[136]

An ion that has recently come into focus with respect to hypertension is the bicarbonate ion. The bicarbonate ion attracts interest because plasma pH (and HCO_3^-) affects peripheral resistance (vascular smooth muscle tone) and because HCO_3^- reabsorption in the kidneys involves renal Na^+ handling. Furthermore, it has been suggested that transmembrane HCO_3^- movements may represent a link in the transduction of growth stimuli.[116,117] Therefore, because vascular smooth muscle tone, vascular smooth muscle growth, and renal Na^+ handling are central to any hypothesis generated about the pathogenesis of hypertension, an understandable interest in the regulation of HCO_3^- transport has appeared and has led to useful hypotheses.[137,138]

However, the examples given above are intended to illustrate the point that if intracellular ions are to be implicated as a critical component in the development and in the consequences of hypertension, then HCO_3^--dependent transport processes cannot be ignored. This point becomes even more important when peripheral blood cells are used to compare pH_i in hyper- and normotensive subjects, as it is unknown if their pH regulatory mechanisms are similar to those of cells involved in blood pressure regulation. Such differences would not be surprising because the regulation of pH_i is accomplished by several different ion transport systems that vary depending on the cell type being investigated.[3]

Whether the findings of abnormalities in Cl^-/HCO_3^- AE mechanisms are important in the origin and evolution of hypertension remains to be determined; however, they have begun well by taking into account that the presence of HCO_3^- allows for a more physiological regulation of pH_i.

REFERENCES

1. **Thomas, R. C.,** Cell growth factors, bicarbonate and pHi response, *Nature,* 337, 601, 1989.
2. **Ross, A. and Boron, W. F.,** Intracellular pH, *Physiol. Rev.,* 61, 296, 1981.
3. **Frelin, C., Vigne, P., Ladoux, A., and Lazdunski, M.,** The regulation of the intracellular pH in cells from vertebrates, *Eur. J. Biochem.,* 174, 3, 1988.
4. **Moolenaar, W. H.,** Effects of growth factors on intracellular pH regulation, *Annu. Rev. Physiol.,* 48, 363, 1986.
5. **Thomas, R. C.,** The role of bicarbonate, chloride and sodium ions in the regulation of intracellular pH in snail neurones, *J. Physiol. (London),* 273, 317, 1977.
6. **Russel, J. M., Boron, W. F., and Brodwick, M. S.,** Intracellular pH and Na fluxes in barnacle muscle with evidence for reversal of the ionic mechanism of intracellular pH regulation, *J. Gen. Physiol.,* 82, 47, 1983.
7. **Jentsch, T. J., Stahlknecht, T. R., Hollwede, H., Fischer, D. G., Keller, S. K., and Wiederhold, M.,** A bicarbonate-dependent process inhibitable by disulfonic stilbenes and a Na^+/H^+ exchange mediate[22] Na^+ uptake into cultured bovine corneal endothelium, *J. Biol. Chem.,* 260, 795, 1985.

8. **L'Allemain, G., Paris, S., and Pouysségur, J.,** Role of a Na^+-dependent Cl^-/HCO_3^- exchange in regulation of intracellular pH in fibroblasts, *J. Biol. Chem.*, 260, 4877, 1985.
9. **Boyarsky, G., Ganz, M. B., Sterzel, R. B., and Boron, W. F.,** pH regulation in single glomerular mesangial cells. II. Na^+-dependent and -independent Cl^-/HCO_3^- exchangers, *Am. J. Physiol.*, 255, C857, 1988.
10. **Olsnes, S., Tonnessen, T. I., and Sandvig, K.,** pH-regulated anion antiport in nucleated mammalian cells, *J. Cell Biol.*, 102, 967, 1986.
11. **Simchowitz, L. and Roos, A.,** Regulation of intracellular pH in human neutrophils, *J. Gen. Physiol.*, 85, 443, 1985.
12. **Boron, W. F. and Boulpaep, E. L.,** Intracellular pH regulation in the renal proximal tubule of the salamander, *J. Gen. Physiol.*, 81, 53, 1983.
13. **Grassl, S. M. and Aronson, P. S.,** Na^+/HCO_3^- co-transport in basolateral membrane vesicles isolated from rabbit renal cortex, *J. Biol. Chem.*, 261, 8778, 1986.
14. **Bierman, A. J., Cragoe, E. J., Jr., deLaat, S. W., and Moolenaar, W. H.,** Bicarbonate determines cytoplasmic pH and suppresses mitogen-induced alkalinization in fibroblastic cells, *J. Biol. Chem.*, 263, 15253, 1988.
15. **Tonnessen, T. I., Sandvig, K., and Olsnes, S.,** Role of Na^+-H^+ and Cl/HCO_3^- antiports in the regulation of cytoplasmic pH near neutrality, *Am. J. Physiol.*, 258, C1117, 1990.
16. **Fairbanks, G., Steck, T. L., and Wallach, D. F. H.,** Electrophoretic analysis of the major polypeptides of the human erythrocyte membrane, *Biochemistry,* 10, 2006, 1971.
17. **Passow, H.,** Molecular aspects of band 3 protein-mediated anion transport across the red blood cell membrane, *Rev. Physiol. Biochem. Pharmacol.*, 103, 61–203, 1986.
18. **Steck, T. L., Ramos, B., and Strapazon, E.,** Proteolytic dissection of band 3, the predominant transmembrane polypeptide of the human erythrocyte membrane, *Biochemistry,* 15, 1154, 1976.
19. **Steck, T. L., Koziard, J. J., Singh, M. K., Reddy, G., and Kohler, N.,** Preparation and analysis of seven major, topographically defined fragments of band 3, the predominant transmembrane polypeptide of the human erythrocyte membrane, *Biochemistry,* 17, 1216, 1978.
20. **Low, P. S.,** Structure and function of the cytoplasmic domain of band 3: center of erythrocyte membrane peripheral protein interactions, *Biochim. Biophys. Acta,* 864, 145, 1986.
21. **Bennett, V. and Stenbuck, P. J.,** Association between ankyrin and the cytoplasmic domain of band 3 isolated from the human erythrocyte membrane, *J. Biol. Chem.*, 255, 6424, 1980.
22. **Bennett, V.,** The membrane skeleton of human erythrocytes and its implications for more complex cells, *Annu. Rev. Biochem.*, 54, 273, 1985.
23. **Pasternack, G. R., Anderson, R. A., Leto, T. L., and Marchesi, V. T.,** Interactions between protein 4.1 and band 3, *J. Biol. Chem.*, 260, 3676, 1985.
24. **Kay, M. M. B.,** Localization of senescent cell antigen on band 3, *Proc. Natl. Acad. Sci. U.S.A.*, 81, 5753, 1984.
25. **Low, P. S., Waugh, S. M., Zinke, K., and Drenckhahn, D.,** The role of hemoglobin denaturation and band 3 clustering in red blood cell aging, *Science,* 277, 531, 1985.
26. **Lepke, S. and Passow, H.,** Effects of incorporated trypsin on anion exchange and membrane proteins in human red blood cell ghosts, *Biochim. Biophys. Acta,* 455, 353, 1976.
27. **Grinstein, S., Ship, S., and Rothstein, A.,** Anion transport in relation to proteolytic dissection of band 3 protein, *Biochim. Biophys. Acta,* 507, 294, 1978.
28. **García, A. M., Kopito, R., and Lodish, H. F.,** Expression of band 3 in *Xenopus laevis* oocytes microinjected with in vitro prepared mRNA, *Biophys. J.*, 51, 567a, 1987.
29. **Jenkins, R. E. and Tanner, M. J. A.,** The structure of the major protein of the human erythrocyte membrane. Characterization of the intact protein and major fragments, *Biochem. J.*, 161, 139, 1977.
30. **Kopito, R. R. and Lodish, H. F.,** Primary structure and transmembrane orientation of the murine anion exchange protein, *Nature,* 316, 234, 1985.
31. **Oikawa, K., Lieberman, D. M., and Reithmeier, R. A. F.,** Conformation and stability of the anion transport protein of human erythrocyte membranes, *Biochemistry,* 24, 2843, 1985.

32. **Lux, S. E., John, K. M., Kopito, R. R., and Lodish, H. F.,** Cloning and characterization of band 3. The human erythrocyte anion-exchange protein (AE1), *Proc. Natl. Acad. Sci. U.S.A.,* 86, 9089, 1989.
33. **Alper, S. L., Kopito, R. R., and Lodish, H. F.,** A molecular biological approach to the study of anion transport, *Kidney Int.,* 32, S117, 1987.
34. **Jennings, M. L., Adams-Lackey, M., and Denney, G. H.,** Peptides of human erythrocyte band 3 protein produced by extracellular papain cleavage, *J. Biol. Chem.,* 259, 4652, 1984.
35. **Jennings, M. L.,** The anion transport protein. Structure and function, in *The Red Cell Membrane,* Raess, B. V. and Tunnicliff, G., Eds., Humana Press, Clifton, NJ, 1989, 143.
36. **Cox, J. V. and Lazarides, E.,** Alternative primary structures in the transmembrane domain of the chicken erythroid anion transporter, *Mol. Cell. Biol.,* 8, 1327, 1988.
37. **Kim, H. R. C., Yew, N. S., Ansorge, W., Voss, H., Schwager, C., Vennström, B., Zenke, M., and Engel, J. D.,** Two different mRNAs are transcribed from a single genomic locus encoding the chicken erythrocyte anion transport (band 3), *Mol. Cell. Biol.,* 8, 4416, 1988.
38. **Tanner, M. J. A., Martin, P. G., and High, S.,** The complete amino acid sequence of the human erythrocyte membrane anion transport protein deduced from the cDNA sequence, *Biochem. J.,* 256, 703, 1988.
39. **Kudrycki, K. E. and Shull, G. E.,** Primary structure of the rat kidney band 3 anion exchange protein deduced from a cDNA, *J. Biol. Chem.,* 264, 8185, 1989.
40. **Alper, S. L., Kopito, R. R., Libresco, S. M., and Lodish, H. F.,** Cloning and characterization of a murine band 3-related cDNA from kidney and from a lymphoid cell line, *J. Biol. Chem.,* 263, 17092, 1988.
41. **Kudrycki, K. E., Newman, P. R., and Shull, G. E.,** cDNA, cloning and tissue distribution of mRNAs for two proteins that are related to the band 3 Cl^-/HCO_3^- exchanger, *J. Biol. Chem.,* 265, 462, 1990.
42. **Lindsey, A. E., Schneider, K., Simmons, D. M., Baron, R., Lee, B. S., and Kopito, R. R.,** Functional expression and subcellular localization of an anion exchanger cloned from choroid plexus, *Proc. Natl. Acad. Sci. U.S.A.,* 87, 5278, 1990.
43. **Demuth, D. R., Showe, L. C., Ballantine, M., Palumbo, A., Fraser, P. J., Cioe, L., Rovera, G., and Curtis, P. J.,** Cloning and structural characterization of a human non-erythroid band 3-like protein, *EMBO J.,* 5, 1205, 1986.
44. **Chow, A., Dobbins, J. W., Hildebrandt, F., Aronson, P. S., and Igaraski, P.,** Cloning of a rabbit ileum cDNA related to erythroid band 3, *Gastroenterology,* 96, A87, 1989.
45. **Kopito, R. R., Lee, B. S., Simmons, D. M., Lindsey, A. E., Morgans, C. W., and Schneider, K.,** Regulation of intracellular pH by a neuronal homolog of the erythrocyte anion exchanger, *Cell,* 59, 927, 1989.
46. **Showe, L. C., Ballantine, M., and Huebner, K.,** Localization of the gene for the erythroid anion exchange protein, band 3, to human chromosome 17, *Genomics,* 1, 71, 1987.
47. **Palumbo, A. P., Isobe, M., Huebner, K., Shane, S., Rovera, G., Demuth, D. R., Curtis, P. J., Ballantine, M., Croce, C. M., and Showe, L. C.,** Chromosomal localization of a human band 3-like gene to region 7q35-7q36, *Am. J. Hum. Gen.,* 39, 307, 1986.
48. **Kopito, R. R.,** Molecular biology of the anion exchanger gene family, *Int. Rev. Cytol.,* 123, 177, 1990.
49. **Alper, S. L.,** The band 3-related anion exchanger (AE) gene family, *Annu. Rev. Physiol.,* 53, 549, 1991.
50. **Wagner, S., Vogel, P. E., Lietzke, R., Koob, R., and Drenckhahn, D.,** Immunochemical characterization of a band 3-like anion exchanger in collecting duct of human kidney, *Am. J. Physiol.,* 253, F213, 1987.
51. **Alper, S. L., Natale, J., Gluck, S., Lodish, H. F., and Brown, D.,** Subtypes of intercalated cells in rat kidney collecting duct defined by antibodies against erythroid band 3 and renal vacuolar H^+-ATPase, *Proc. Natl. Acad. Sci. U.S.A.,* 86, 5429, 1989.
52. **Alper, S. L., Stuart-Tilley, A., and Brown, D.,** Tissue distribution of the Cl^-/HCO_3^- exchanger AE2: abundant expression in the choroid plexus, *J. Am. Soc. Nephrol.,* 1, 711a, 1990.

53. **Thomas, H. A., Machen, T. E., Smolka, A., Baron, R., and Kopito, R. R.,** Identification of a 185 kDa band 3-related polypeptide in oxyntic cells, *Am. J. Physiol.*, 257, C537, 1989.
54. **Gunn, R. B., Fröhlich, O., King, P. A., and Shoemaker, D. G.,** Anion transport, in *Red Blood Cell Membranes. Structure. Function. Clinical Implications,* Agre, P. and Parker, J. C., Eds., Marcel Dekker, New York, 1989, 563.
55. **Dalmark, M.,** Effects of halides and bicarbonate on chloride transport in human red blood cells, *J. Gen. Physiol.*, 67, 223, 1976.
56. **Knauf, P. A.,** Erythrocyte anion exchange and the band 3 protein: transport kinetics and molecular structure, *Curr. Topics Membr. Transport,* 12, 249, 1979.
57. **Ku, C. P., Jennings, M. L., and Passow, H.,** A comparison of the inhibitory potency of reversibly acting inhibitors of anion transport on chloride and sulfate movements across the human red cell membrane, *Biochim. Biophys. Acta,* 553, 132, 1979.
58. **Obaid, A. L., Leininger, T. F., and Crandall, E. D.,** Exchange of HCO_3^- for monovalent anions across the human erythrocyte membrane, *J. Membr. Biol.*, 52, 173, 1980.
59. **Salhany, J. M. and Rauenbuehler, P. B.,** Kinetics and mechanism of erythrocyte anion exchange, *J. Biol. Chem.*, 258, 245, 1983.
60. **Milanick, M. A. and Gunn, R. B.,** Proton-sulfate cotransport: external proton activation of sulfate influx into human red blood cells, *Am. J. Physiol.*, 247, C247, 1984.
61. **Milanick, M. A. and Gunn, R. B.,** The selectivity of the external anion exchange transport site of red blood cells, *Biophys. J.*, 33, 47a, 1981.
62. **Wieth, J. O.,** Bicarbonate exchange through the human red cell membrane determined with [^{14}C] bicarbonate, *J. Physiol.*, 294, 521, 1979.
63. **Gunn, R. B. and Fröhlich, O.,** Asymmetry in the mechanism for anion exchange in human red blood cell membranes. Evidence for reciprocating sites that react with one transported anion at a time, *J. Gen. Physiol.*, 74, 351, 1979.
64. **Fröhlich, O. and Gunn, R. B.,** Erythrocyte anion transport: the kinetics of a single-site obligatory exchange system, *Biochim. Biophys. Acta,* 864, 169, 1986.
65. **Wieth, J. O. and Bjerrum, P. J.,** Titration of transport and modifier sites in the red cell anion transport system, *J. Gen. Physiol.*, 79, 253, 1982.
66. **Jennings, M. L.,** Proton fluxes associated with erythrocyte membrane anion exchange, *J. Membr. Biol.*, 28, 187, 1976.
67. **Gunn, R. B.,** H^+ (or OH^-) fluxes activated by inorganic ions on the anion exchanger (band 3) of human red blood cells, *Biophys. J.*, 49, 579a, 1986.
68. **Funder, J., Tosteson, D. C., and Wieth, J. O.,** Effects of bicarbonate on lithium transport in human red cells, *J. Gen. Physiol.*, 71, 721, 1978.
69. **Duhm, J. and Becker, B. F.,** Studies on Na^+-dependent Li^+ countertransport and bicarbonate stimulated Li^+ transport in human erythrocytes, in *Cell Membrane Receptors for Drugs and Hormones: A Multidisciplinary Approach,* Straub, R. W. and Bolis, L., Eds., Raven Press, New York, 1978, 281.
70. **Wieth, J. O. and Brahm, J.,** The inhibitory effect of salicylate on chloride and bicarbonate transport in human red cells. A hypothesis for the stimulatory effect of salicylate on the respiration, *Ugeskr. Laeg.*, 140, 1859, 1978.
71. **Brazy, P. C. and Gunn, R. B.,** Furosemide inhibition of chloride transport in human red blood cells, *J. Gen. Physiol.*, 68, 583, 1976.
72. **Gunn, R. B.,** Bumetanide inhibition of anion exchange in human red blood cells, *Biophys. J.*, 47, 326a, 1985.
73. **Gunn, R. B., Feldman, S. T., and Horton, J. M.,** Inhibition of chloride transport in human red cell by diuretics, *Fed. Proc.*, 36, 564, 1977.
74. **Nazaret, C., Díez, J., Hannaert, P., Christen, M. O., Wierzbicki, N., and Garay, R. P.,** Inhibition of the $Cl^-/NaCO_3^-$ anion exchanger by xipamide in human red blood cells, *Eur. J. Pharmacol.*, 144, 353, 1987.
75. **Gunn, R. B. and Cooper, J. A.,** Effect of local anesthetics on chloride transport in erythrocytes, *J. Membr. Biol.*, 25, 311, 1975.

76. **Stone, D. K., Seldin, D. W., Kokko, J. P., and Jacobson, H. R.,** Anion dependence of medullary collecting duct acidification, *J. Clin. Invest.*, 71, 1505, 1983.
77. **Paradiso, A. M., Tsien, R. Y., and Machen, T. E.,** Digital image processing of intracellular pH in gastric oxyntic and chief cells, *Nature,* 325, 447, 1987.
78. **Grinstein, S.,** Intracellular chloride concentration: determinants and consequences, *Progr. Clin. Biol. Res.*, 254, 31, 1987.
79. **Grinstein, S. and Foskett, J. K.,** Ionic mechanisms of cell volume regulation in leucocytes, *Annu. Rev. Physiol.*, 52, 399, 1990.
80. **Ganz, M. B., Boyarsky, G., Sterzl, R. B., and Boron, W. F.,** Arginine vasopressin enhances pH_i regulation in the presence of HCO_3^- by stimulating the three acid-base transport systems, *Nature,* 337, 648, 1989.
81. **Reinertsen, K. V., Tonnessen, T. I., Jacobsen, J., Sandvig, K., and Olsnes, S.,** Role of chloride/bicarbonate antiport in the control of cytosolic pH: cell-line differences in activity and regulation of antiport, *J. Biol. Chem.*, 263, 11117, 1988.
82. **Tonnessen, T. I., Aas, A. T., Ludt, J., Blomhoff, H. K., and Olsnes, S.,** Regulation of Na^+/H^+ and Cl^-/HCO_3^- antiports in Vero cells, *J. Cell. Physiol.*, 143, 178, 1990a.
83. **Grinstein, S., Rotin, D., and Mason, M. J.,** Na^+/H^+ exchange and growth factor-induced cytosolic pH changes. Role in cellular proliferation, *Biochim. Biophys. Acta,* 988, 73, 1989.
84. **Schuster, V. L. and Stokes, J. B.,** Chloride transport by the cortical and outer medullary collecting duct, *Am. J. Physiol.*, 253, F203, 1987.
85. **Harada, H., Kanai, Y., Anzai, M., and Suketa, Y.,** cAMP activates Cl^-/HCO_3^- exchange for regulation of intracellular pH in renal epithelial cells, *Biochim. Biophys. Acta,* 1092, 404, 1991.
86. **Vigne, P., Breittmayer, J. P., Frelin, C., and Lazdunski, M.,** Dual control of the intracellular pH in aortic smooth muscle cells by a cAMP-sensitive HCO_3^-/Cl^- antiporter and a protein kinase C-sensitive Na^+/H^+ antiporter, *J. Biol. Chem.*, 263, 18023, 1988.
87. **Creen, J., Yamaguchi, D. T., Kleeman, C. R., and Muallem, S.,** Cytosolic pH regulation in osteoblasts. Regulation of anion exchange by intracellular pH and Ca^{2+} ions, *J. Gen. Physiol.*, 95, 121, 1990.
88. **Preisig, P. A. and Alpern, R. J.,** Basolateral membrane H/HCO_3 transport in renal tubules, *Kidney Int.*, 39, 1077, 1991.
89. **Guggino, W. B. and Guggino, S. E.,** Renal anion transport, *Kidney Int.*, 36, 385, 1989.
90. **Alpern, R. J.,** Mechanisms of basolateral $H^+/OH^-HCO_3^-$ transport in the rat proximal convoluted tubule: a sodium-coupled electrogenic process, *J. Gen. Physiol.*, 86, 613, 1985.
91. **Preisig, P. A. and Alpern, R. J.,** Chronic metabolic acidosis causes an adaptation in basolateral $Na(HCO_3)_3$ symport in rat proximal convoluted tubule, *J. Clin. Invest.*, 82, 1445, 1988.
92. **Friedman, P. A. and Andreoli, T. E.,** CO_2-stimulated NaCl absorption in the mouse renal cortical thick ascending limb of Henle. Evidence for synchronous Na^+/H^+ and Cl^-/HCO_3^- exchange in apical plasma membranes, *J. Gen. Physiol.*, 80, 683, 1982.
93. **Krapf, R.,** Basolateral membrane $H/OH/HCO_3$ transport in the rat cortical thick ascending limb, *J. Clin. Invest.*, 82, 234, 1988.
94. **Weinberger, M. H., Miller, J. Z., Luft, F. C., Grim, C. E., and Fineberg, N. S.,** Definitions and characteristics of sodium sensitivity and blood pressure resistance, *Hypertension,* 8(Suppl. II), II-127, 1986.
95. **Kunau, R. T., Jr., Hart, J. I., and Walker, K. A.,** Effect of metabolic acidosis on proximal tubular total CO_2 absorption, *Am. J. Physiol.*, 249, F62, 1985.
96. **Sharma, A. M., Kribben, A., Shattenfroch, S., Cetto, C., and Distler, A.,** Salt sensitivity in humans is associated with abnormal acid-base regulation, *Hypertension,* 16, 407, 1990.
97. **Preisig, P. A. and Alpern, R. J.,** Increased Na/H antiporter and Na/HCO_3 symporter activities in chronic hyperfiltration: a model of cell hypertrophy, *J. Gen. Physiol.*, 97, 195, 1990.
98. **Schmieder, R. E., Messerli, F. H., Garavaglia, G., and Nunez, B.,** Glomerular hyperfiltration indicates early target organ damage in essential hypertension, *JAMA,* 264, 2775, 1990.

99. **Aalkjaer, C.,** Regulation of intracellular pH and its role in vascular smooth muscle function, *J. Hypertension,* 8, 197, 1990.
100. **Aickin, C. C.,** Direct measurement of intracellular pH and buffering power in smooth muscle cells of guinea-pig vas deferens, *J. Physiol.*, 349, 571, 1984.
101. **Aickin, C. C. and Brading, A. F.,** The role of chloride-bicarbonate exchange in the regulation of intracellular chloride in guinea pig vas deferens, *J. Physiol.*, 349, 587, 1984.
102. **Gerstheimer, F. P., Muhleisen, M., Nehring, D., and Kreye, V. A. W.,** A chloride-bicarbonate exchanging anion carrier in vascular smooth muscle of the rabbit, *Pfluegers' Arch.*, 409, 60, 1987.
103. **McMahon, E. G. and Jones, A. W.,** Altered chloride transport in arteries from aldosterone salt-hypertensive rats, *J. Hypertension,* 6, 593, 1988.
104. **Aalkjaer, C., and Cragoe, E. J., Jr.,** Intracellular pH regulation in resting and contracting segments of rat mesenteric resistance vessels, *J. Physiol.*, 402, 391, 1988.
105. **Korbmacher, C., Helbig, H., Stahl, F., and Wiederholt, M.,** Evidence for Na/H exchange and Cl-HCO_3 exchange in A10 vascular smooth muscle cells, *Pfluegers' Arch.*, 412, 29, 1988.
106. **Aalkjaer, C. and Mulvany, M. J.,** Angiotensin II and noradrenaline induced contraction and intracellular pH in segments of rat resistance vessels, in *Resistance Arteries,* Halpern, W., Pegram, B., and Brayden, J., Eds., Perinatology Press, New York, 1988, 229.
107. **Aalkjaer, C. and Nielsen, H.,** Activation of Na, HCO_3-cotransport and Na,H-exchange with vasopressin in isolated rat mesenteric small arteries, *Acta Physiol. Scand.*, 136, 8A, 1989.
108. **Zhang, A., Altura, B. T., and Altura, B. M.,** Effect of disulfonic stilbene anion-channel blockers on contractility of vascular smooth muscle, *Ann. N.Y. Acad. Sci.*, 574, 123, 1989.
109. **Batlle, D. C., Saleh, A., and Rombola, G.,** Reduced intracellular pH in lymphocytes from the spontaneously hypertensive rat, *Hypertension,* 15, 97, 1990.
110. **Blaustein, M. P.,** Sodium ions, calcium ions, blood pressure regulation, and hypertension: a reassessment and a hypothesis, *Am. J. Physiol.*, 232, C165, 1977.
111. **Folkow, B.,** Physiological aspects of primary hypertension, *Physiol. Rev.*, 62, 347, 1982.
112. **Aalkjaer, C., Heagerty, A. M., Petersen, K. K., Swales, J. D., and Mulvany, M. J.,** Evidence for increased media thickness, increased neuronal amine uptake, and depressed excitation-contraction coupling in isolated resistance vessels from essential hypertensives, *Circ. Res.*, 61, 181, 1987.
113. **Campbell-Boswell, M. and Robertson, A. L.,** Effects of angiotensin II and vasopressin on human smooth muscle cells "in vitro", *Exp. Mol. Pathol.*, 35, 265, 1981.
114. **Lyall, F., Lever, A. F., and Morton, J. J.,** Vascular hypertrophy and hypertension: a role for growth factors?, *Acta Physiol. Scand.*, 133(Suppl. 571), 189, 1988.
115. **Blaes, N. and Boissel, J. P.,** Growth-stimulating effect of catecholamines on rat aortic smooth muscle cells in culture, *J. Cell. Physiol.*, 116, 167, 1983.
116. **Moolenaar, W. H., Yarden, Y., deLaat, S. W., and Schlessinger, J.,** Epidermal growth factor induces electrically silent Na^+ influx in human fibroblasts, *J. Biol. Chem.*, 257, 8502, 1982.
117. **Pouysségur, J., Chambard, J. C., Franchi, A., Paris, S., and Van Obberrghen-Schilling, E.,** Growth factor activation of an amiloride sensitive Na^+/H^+ exchange system in quiescent fibroblasts: coupling to ribosomal protein S6 phosphorilation, *Proc. Natl. Acad. Sci. U.S.A.*, 79, 3935, 1982.
118. **Moolenaar, W. H., Tsien, R. Y., Saag, P. T., and deLaat, S. W.,** Na^+/H^+ exchange and cytoplasmic pH in the action of growth factors in human fibroblasts, *Nature,* 304, 645, 1983.
119. **Pouysségur, J., Franchi, A., L'Allemain, G., and Paris, S.,** Cytoplasmic pH, a key determinant of growth factor-induced DNA synthesis in quiescent fibroblasts, *FEBS Lett.*, 190, 115, 1985.
120. **L'Allemain, G., Franchi, A., Cragoe, E., and Pouysségur, J.,** Blockade of the Na^+/H^+ antiport abolishes growth factor-induced DNA synthesis in fibroblasts, *J. Biol. Chem.*, 259, 4313, 1984.
121. **Hogg, M., Ng, L. L., and Davies, J. E.,** Chloride influx in human leucocytes: a triple-isotope technique for the assessment of chloride transporters, *Clin. Sci.*, 81, 405, 1991.

122. **Grinstein, S. and Dixon, S. J.**, Ion transport, membrane potential and cytoplasmic pH in lymphocytes: changes during activation, *Physiol. Rev.*, 69, 417, 1989.
123. **Gulak P. V., Orlov, S. N., Pokudin, N. I., Postnov, Y. V., Litvinov, I. S., Orlov, N. I., and Shnyrov, M. V.**, Microcalorimetry and electrophoresis of the erythrocyte membrane of spontaneously hypertensive rats, *J. Hypertension,* 2, 81, 1984.
124. **Jones, A. W.**, Altered chloride transport in vascular smooth muscle from spontaneously hypertensive rats. Influence of aldosterone, norepinephrine and angiotensin, *Circ. Res.*, 33, 563, 1973.
125. **Izzard, A. S. and Heagerty, A. M.**, The measurement of internal pH in resistance arterioles: evidence that intracellular pH is more alkaline in SHR than WKY animals, *J. Hypertension,* 7, 173, 1989.
126. **Izzard, A. S. and Heagerty, A. M.**, Resting intracellular pH in mesenteric resistance arteries from spontaneously hypertensive and Wistar-Kyoto rats: effects of amiloride and, 4,4′-diisothiocyanatostilbene-2,2′-disulfonic acid, *J. Hypertension,* 7(Suppl. 6), S128, 1989.
127. **Lucas, P. A., Mansour, A. B., Lacour, B., McCarron, D. A., Desjeux, J. F., and Druecke, T.**, Defective epithelial HCO_3^- transport in spontaneously hypertensive rats: possible role of abnormal Cl^-/HCO_3^- exchange, *Am. J. Hypertension,* 1, 66A, 1988.
128. **Izzard, A. S., Cragoe, E. J., Jr., and Heagerty, A. M.**, Intracellular pH in human resistance arteries in essential hypertension, *Hypertension,* 17, 780, 1991.
129. **Izzard, A. S., MacIver, D. H., Cragoe, E. J., and Heagerty, A. M.**, Intracellular pH in rat resistance arteries during the development of experimental hypertension, *Clin. Sci.*, 81, 65, 1991.
130. **Postnov, Y. V. and Orlov, S. N.**, Ion transport across plasma membrane in primary hypertension, *Physiol. Rev.*, 65, 904, 1985.
131. **Díez, J., Arrazola, A., Castiella, J., Iñigo, B., and Cía, P.**, Increased activity of the Na^+-dependent Cl^-/HCO_3^- anion exchanger. A new abnormality of red blood cell Na^+ transport in essential hypertension, *Am. J. Hypertension,* 4, 95A, 1991.
132. **Díez, J., Arrazola, A., Castiella, J., Iñigo, B., and Cía, P.**, Increased activity of the Na^+-dependent Cl^-/HCO_3^- anion exchanger in red cells of patients with essential hypertension, *J. Hypertension,* 10, 579, 1992.
133. **Díez, J.**, Diuretics and transmembrane ionic exchanges: structure-activity relations and clinical applications, *Am. J. Cardiol.*, 65, 55H, 1990.
134. **Diez, J., Esparza, N., Arrázola, A., Alonso, A., and Garciandía, A.**, Hyperactivity of Cl^-/HCO_3^- anion exchanger (AE) in normotensive men with family history of hypertension. Pathophysiological implications, *Am. J. Hypertension,* 5, 66A, 1992.
135. **Alonso, A., Arrázola, A., Garciandía, A., Esparza, N., Gomez-Alamillo, C., and Diez, J.**, Erythrocyte anion exchanger activity and intercellular pH in essential hypertension, *Hypertension,* in press.
136. **Fenous, K., Berthlet, P. H., and Garay, R. P.**, Opposite effects of cell growth factors and the sulfo-conjugate metabolite of cicletanine on Na^+ independent Cl^-/HCO_3 exchange in A1O vascular smooth muscle cells, *Am. J. Hypertension,* 5, 45A, 1992.
137. **Lever, A. F.**, Slow pressor mechanisms in hypertension: a role for hypertrophy of resistance vessels?, *J. Hypertension,* 4, 515, 1986.
138. **Aviv, A.**, The link between cytosolic Ca^{2+} and the Na^+/H^+ antiport: a unifying factor for essential hypertension, *J. Hypertension,* 6, 685, 1988.
139. **Knauf, P.**, Kinetics of anion transport, in *The Red Cell Membrane,* Raess, B. V. and Tunnicliff, G., Eds., Humana Press, Clifton, NJ, 1989, 171.

Chapter 8

ENDOGENOUS DIGITALIS-LIKE FACTORS: PAST PROGRESS AND FUTURE PROSPECTS

Kenneth A. Gruber

TABLE OF CONTENTS

I. Introduction 158

II. The Natriuretic Hormone Hypothesis 158
  A. Physiological Evidence 158
  B. Mechanism of Action 159

III. The Hypertensive Factor Hypothesis 159
  A. Physiological Evidence 159
  B. Mechanism of Action 160

IV. Merging of the Natriuretic Hormone and Hypertensive Factor Hypotheses 161

V. Characteristics of Digitalis-Like Factors 162
  A. Criteria 162
  B. Sources 164
    1. Urine 164
    2. Plasma 165
      a. General Approaches 165
      b. Studies Related to Renal Function 166
      c. Studies Related to Cardiovascular Function 168
    3. Tissue 172
    4. Cerebrospinal Fluid 175

VI. Conclusions 175

References 176

0-8493-5474-9/94/$0.00 + $.50

I. INTRODUCTION

In the late 1970s and early 1980s several lines of investigation in the fields of body fluid homeostasis regulation and hypertension converged to support the existence of a circulating factor with both natriuretic and blood pressure elevating activities. The apparent mechanism of action of this putative hormone was inhibition of the Na pump (Na,K-ATPase), a mechanism held in common with the cardiac glycoside class of drugs. This similarity led to the use of the terms endogenous "ouabain-like" or "digitalis-like" when reference to this putative hormone was made.

It is now over a decade since this unifying concept was first advanced. This chapter briefly describes the work that contributed to the formulation of this hypothesis, the data that provided the first direct evidence, a brief synopsis of the extensive number of publications that have subsequently appeared supporting the existence of an endogenous hormonal substance with digitalis-like activity, problems encountered in the selection of material sources or assays, and prospects for future advances in this field. This chapter is not intended to be inclusive of all work in this field, but rather to highlight the major lines of evidence that support this hypothesis (for more extensive reviews of specific areas of research in this field see References 1 to 3).

II. THE NATRIURETIC HORMONE HYPOTHESIS

A. PHYSIOLOGICAL EVIDENCE

Numerous studies support the ability of the kidney to excrete sodium loads independent of changes in renal blood flow or glomerular filtration rate.[4-6] The possibility that alterations in the circulating levels of sodium-retaining hormones (aldosterone or angiotensin II) accounted for these effects was also eliminated in these experiments. Indeed, the excretion of sodium loads could occur in the face of the exogenous administration of sodium-retaining hormones. The evidence appeared to indicate that saline loads produced a change in the tubular reabsorption of sodium.

Although Homer Smith originally predicted that the ability to excrete sodium loads was due to decreased circulating levels of a antinatriuretic hormone, studies with extracts from plasma or urine of saline-expanded subjects provided evidence for the opposite hypothesis (i.e., increased levels of a natriuretic hormone).[8-10]

Studies of fluid homeostasis mechanisms suggested that the brain was an essential component in the renal response to extracellular fluid expansion. Both hypothalamic lesions[11] and total elimination of the supraspinal central nervous system[12] have been shown to inhibit the renal response to acute extracellular volume expansion. Buckalew et al.[9] demonstrated higher levels of sodium transport inhibitory activity in jugular vs. femoral vein blood during volume expansion in the dog. These early studies clearly influenced subsequent investigations of the tissue origin of digitalis-like factors.

B. MECHANISM OF ACTION

The first suggestion that the putative natriuretic hormone could function as an inhibitor of Na,K-ATPase was in a preliminary report by Kramer et al.[13] Subsequent work by Gonick and associates[14] clearly demonstrated that Na,K-ATPase activity was inhibited in the kidneys of volume-expanded animals, and that extracts of kidneys from volume-expanded animals contained Na,K-ATPase inhibitory activity. This transport system is located in the distal renal tubule and collecting duct, and is responsible for a considerable fraction of total renal sodium reabsorption.

In 1980 Gruber et al.[15] presented evidence that extracts of plasma from saline-expanded dogs contained Na,K-ATPase inhibitory activity and could compete with digoxin (a cardiac glycoside) for binding to antidigoxin antibodies. These activities appeared to comigrate on high performance liquid chromatography (HPLC), suggesting that both activities could reside in a single substance. Due to its potential immunological similarity to digoxin, this endogenous digoxin-like factor was termed "endoxin".

The isolated activities appeared to be sensitive to acid hydrolysis, unlike other known Na,K-ATPase inhibitors such as polyamines,[16] vanadate,[17] or steroids.[18] In addition, the activities had the same HPLC retention time as an inhibitor of toad bladder sodium transport (the anuran bladder is an analog of the mammalian distal tubule and collecting duct) we had previously isolated from the plasma of saline-loaded dogs.[19]

From a historical perspective it is interesting to note that during the development of clinical laboratory assays for cardiac glycosides in blood, endogenous interference was detected in patients with congestive heart failure or fluid balance problems.[20-22] This interference appeared to be present for transport, enzymatic, and radioimmunoassays. Subsequent work on endogenous digitalis-like substances has confirmed and extended these observations.

III. THE HYPERTENSIVE FACTOR HYPOTHESIS

A. PHYSIOLOGICAL EVIDENCE

Beginning in the 1940s evidence appeared in the literature for the presence of a pressor factor in the blood of hypertensive animal subjects, other than angiotensin II.[23-25] The forms of hypertension in which this factor could best be detected were those with some renal impairment. Unlike angiotensin II, the activity attributed to this factor produced a relatively slow increase in blood pressure, accompanied by a potentiation of the responses of known pressor substances (e.g., angiotensin II and norepinephrine). Further, in at least one report the hypertensive effect was potentiated by renal impairment in the recipient or test animal.[23]

Evaluation of known pressor substances, such as vasopressin, catecholamines, prostaglandins, etc., did not produce the presence of the spectrum of activities which appeared to be associated with this unknown factor (see Reference 3 for a historical review).

B. MECHANISM OF ACTION

The possibility that abnormalities in cation transport mechanisms might be associated with renal hypertension was first suggested by Overbeck.[26] This work investigated the vascular responses to brachial artery infusions of various ions, sugar, and vasoactive agents in renal hypertensive dogs. The most striking finding was a decrease in the vasodilatory effect of potassium. The mechanism through which potassium produced its vasodilatory effect was thought to be stimulation of an electrogenic Na pump.[27] Thus, Overbeck proposed the possibility that an electrogenic Na pump defect was present in the vascular smooth muscle of renal hypertensive dogs.

Direct evidence for this hypothesis was provided by subsequent work from Overbeck and colleagues,[28] in which they measured total and ouabain-sensitive rubidium (Rb) uptake during *in vitro* incubation of the veins and arteries of renal hyper- and normotensive dogs. Only ouabain-sensitive Rb uptake was depressed. Because ouabain is an established inhibitor of Na,K-ATPase, they concluded that the activity of this cation transport mechanism was specifically reduced in this form of hypertension.

The mechanism by which this effect was produced appeared to be humorally mediated, as arteries from hypertensive dogs showed inhibition of ouabain-sensitive rubidium uptake only if the incubation was performed in plasma from a hypertensive dog.

The possibility of a hypertensive hormone with a ouabain-like mechanism of action was not inconsistent with the established cardiovascular effects of cardiac glycoside administration. For example, while hypertension is not encountered in cardiac glycosides therapy, their use is frequently accompanied by a reduction in blood volume due to their natriuretic and diuretic effect.[29] Maintenance of circulating blood volume during cardiac glycoside administration results in an increase in arterial pressure, which is due to a rise in total peripheral resistance. Cardiac glycosides have also been shown to potentiate the effects of other pressor agents.[30] Thus, some of their effects are not unlike the hypothesized unknown pressor factor referred to previously. However, it was acknowledged by the proponents of this theory that the analogy to cardiac glycosides was not to be taken too strictly because the hypertensive actions proposed for this putative hormone were quite different than the spectrum of cardiovascular activities present in the cardiac glycoside class of drugs.

At the time Overbeck et al. performed these experiments the potential significance of the depressed function of the Na pump was suggested to be a depolarization of the vascular smooth muscle cell membrane, producing vasoconstriction and/or a reduction in the response threshold to vasoconstrictor stimuli. While considerable progress has been made in the concepts of the ionic mechanisms associated with vascular smooth muscle constriction over the past decade, depression of the Na pump would still be considered a factor that predisposes a vascular smooth muscle cell toward a vasoconstrictor state.

Subsequent work by Haddy, Overbeck, and colleagues (reviewed in Reference 31) demonstrated numerous forms of experimental and genetic forms of hypertension in which inhibition of cardiac and/or vascular smooth muscle Na,K-ATPase could be detected. This work has generally been confirmed, and extended to other physiological states that relate to hypertension (see below).

IV. MERGING OF THE NATRIURETIC HORMONE AND HYPERTENSIVE FACTOR HYPOTHESES

In a 1976 review Haddy and Overbeck[3] noted the similarity in the mechanism of action of the putative natriuretic hormone and the hypertensive factor which they and their colleagues had detected in "volume-dependent" forms of hypertension, and hypothesized that a common substance may account for the biological activities attributed to these factors. In their scenario, a renal sodium excretory defect would produce elevated levels of natriuretic hormone as a compensatory action. A potential secondary effect of these elevated levels could be effects on the Na pump in cardiac or vascular smooth muscle.

As part of the evidence in support of their hypothesis, they noted that a uremic state produced a general depression of Na pump activity in different tissues, and that plasma from uremic patients produced a depression of Na pump activity in normal red blood cells (RBC). Their conclusion from these data was that decreased renal function resulted in the appearance of humoral Na pump inhibitory activity.

Subsequent work by several groups of investigators, most notably Poston et al.,[32,33] clearly demonstrated that different states of body fluid imbalance (e.g., cirrhosis) produced a humorally mediated inhibition of blood cell Na pump activity. When considered with the other work in this field, these data suggest that a generalized depression in Na pump activity accompanies many states of disturbed fluid/electrolyte homeostasis and some forms of hypertension.

To be historically accurate, it should be noted that the first suggestion of the existence of a natriuretic hormone which could produce hypertensive effects was from the work of Dahl and colleagues[34] almost a decade prior to the suggestion of Haddy and Overbeck. In their study, Dahl et al. provided evidence that a salt-sensitive hypertensive strain of rats possessed a humoral factor which could produce hypertension. They suggested that the physiological role of this factor was to promote sodium excretion, but that a renal sodium excretory defect resulted in the compensatory elevation of the levels of this substance, which had a secondary action as a hypertensive factor.

Independent evidence in support of the Haddy and Overbeck hypothesis was due to a collaborative effort between our group and that of Brody and Johnson at the University of Iowa. Brody, Johnson, and their collaborators demonstrated that electrolytic lesions of the periventricular tissue surrounding the third ventricle (the anteroventral third ventricle or AV3V) in rats produced animals that were refractory to the development of many forms of hypertension,[35] including forms that Haddy and Overbeck suggested should have a humoral Na pump inhibitor. In preliminary experiments Brody et al. observed that AV3V lesioned rats appeared to have a sodium excretory defect. We then performed a collaborative experiment in which we demonstrated that AV3V lesioned rats not only failed to produce an appropriate natriuretic response to saline expansion, but that they also lacked appropriate circulating levels (compared to saline-expanded controls) of a toad bladder sodium transport inhibitor.[36] In a subsequent communication[37] we suggested that the failure of AV3V lesioned rats to develop hypertension was their inability to produce elevated levels of a Na pump inhibitor. The essential elements of this work were confirmed by Haddy et al.,[38] when they showed that plasma from saline-loaded AV3V lesioned rats did not have the ability to inhibit ouabain-sensitive Rb uptake in vascular tissue.

Further evidence in support of the unitary factor hypothesis was our demonstration (detailed in a subsequent section) that two forms of hypertension in non-human primates were associated with elevated circulating levels of digoxin-like immunoactivity.

To directly test the hypothesis that the natriuretic Na pump inhibitor which we were attempting to isolate had cardiovascular actions, we examined its ability to potentiate the vasoconstrictive actions of known pressor agents (i.e., vascular sensitization) as well as increase mean arterial pressure. Vascular sensitizing and (slow and prolonged) pressor activity were only found in HPLC fractions of plasma from saline-loaded dogs, whereas control plasma extracts had no effects.[39] Because this HPLC fraction had natriuretic, Na pump inhibitory, and digoxin-like activities, we hypothesized that all of these activities might reside in a single substance. The chemical nature of this substance appeared to be peptidic because it was destroyed by acid treatment or enzyme digestion.[15,40]

Subsequent to the above experiments, an enormous body of evidence has appeared examining the existence of endogenous Na pump inhibitors, and their potential relationship to various disease states. The length of this chapter precludes an in-depth examination of the contributions of all the laboratories involved in this field. Rather, the remainder of this chapter reviews the evidence for the types of Na pump inhibitory or digoxin-like factors that have been detected, and the physiological states with which these factors are associated. We further suggest additional lines of research which could strengthen the evidence for endogenous digitalis-like substances.

V. CHARACTERISTICS OF DIGITALIS-LIKE FACTORS

A. CRITERIA

Any discussion of this topic contains both "liberal" and "conservative" points of view (as well as a wide spectrum in between). In this case the conservative view, in essence, demands virtually all the mechanistic actions of a cardiac glycoside before a factor can be granted the title of endogenous digitalis or ouabain-like. The diametrically opposed position would be that anything that could produce inhibition of the Na pump in a given experimental situation could, for those circumstances, produce an effect which might be characterized as ''digitalis-like''. A true digitalis-like factor should inhibit Na,K-ATPase in its isolated form or in an intact cell. A less-frequently used assay is inhibition of ouabain binding to either the isolated enzyme or an isolated cell (or cell membrane). However, the latter assay suffers from a universal drawback of all receptor binding assays, which is the inability to distinguish true agonist competition from a competitive antagonist.

The assays used to detect digitalis or ouabain-like activity include inhibition of isolated Na, K-ATPase, inhibition of sodium or rubidium (an analog of potassium) transport in isolated cells, inhibition of rubidium uptake in isolated blood vessels, binding assays (using ouabain as the competitive ligand), inhibition of sodium transport in isolated anuran bladder, and, perhaps the most controversial, inhibition of digoxin binding to antidigoxin antibodies or the *in vivo* administration of these antibodies to lower blood pressure in hypertensive models. In most of the transport models the specificity of the effect is assessed by demonstrating that the effect is limited to cation transport that is sensitive to cardiac glycoside inhibition (i.e., the Na pump).

One of the earliest sodium transport assays used in this work was the anuran bladder, regarded as a model of the mammalian distal tubule and collecting duct. This assay requires fairly complicated electronics because the bladder is used to form a semipermeable membrane between both sides of an Ussing chamber. An electrical potential difference is generated by the ion transport mechanisms in the bladder cells, and effects in the transport rate are measured as the current required to null the potential difference between both sides of the chamber (i.e., short circuit current). While this assay system is typically not calibrated with ouabain, evidence exists that the majority of electrogenic sodium transport in this tissue is ouabain-sensitive.[15] Problems in the use of this assay are widely differing sensitivities to regulatory factors in the bladders from different animals, the need for stringent requirements in the magnitude and stability of the potential differences generated by a bladder, and problems in performing repeated assays on a single bladder.

Analysis of Na,K-ATPase activity can involve direct measurements of the isolated activity of the enzyme via the hydrolysis of adenosine triphosphate (ATP), or cation transport in intact cells. While it is not difficult to perform consistent assays with these procedures, potential artifacts exist with either method. Solubilization of the enzyme increases its susceptibility to nonreceptor-mediated regulation of activity.[40] While such effects are minimized through the use of intact cells, factors (including hormones; see, e.g., Reference 42) that can alter the intracellular sodium concentration independent of the Na pump will produce changes in Na pump activity. This is because intracellular sodium is an important regulator of Na pump activity.

While the use of a digoxin radioimmunoassay has been considered by some investigators to be prone to potential artifacts, there appear to be a variety of physiological states in which elevated levels of digoxin-like immunoactivity have been detected (discussed in detail below). While detection of endogenous digoxin-like substances should always be confirmed with enzyme or transport inhibition assays (as we did in our original studies[15]), this has not always been the case. Indeed, some authors have suggested that these assays do not correlate, or that known constituents in plasma can account for the "apparent" endogenous digoxin levels reported by investigators. Lau and Valdes[43] have investigated a variety of compounds which have been suggested to account for digoxin-like activity, including fatty acids, phospholipids, and steroid hormones. Under appropriate measurement conditions which can detect endogenous digoxin, none of these substances produced detectable interaction with antidigoxin antibodies or Na,K-ATPase.

Criteria that are often ignored during the isolation of digitalis-like factors are physiological regulation of its presence, and an *in vivo* biological effect at a physiologically relevant concentration. While the latter criteria are not directly related to digitalis-like activity, they would appear to be important if the goal is to isolate a physiological regulator of the Na pump.

Some investigators maintain that appropriate biological testing will occur after the substance they are isolating is identified, i.e., they need all their material for biochemical analysis. However, this point of view has led to an attempt to determine the action of a digitalis-like factor on the conformation of the Na,K-ATPase molecule before evidence for *in vivo* biological activity had been presented,[44] and even prior to definitive knowledge that only one substance was present in the extract being tested. It seems almost axiomatic to suggest that the relative significance of a substance with Na pump inhibitory activity is not necessarily related to how similar its molecular effects are to cardiac glycosides, but rather is dependent on if its effects on sodium transport play a role in physiological or pathophysiological processes.

B. SOURCES

1. Urine

The initial isolation attempts of DeWardener and colleagues[4] and Bricker et al.[53] used urine from saline-loaded or uremic subjects, with inhibition of renal tubule or anuran bladder sodium transport as the assay system. The apparent advantages in using urine as a source of material, e.g., ease of collection and the ability to obtain large amounts of material on a repeated basis, have to be weighed against the disadvantages. Urine is necessarily collected over long periods of time (at least hours), increasing the possibility that the compound of interest might degrade. Further, many hormones are metabolically altered when they appear in urine, often with a consequential loss in biological activity.

Despite these potential difficulties, Kramer and associates[45] have used antidigoxin antibodies to isolate natriuretic activity from the urine of salt-loaded humans. This material appeared to be peptidic in nature, however, it did not inhibit the activity of isolated Na,K-ATPase. In addition, these investigators have reported the existence of two sodium transport inhibitors in their urinary extracts, one of which crossreacted with digoxin antibodies. Both of these inhibitors were elevated after salt loading, and they were able to increase intracellular pH and calcium in isolated vascular smooth muscle, an effect similar to ouabain. The chemical nature of the activity appeared to be peptidic because it was destroyed by enzyme digestion.

Cloix and collaborators[46] have reported the detection and preliminary isolation of digitalis-like activity from urine and plasma in normo- and hypertensive patients, which appeared to be elevated in the hypertensives. Their extract had the ability to inhibit isolated Na,K-ATPase, ouabain binding, active sodium transport, and to crossreact with antidigoxin antibodies. Chemical analysis suggested that the compound responsible for these activities was a glucurosteroid, though no structure was ever proposed. Confirmation of some of this work may be found in the report of Morise et al.,[47] which found that urinary digoxin immunoactivity positively correlated with sodium intake in patients.

Most recent work in this field has moved away from utilizing urine as a starting material to using plasma and tissue instead. However, the latter source has at least one of the disadvantages of urine in that it is difficult to draw a direct relationship to a physiological state (see below).

2. Plasma

a. General Approaches

In contrast to urine, plasma offers the advantage of allowing the immediate monitoring of a biologically relevant amount of sample in a given physiological state. By this we mean that if it is possible to assay for the presence of biological activity in a small volume of plasma, then the factor(s) responsible for the effect are probably present at a concentration which has potential physiological relevance. Such a conclusion is not possible if the starting material for the assay is an extract from a large volume or weight of material.

This analogy points out a potential danger when ''scaling up'' an isolation for large amounts of material. The physiological controls that were initially considered crucial to demonstrating the specificity of the activity being measured are often neglected because their inclusion would in essence double the work load. Substances that would not be detected in small-scale isolations, due to their extremely low levels and/or their absolute loss during extraction, can suddenly appear in apparently significant quantities. The failure to maintain appropriate physiological controls, or to incorporate knowledge of the chemical characteristics of the activities gained from physiologically relevant samples, appears to be a common occurrence when investigators in this area make the transformation from measuring digitalis-like activity in specific physiological states to large-scale isolation procedures.

A recent report from Mathews et al.[48] may be an example of the above problems. They claim to have isolated digitalis-like activity from a large volume of human plasma, which appears to be indistinguishable from ouabain based on mass spectrometric techniques. They further suggest that the natriuretic/hypertensive hormone that other groups have sought to isolate and identify is in fact ouabain synthesized in mammalian tissues (probably the adrenal). While Mathews et al. may well have isolated authentic ouabain from a large quantity of plasma, it has long been appreciated that the organ-specific spectrum of activities that would be needed in a natriuretic/hypertensive hormone are totally different from that present in the cardiac glycoside class of drugs. In particular, based on half-life alone, ouabain could not account for the effects seen in the various *in vivo* assays that investigators in this field have utilized. This is to say nothing of the poor therapeutic index displayed by all cardiac glycosides, a factor that makes them doubtful candidates for physiological regulators.

Finally, in a related article by Harris et al.,[49] the circulating endogenous levels of ouabain in humans are reported to be slightly greater than 100 fmol/ml of plasma. Comparison of this concentration to reports of the plasma concentration of ouabain required for a minimal biological effect clearly suggests a problem of potency. For example, Hougen and Smith[50] have shown that the minimum plasma concentration of ouabain which will effect active cation transport in the heart is approximately 10 pmol/ml, i.e., 100-fold higher than the levels reported by Harris et al. Further review of the literature (see Reference 51 for an excellent discussion of the therapeutic levels of ouabain) indicate that even higher circulating levels of ouabain are needed to produce minimally measurable effects on Na, K-ATPase activity. Thus, it is difficult to believe that the ouabain apparently isolated and assayed by Mathews et al. could account for the effects on vascular Rb uptake seen in the work of Haddy et al.[3,31] or the effects on lymphocyte Rb transport reported by Poston et al.,[32,33] to cite but two examples. Indeed, this is the reason that both our laboratory[15] and that of Godfraind[52] have suggested and provided some evidence that the potency of an endogenous digitalis-like factor would be approximately 1000-fold greater than ouabain.

The initial studies demonstrating the presence of a sodium transport inhibitor were performed with plasma from saline-loaded or uremic subjects.[53,54] A link between many of these studies was the finding that the activity appeared to elute on Sephadex® or Biogel® columns in a postsalt peak fraction, suggesting it was bound on the column rather than being solely retained by molecular sieving.[55] However, dialysis or membrane filtration procedures clearly established that the activity was present in a fraction with a molecular weight <1000.

Subsequent to our demonstration that the anuran bladder sodium transport inhibitor (i.e., the putative natriuretic/hypertensive hormone) eluted in a HPLC fraction that contained pressor agent potentiating, Na,K-ATPase inhibitory, and digoxin-like immunological activity, most work in this field has used some modification of the latter two assays (see subsequent sections), with a concomitant lack of *in vitro* assay verification in an appropriate *in vivo* test system. This has led to the curious situation in which investigators claim to be isolating a natriuretic and/or hypertensive hormone without performing assays that measure sodium excretion or blood pressure.

Nevertheless, a large body of evidence has accumulated that confirms and expands upon the original observations of elevated digitalis-like activity in renal and cardiovascular system-related physiological states.

b. Studies Related to Renal Function

Subsequent to our demonstration of digitalis-like activity in the plasma of volume-expanded dogs,[15] other groups confirmed elevated levels of one or both of these activities in saline expansion, high-salt diets, or renal disease. Gault et al.[56] initially presented evidence that either an intravenous saline load or 5 d of a high-salt diet produced an elevation in plasma digoxin-like immunoactivity. Plasma levels of digoxin-like activity showed a positive and significant correlation with urinary sodium excretion and an inverse correlation with plasma renin activity or aldosterone. Though subsequent work by this group[57] suggested that certain steroids (e.g., dehydroepiandrosterone) could account for some of this activity, studies by Lau and Valdes (discussed previously) indicate that this is unlikely. Work by Hamlyn et al.[58] appeared to confirm some aspects of the relationship between digoxin-like activity and sodium-retaining hormones because they also reported an inverse relationship between plasma digoxin-like activity and aldosterone.

Another approach to the demonstration of a digitalis-like factor in response to saline loading is found in the work of Poston et al.[33] They found lower leukocyte Na pump activity in patients undergoing volume expansion, with the ion transport characteristics of the lymphocytes mediated by the plasma (volume expanded or control) in which the transport incubation was performed. This type of study is perhaps the most direct approach to demonstrating a humoral mediator of ion transport, which can function at a physiological concentration.

Another experimental model that has been used to demonstrate the presence of digitalis-like factors is impaired renal function. Studies of this state are clearly an extension of the work of Bourgoignie and associates[10] on a natriuretic factor which could be isolated from the plasma or urine of uremic subjects. Valdes[59] was the first to systematically examine the ability of digoxin radioimmunoassays to detect an interfering substance in patients with renal impairment who were not receiving digoxin therapy. They found that up to 50% of patients with renal impairment had significant levels of endogenous digoxin, while this substance could be found in only 10% of normal controls. Because the degree of renal dysfunction was not directly related to the presence of the immunoactivity, mere accumulation of an uncleared substance could not account for the effect. Izumo et al.[60] found suppressed erythrocyte Na pump activity in patients with uremia, and were able to correct the defect by hemodialysis, suggesting that the effect was humorally mediated.

Digitalis-like activity, in particular digoxin immunoactivity, has been found in other physiological states that are associated with body fluid imbalance, including pregnancy and liver disease. Many of these investigations were stimulated by the evidence for altered natriuretic hormone levels in models directly or indirectly related to these conditions.

The association of hepatic failure with fluid retention was the initial impetus to examine natriuretic hormone levels in this state. Both Kramer[61] and Favre[62] have shown that edematous (i.e., decompensated), cirrhotic patients do not have natriuretic hormone levels appropriate for their state of volume expansion. Further work by Naccarato et al.[63] in "compensated" cirrhosis (i.e., no history of edema) showed that these patients did not have an appropriate natriuretic response to acute saline loading and lacked appropriate natriuretic hormone levels. Thus, the significance of elevated digoxin-like immunoactivity in several different forms of liver disease[64] (including alcoholic cirrhosis) is potentially confusing because no physiological explanation of what would link these different forms of the disease was provided. While it is conceivable that the radioimmunoassay detects an inactive form of a natriuretic hormone, these data are difficult to interpret without further physiological information on these patients.

Valdes and collaborators[65,66] were the first to report elevated digoxin-like immunoactivity in the blood of pregnant women and newborn infants. Pregnancy is a state that is associated with a considerable degree of volume expansion, and the circulating levels of digoxin-like factor were reduced soon after parturition. The rationale for the elevated levels in infants was not clear.

Other states of elevated endogenous digitalis-like activity related to renal function involve experimental forms of hypertension, and are therefore discussed in the next section.

c. *Studies Related to Cardiovascular Function*

The studies of Haddy and associates[3,31] were the first to systematically investigate the presence of a humorally mediated depression in vascular tissue Na pump activity which accompanied many forms of experimental hypertension. They showed that plasma extracts from different forms of renal hypertension could inhibit ouabain-sensitive potassium transport (i.e., Na,K-ATPase) in vascular tissue. Confirmation and extension of this type of experiment may be found in the work of Poston et al.,[33] who demonstrated that plasma from essential hypertensives had the ability to depress leukocyte Na pump activity.

Given the evidence that endogenous digoxin-like immunoactivity eluted in the same HPLC fraction as Na pump inhibitory and vascular sensitizing/pressor activities, we had some confidence that the immunoactivity measured in our studies was representative of a biologically active substance. We therefore examined the relationship of digoxin-like immunoactivity and arterial pressure in several species of hypertensive nonhuman primates.[67]

In rhesus monkeys, plasma digoxin immunoactivity had a significant and positive correlation ($r > 0.9$) with both systolic and diastolic pressure (Figures 1 and 2). The remarkably strong relationship between this humoral factor and blood pressure in the rhesus suggested that a similar correlation should exist between the transport system supposedly controlled by the factor (i.e., the Na pump) and arterial pressure. In a collaborative series of studies with Ricardo Garay's laboratory[68] we demonstrated that rhesus erythrocyte intracellular sodium, which is mainly controlled by Na pump activity, had a significant correlation with mean arterial pressure (Figure 3).

An unexpected finding in these studies was that the Na pump rate was also directly related to arterial pressure (Figure 4). While the correlation of elevated arterial pressure with high pump activity would initially appear to be the antithesis of the circulating Na pump inhibitor hypothesis, one potential explanation for this was that a humoral factor (presumably endogenous digoxin) inhibited the Na pump on erythrocytes *in vivo,* producing an increase in intracellular sodium. Isolating and

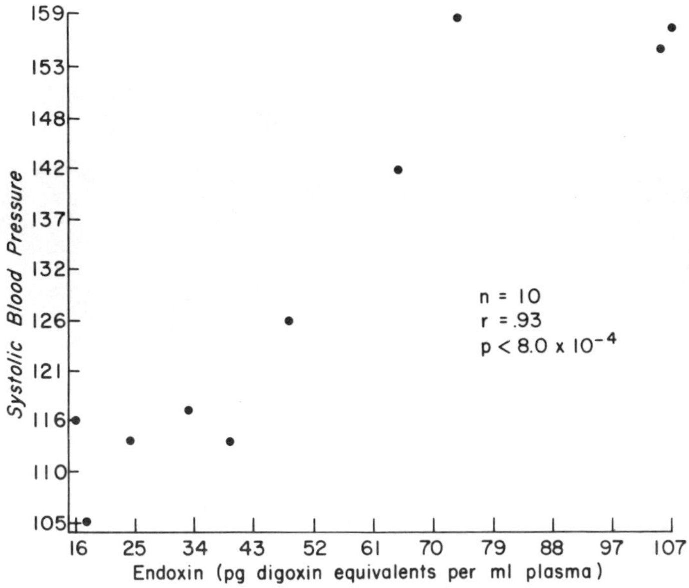

FIGURE 1. Endogenous digoxin immunoactivity in rhesus monkey plasma is plotted against systolic pressure. The correlation coefficient is >0.9.

washing the cells prior to our studies could have removed the inhibitor from the pump, leaving a cell with a high intracellular sodium concentration which in turn acted as a stimulus for pump activity. This hypothesis was strengthened by the fact that the rhesus erythrocyte contains no other sodium transport systems, such as Na-K cotransport. Further, neither Na pump unit number nor passive sodium permeability showed any correlation with arterial pressure.

A second nonhuman primate model of hypertension which we investigated was chronic 2 kidney-1 clip (2K1C) in African green vervets.[67] Our data indicated that the presence of a renal artery clip consistently elevated plasma digoxin-like activity, although only 50% of clipped monkeys presented with hypertension. Initially, critics of the endogenous digoxin-hypertension hypothesis cited the failure of all the clipped monkeys to develop hypertension as evidence against this concept. However, in further work with these monkeys, we showed that both normo- and hypertensive 2K1C monkeys had renal and cardiovascular deficits.[69]

For example, compared to sham-operated controls, the 2K1C groups had an inhibited cardiac baroreceptor reflex, a dependence of arterial pressure on angiotensin II in the face of normal renin activity, and significant azotemia. In retrospect, this work was consistent with the previous reports of elevated levels of a sodium transport inhibitor in renal failure,[10] and was the harbinger of subsequent studies (cited previously) describing elevated endogenous digoxin-like activity in patients with renal disease.

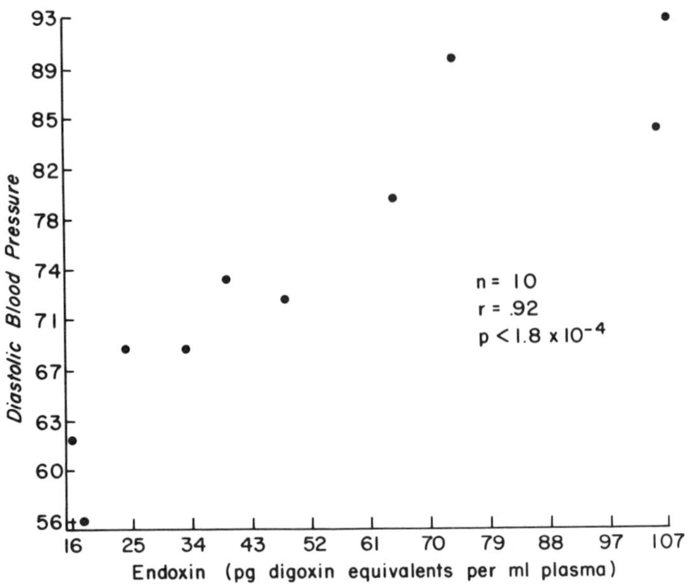

FIGURE 2. Endogenous digoxin immunoactivity in rhesus monkey plasma is plotted against diastolic pressure. The correlation coefficient is >0.9.

Concurrent with our work in rhesus monkeys, Schreiber et al.[70] reported elevated levels of endogenous digoxin in the aortic coarctation model of hypertension in rats. Significant correlations were found between serum digoxin immunoactivity and heart weight when comparing different post-coarctation time groups. The concept of endogenous digoxin as a causative factor in hypertension was strengthened by the approach of Kojima et al.,[71] who demonstrated a marked decrease in blood pressure following the administration of antidigoxin antisera in mineralocorticoid-salt hypertension in rats. While an immune response to the antisera could account for such an effect, administration of the antisera to normotensive controls did not result in a depressor effect. The use of digoxin antibody administration was extended by Huang and Smith[72] to the aortic coarctation model in rats, and once again only the hypertensive group had a depressor response to the antibody. Subsequent work by Kojima[73] in rats with mineralocorticoid-salt hypertension showed elevated ouabain-binding activity in plasma. Chromatographic purification of the binding activity demonstrated that Na,K-ATPase was inhibitory and digoxin-like activities coeluted with it.

Hamlyn et al.[74] were the first to directly measure elevated circulating levels of a Na,K-ATPase inhibitor in essential hypertensives. While the level of activity that they measured correlated with erythrocyte intracellular sodium content, no relationship with plasma digoxin-like activity was apparent. This seeming failure to support a role for endogenous digoxin in hypertension should be assessed in light

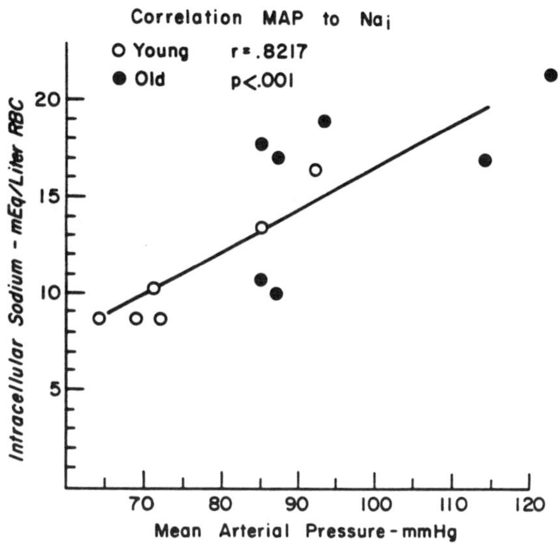

FIGURE 3. The relationship between rhesus monkey erythrocyte intracellular sodium concentration is plotted against the indirect mean arterial pressure taken at the time of sample collection. The linearity of the relationship is >0.8. Young monkeys averaged 3.3 ± 0.3 years, while old monkeys were 15.4 ± 1.0 years.

of the fact that subsequent work from Hamlyn et al.[58] found correlations between digoxin immunoactivity in plasma and aldosterone (an inverse relationship) or catecholamines (a positive relationship) that are consistent with a natriuretic hormone that also has the ability to activate the sympathetic nervous system. A potential explanation for the reported discrepancy is that their radioimmunoassay may have detected biologically active and inactive forms of the same substance. Subsequent work from other laboratories (discussed below) provides evidence that Na,K-ATPase inhibitory activity and digoxin-like immunoactivity in blood can correlate and be related to blood pressure and urinary sodium excretion.

A large body of evidence from China and Japan suggests a relationship between digitalis-like activity with blood pressure or dietary sodium. For example. Liu et al.[75] have reported that digoxin immunoactivity was significantly elevated in Chinese children above the 75th percentile of blood pressure as compared to the lower half of the population. Significant relationships in the entire population studied were also found between the immunoactivity and blood pressure or erythrocyte intracellular sodium content. Takahashi et al.[76] used both a digoxin radioimmunoassay and a Na,K-ATPase assay to examine an adult population in Japan. Endogenous digoxin could be correlated with blood pressure, and this relationship was confirmed by the Na,K-ATPase inhibition assay.

A unique approach to delineating a role for a digitalis-like factor in blood pressure regulation was presented by Graves et al.[77] A potential complication of bone marrow transplants and alkylating agent therapy is severe hypertension. This

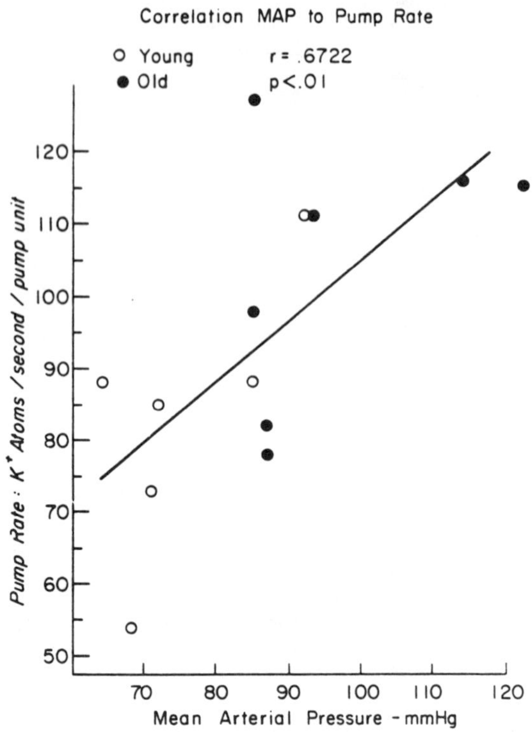

FIGURE 4. The correlation of erythrocyte sodium pump rate to mean arterial pressure is shown. The strongly linear relationship is probably related to the stimulatory effect of elevated intracellular sodium (see Figure 3) on the activity of the sodium pump.

is a unique model because patients can be followed from normo- to hypertension. The changes in mean arterial pressure produced by the treatment could be significantly and positively correlated with the changes in circulating digoxin-like immunoactivity. In addition, the immunoassay in patients was confirmed by a Na,K-ATPase assay, with a highly significant correlation. These data comprise the first longitudinal analysis of digitalis-like activity in hypertension, and strongly suggest that a causal relationship is present.

3. Tissue

Gonick et al.[78] were the first to extract a Na,K-ATPase inhibitor from tissue, using kidneys from saline-loaded animals as the source. This factor appeared to be a peptide because it was destroyed by proteolytic enzymes, and qualified as a candidate for a natriuretic hormone because it was natriuretic and not present in control kidneys. It may be important to note that the spectrum of enzyme susceptibility of this factor reported by Raghavan and Gonick,[79] i.e., sensitive to trypsin and insensitive to chymotrypsin, are identical to what we reported for a sodium transport inhibitor isolated from plasma.[40]

While a variety of groups were attempting to isolate a sodium transport inhibitor due to its potential role as a natriuretic/hypertensive hormone, others were intrigued by the fact that Na,K-ATPase appeared to function as a high affinity receptor for the cardiac glycoside class of drugs. Clearly influenced by the fact that the enkephalins appeared to be the endogenous ligands for opioid receptors, several groups hypothesized that a naturally occurring ligand may exist for the cardiac glycoside binding site on Na,K-ATPase. Both Haupert and Sancho[80] and Fishman[81] reported the preliminary isolation of a substance in the hypothalamus or brain that appeared have digitalis-like properties, including inhibition of ouabain binding, erythrocyte Rb transport, and Na,K-ATPase activity. Lichtstein and Samuelov[82] confirmed these initial observations. However, the digitalis-like factor isolated by all of these groups did not crossreact with antidigoxin antibodies, nor did it appear to be a peptide.

These reports therefore must be contrasted to that of Akagawa et al.,[83] who isolated digitalis-like activity (using inhibition of Na,K-ATPase and ouabain binding as criteria) from bovine hypothalamus which appeared to be sensitive to carboxypeptidase A. Based on the enzyme sensitivity evidence, the digitalis-like substance found by Morgan and colleagues[84] in the medium from cultured rat hypothalamic cells would appear to be quite similar. Carboxypeptidase A was one of several proteolytic enzymes which could destroy Na,K-ATPase inhibitory activity in their extracts. The spectrum of activities that appeared to be associated with this factor included inhibition of the Na pump in erythrocytes and ouabain binding.

Godfraind and Castaneda Hernandez[52] was the first group to report the extraction of a digoxin-like Na,K-ATPase inhibitor from brain (guinea pig). Using a digoxin radioimmunoassay as the basis for calculating molar concentrations, an affinity constant for Na,K-ATPase inhibition approximately 1000-fold higher than digoxin was calculated. This is similar to the potency of the digoxin-like substance that we isolated from the plasma of saline-loaded dogs.[15] Further work by Godfraind's laboratory[85] examined the effect of a high-salt diet in rats on the concentrations of digoxin-like immunoactivity in tissues and serum. While significant levels of immunoactivity were found in all tissues studied, by far the highest levels were present in adrenals. However, increased levels in response to a high-salt diet were found only in serum.

Somewhat different results have been reported by Takahashi and collaborators. They initially reported that digoxin-like immunoactivity was highly localized in the brain, with the highest levels present in the pituitary and hypothalamus.[86] Digoxin immunoactivity was also detected in the plasma and urine. A high-salt diet produced a decrease in hypothalamic levels while markedly increasing concentrations in pituitary and urine. Central administration of colchicine, a drug that blocks axonal transport, produced an increase in hypothalamic immunoactivity and a decrease in plasma levels. In a subsequent study[87] this group found that adrenalectomy did not decrease plasma or the hypothalamic content of digoxin-like immunoactivity. In fact, adrenalectomized rats on a high-salt diet were able to increase their hypothalamic and plasma levels, with a high correlation between assays for tissue content vs. circulating levels. The possibility that a digitalis-like hormone that appears to be activated by changes in sodium balance is released by the pituitary is consistent with the early report of Lichardus and co-workers,[88] suggesting that hypophysectomy impaired the renal response to volume expansion in rats.

The possibility that antidigoxin antibodies recognize a digitalis-like substance has led to the use of these antibodies in immunohistochemical studies. Yamada et al.[89] first reported the presence of immunoreactive material in cell bodies and nerve tracts of the supraoptic and paraventricular nuclei of the hypothalamus. The major projection appeared to be to the posterior pituitary and hypophyseal portal vessels. No immunoactivity was seen in sections of the anterior pituitary, adrenal gland, or kidney. A subsequent study from these investigators[90] suggested that some of the digoxin immunoactivity coexisted in neurons which also stained for vasopressin or oxytocin. Colchicine treatment was again able to increase the apparent hypothalamic content of digoxin immunoactivity, suggesting it was normally moved away from these areas by axonal transport. Finally, antibodies against a different cardiac glycoside, digitoxin, were unable to detect any immunoactive neurons in the hypothalamus.

The ability of certain adrenal steroids to produce "false" digoxin immunoactivity has long been appreciated. While known steroid hormones do not circulate in levels which, based on their relative crossreactivity with antidigoxin antibodies, could account for the reported levels of endogenous digoxin, the existence of an unknown adrenal steroid has been postulated. LaBella et al.[91,92] have been particularly active in assessing the structural requirements for binding to Na,K-ATPase and for the production of a positive inotropic action. They have presented evidence that progesterone derivatives can interact with the cardiac glycoside binding site on Na,K-ATPase, producing varying degrees of inotropy. However, no evidence can be found that these compounds are candidates for a putative natriuretic/pressor hormone.

Other approaches for investigating the possible adrenal origin of an endogenous digitalis have included the assay of adrenal extracts, or combining pharmacological manipulation of adrenal steroid secretion with assays for circulating digitalis-like activity. Schreiber and colleagues[93] detected digitalis-like activity in adrenal extracts using both digoxin immunoassays and inhibition of Rb uptake by erythrocytes. Shilo et al.[94] have manipulated circulating levels of digoxin immunoactivity in normal patients with dexamethasone (an inhibitor of adrenocortical secretion) and adrenocorticotrophic hormone (ACTH). The reported effects were consistent with an adrenal origin for an endogenous digoxin.

Doris[95] also used a digoxin radioimmunoassay to assess the levels of endogenous digoxin immunoactivity in extracts of various organs of the rat. Only the adrenal produced consistent displacement of digoxin tracer. Further, plasma levels of digoxin-like immunoactivity were significantly reduced following bilateral adrenalectomy. However, in subsequent studies, Doris and Stocco[96] reported that aminoglutathimide (a steroid hormone synthesis antagonist) was unable to inhibit the release of digoxin-like immunoactivity from incubated rat adrenal slices, and that ether stress (a stimulator of corticosterone secretion) lowered plasma levels of endogenous digoxin. Though these investigators presented evidence that the immunoactivity released by adrenals *in vitro* could compete with ouabain in a binding assay at some dilutions, an incomplete binding curve was performed. Thus, it was impossible to assess if competitive binding was being detected. In addition, a comparison of the antibody displacement curves comparing adrenal extracts to cold digoxin indicates that parallel displacement was not always seen (compare to References 95 and 96).

4. Cerebrospinal Fluid

Hormones that are synthesized and released by the central nervous system often appear in significant quantities in cerebrospinal fluid (CSF). Changes in the CSF levels of these hormones can be reflective of alterations in circulating levels. In consideration of this and the evidence for a central nervous system origin of circulating digitalis-like activity, Halperin et al.[97] investigated the presence of digitalis-like activity in CSF via isolated Na,K-ATPase and erythrocyte Rb uptake studies. Activity was detected in CSF, and was shown to be increased during extracellular saline expansion. Purification of the activity suggested that it was a low molecular weight peptide because the purified activity appeared to be sensitive to proteolytic enzymes.[98]

One potential action of a digitalis-like substance in the CSF is regulation of CSF composition. Most solute transport into the CSF is via the choroid plexus, and the secretory rate and composition of CSF from choroid plexus epithelial cells is directly linked to the Na pump activity of the cell. The anatomical location of the Na pump is on the CSF surface of these epithelial cells, allowing potential regulatory influence from CSF factors.

VI. CONCLUSIONS

The evidence discussed above strongly suggests the existence of at least two classes of endogenous digitalis-like substances, one of which appears to be peptidic. Based on the available data, the best candidate for a natriuretic/hypertensive hormone would appear to be a peptide(s) that is synthesized in the hypothalamus and released through transport to the posterior pituitary. The circulating levels and urinary excretion appear to be affected by changes in sodium balance.

This substance may at times exist in a form that has antigenic determinants which allow it to be recognized by antidigoxin antibodies. A potential explanation for this is that the chemical groups contributing to the recognition may be important for binding to transport proteins in blood. The basis for this hypothesis is that the 12β hydroxyl group of digoxin is the only point in its structure in which it differs from digitoxin, yet this hydroxyl group governs the large difference in plasma protein binding between these two cardiac glycosides. If antibodies that are specific for digoxin, but not digitoxin, recognize an endogenous factor, then it is likely that the antigenic determinant in digoxin which is recognized by the antibody includes the 12β hydroxyl. Rather than the antibody serving as a model of the Na,K-ATPase binding site, as we initially hypothesized, it may be serving as a model of the plasma protein binding site for digoxin.

However, the data do not exclude the additional possibility of a nonpeptidic digitalis-like substance. This concept excludes clear artifacts such as lipids and fatty acids, but includes the potential of an adrenal steroid with some digitalis-like properties. However, while several groups appear to have isolated a nonpeptidic ouabain-like substance, little evidence exists for physiological alterations in the tissue or circulating levels of this substance(s).

In contrast, the substance or substances that have the properties of a peptide have consistently been shown to be elevated in states of body fluid imbalance. Whether the peptide-like substance has as many ouabain-like properties as the nonpeptide factor remains to be determined, but its physiological significance would appear to be more firmly established.

One of the potential difficulties in the isolation of substances with digitalis-like properties is the existence in biological extracts of many substances which can produce "apparent" digitalis-like actions. Performing experiments with all the appropriate biochemical controls can result not only in a large number of assays, but also in the use of most (if not all) of the material of interest. It is for this reason that physiological controls (discussed above) offer an attractive alternative to rapidly eliminate fractionated material which appears to have some digitalis-like properties, but whose level of activity fails to change after appropriate physiological manipulation.

It is also possible to use the chemical properties (e.g., enzyme or acid lability) of the crude extract from physiological studies as a standard which must be met by a potentially interesting fraction during large-scale isolation procedures.

In conclusion, despite the enormous literature that has been produced in this field during the 1980s, it is clear that the final chapter has yet to be written on the existence and physiological significance of digitalis-like substances.

REFERENCES

1. **DeWardener, H. E. and Clarkson, E. M.,** Concept of a natriuretic hormone, *Physiol. Rev.*, 65, 658, 1985.
2. **Kelly, R. A.,** Endogenous cardiac glycosidelike compounds, *Hypertension,* 10(Suppl. I), I-87, 1987.
3. **Haddy, F. J. and Overbeck, H. W.,** The role of humoral agents in volume-expanded hypertension, *Life Sci.*, 19, 935, 1976.
4. **DeWardener, H. E., Mills, I. H., Clapham, W. F., and Hayter, C. J.,** Studies on the efferent mechanism of the sodium diuresis which follows the administration of intravenous saline in the dog, *Clin. Sci.*, 21, 249, 1961.
5. **Levinski, N. S. and Lalone, R. C.,** The mechanism of sodium diuresis after saline infusion in the dog, *J. Clin. Invest.*, 42, 1261, 1963.
6. **Johnston, C. I. and Davis, J. O.,** Evidence from cross circulation studies for a humoral mechanism in the natriuresis of saline loading, *Proc. Soc. Exp. Biol. Med.*, 121, 1058, 1966.
7. **Smith, H. W.,** Salt and water volume receptors: an exercise in physiologic apologetics, *Am. J. Med.*, 23, 623, 1957.

8. **Cort, J. H., Dousa, T., Pliska, V., Lichardus, B., Safarova, J., Vranesik, M., and Rudinger, J.,** Saluretic activity of blood during carotid occlusion in the cat, *Am. J. Physiol.,* 215, 921, 1968.
9. **Buckalew, V. M., Jr., Martinez, F. J., and Green, W. E.,** The effect of dialysates, and ultrafiltrates of plasma of saline loaded dogs on toad blauder sodium transport, *J. Clin. Invest.,* 49, 926, 1970.
10. **Bourgoignie, J. J., Klahr, S., and Bricker, N. S.,** Inhibition of transepithelial sodium transport in the frog skin by a low molecular weight fraction of uremic serum, *J. Clin. Invest.,* 50, 303, 1971.
11. **Keeler, R.,** Effect of chronic preoptic lesions on the renal excretion of sodium in rats, *Am. J. Physiol.,* 228, 1725, 1975.
12. **Kaloyanides, G. J., Balabanian, M. B., and Bowman, R. I.,** Evidence that the brain participates in the humoral natriuretic mechanism of blood volume expansion in the dog, *J. Clin. Invest.,* 62, 1288, 1978.
13. **Kramer, H. J., Gonick, H. C., Paul, W., Lu, E.,** Third factor: inhibitor of Na-K-ATPase?, *Proc. 4th Int. Cong. Nephrol. (Stockholm, 1969),* Abstr. I (Free Communications) S. Karger, Basel, 1970, p. 373.
14. **Gonick, H. C., Kramer, H. J., Paul, W., and Lu, E.,** Circulating inhibitor of sodium potassium activated adenosine triphosphatase after expansion of extracellular fluid volume in rats, *Clin. Sci. Mol. Med.,* 53, 329, 1977.
15. **Gruber, K. A., Whitaker, J. M., and Buckalew, V. M., Jr.,** Endogenous digitalis-like substance in plasma of volume-expanded dogs, *Nature,* 287, 743, 1980.
16. **Ahmed, K. and Williams-Ashman, H. G.,** Studies on the microsomal sodium-plus-potassium ion-stimulated adenosine triphosphatase system in rat ventral prostate, *Biochem. J.,* 113, 829, 1969.
17. **Cantley, L. C.,** Vanadate is a potent (Na,K)-ATPase inhibitor found in ATP derived from muscle, *J. Biol. Chem.,* 252, 7421, 1977.
18. **Flier, J. S.,** Ouabain-like activity in toad skin and its implications for endogenous regulation of ion transport, *Nature,* 274, 285, 1978.
19. **Gruber, K. A. and Buckalew, V. M., Jr.,** Further characterization and evidence for a precursor in the formation of plasma antinatriferic activity, *Proc. Soc. Exp. Biol. Med.,* 159, 463, 1978.
20. **Burnett, G. H. and Conklin, R. L.,** The enzymatic assay of plasma digoxin, *J. Lab. Clin. Med.,* 78, 779, 1971.
21. **Lowenstein, J. M.,** A method for measuring plasma levels of digitalis glycosides, *Circulation,* 31, 228, 1965.
22. **Gibson, T. P. and Nelson, H. A.,** Evidence for accumulation of digoxin metabolites in renal failure, *J. Clin. Res.,* 64, 665A, 1979.
23. **Solandt, D. Y., Nassim, R., and Cowan, C. R.,** Hypertensive effect of blood from hypertensive dogs, *Lancet,* 1, 873, 1940.
24. **McAllister, R. G., Jr., Van Way, C. W., III, Dayani, K. et al.,** Malignant hypertension: effect of therapy on renin and aldosterone, *Circ. Res.,* 29(Suppl. II), 160, 1971.
25. **Mizukoshi, H. and Michelakis, A.,** Evidence for the existence of a sensitizing factor to pressor agents in plasma of hypertensive patients, *J. Clin. Endocrinol. Metab.,* 34, 1016, 1972.
26. **Overbeck, H. W.,** Vascular responses to cations, osmolality, and angiotensin in renal hypertensive dogs, *Am. J. Physiol.,* 223, 1358, 1972.
27. **Chen, W. T., Brace, R. A., Scott, J. B., Anderson, D. K., and Haddy, F. J.,** The mechanism of the vasodilatory action of potassium, *Proc. Soc. Exp. Biol. Med.,* 140, 820, 1972.
28. **Overbeck, H. W., Pamnani, M. B., Akera, T., Brody, T. M., and Haddy, F. J.,** Depressed function of a ouabain-sensitive sodium-potassium pump in blood vessels from renal hypertensive dogs, *Circ. Res.,* 38(Suppl. II), II-48, 1976.
29. **Haddy, F. J. and Scott, J. B.,** Mechanism of the acute pressor action of hypokalemia, hypomagnesemia, and hypoosmolality, *Am. Heart J.,* 85, 655, 1973.
30. **Guthrie, G. P.,** Effects of digoxin on responsiveness to the pressor actions of angiotensin and norepinephrine in man, *J. Clin. Endocrinol. Metab.,* 58, 76, 1984.

31. **Haddy, F. J. and Pamnani, M. B.,** Natriuretic hormones in low renin hypertension, *Klin. Wochenschr.*, 65 (Suppl. VIII), 154, 1987.
32. **Poston, L., Wilkinson, S. P., and Williams, R.,** Inhibition of leukocyte sodium transport by the natriuretic factor of human urine: demonstration of the lack of the factor in cirrhotic patients retaining sodium, in *Hormonal Regulation of Sodium Transport,* Lichardus, B., Schrier, R. W., and Ponec, J., Eds., Elsevier/North-Holland, Amsterdam, 1980, 373.
33. **Poston, L., Wilkinson, S., Sewell, R. B., and Williams, R.,** Sodium transport during the natriuresis of volume expansion: a study using peripheral blood leukocytes, *Clin. Sci.*, 63, 243, 1982.
34. **Knudsen, K. D., Iwai, H., Heine, M., Leitl, G., and Dahl, L. K.,** Genetic influence of the development of renoprival hypertension in parabiotic rats, *J. Exp. Med.*, 130, 1353, 1969.
35. **Brody, M. J., Fink, G. D., Buggy, J., Haywood, J. R., Gordon, F. J., and Johnson, A. K.,** The role of the anteroventral third ventricle (AV3V) region in experimental hypertension, *Circ. Res.*, 43(Suppl. I), I-2, 1978.
36. **Bealer, S. L., Haywood, J. R., Johnson, A. K., Gruber, K. A., Buckalew, V. M., Jr., and Brody, M. J.,** Impaired natriuresis and secretion of natriuretic hormone (NH) in rats with lesions of the anteroventral third ventricle (AV3V) region, *Fed. Proc.*, 38, 1232, 1979.
37. **Bealer, S. L., Haywood, J. R., Gruber, K. A., Buckalew, V. M., Jr., Fink, G. D., Brody, M. J., and Johnson, A. K.,** Preoptic-hypothalamic periventricular lesions reduce natriuresis to volume expansion, *Am. J. Physiol.*, 244 (Reg. Integr. Comp. Physiol. 13), R51, 1983.
38. **Huot, S. J., Pamnani, M. B., Clough, D. L., Buggy, J., Bryant, H. J., Harder, D. R., and Haddy, F. J.,** Sodium-potassium pump activity in reduced renal mass hypertension, *Hypertension,* 5(Suppl. I), 94, 1983.
39. **Plunkett, W. C., Hutchins, P. M., Gruber, K. A., and Buckalew, V. M., Jr.,** Evidence for a vascular sensitizing factor in plasma of saline-loaded dogs, *Hypertension,* 4, 581, 1982.
40. **Gruber, K. A. and Buckalew, V. M., Jr.,** Evidence that natriuretic factor is a cascading peptide hormone system, in *Hormonal Regulation of Sodium Excretion,* Lichardus, B., Schrier, R. W., and Ponec, J., Eds., Elsevier/North-Holland, Amsterdam, 1980, 349.
41. **Ng, Y.-C., Akera, T., Han, C.-S., Braselton, W. E., and Kennedy, R. H.,** Ascorbic acid: an endogenous inhibitor of isolated Na,K ATPase, *Biochem. Pharmacol.*, 34, 2525, 1985.
42. **Kim, D. and Smith, T. W.,** Effect of thyroid hormone on sodium pump sites, sodium content, and contractile response to cardiac glycosides in cultured chick ventricular cells, *J. Clin. Invest.*, 74, 1481, 1984.
43. **Lau, B. W. C. and Valdes, R., Jr.,** Criteria for identifying endogenous compounds as digoxin-like immunoreactive factors in humans, *Clin. Chim. Acta,* 175, 67, 1988.
44. **Haber, E. and Haupert, G. T.,** The search for a hypothalamic Na,K-ATPase inhibitor, *Hypertension,* 9, 315, 1987.
45. **Kramer, H. J., Meyer-Lehnert, H., Michel, H., and Predel, H.-G.,** Endogenous natriuretic and ouabain-like factors, *Am. J. Hypertension,* 4, 81, 1991.
46. **Cloix, J.-F.,** What is new in the chemistry of endogenous digitalis-like compounds, *News Physiol. Sci.*, 5(October), 204, 1990.
47. **Morise, T., Miyamori, I., Hifumi, S. et al.,** Effect of sodium intake on the excretion of urinary natriuretic factor in essential hypertensives, *Endocrinol. Jpn.*, 32, 405, 1985.
48. **Mathews, W. R., DuCharme, D. W., Hamlyn, J. M., Harris, D. W., Mandel, F., Clark, M. A., and Ludens, J. H.,** Mass spectral characterization of an endogenous digitalislike factor from human plasma, *Hypertension,* 17, 930, 1991.
49. **Harris, D. W., Clark, M. A., Fisher, J. F., Hamlyn, J. M., Kolbasa, K. P., Ludens, J. H., and DuCharme, D. W.,** Development of an immunoassay for endogenous digitalislike factor, *Hypertension,* 17, 936, 1991.
50. **Hougen, T. J. and Smith, T. W.,** Inhibition of myocardial monovalent cation active transport by subtoxic doses of ouabain in the dog, *Circ. Res.*, 42, 856, 1978.
51. **Noble, D.,** Mechanism of action of therapeutic levels of cardiac glycosides, *Cardiovasc. Res.*, 14, 495, 1980.

52. **Godfraind, T. and Castaneda Hernandez, G.,** Properties of a digitalis-like factor extracted from guinea pig brain, *Arch. Int. Pharmacodyn. Ther.*, 250, 316, 1981.
53. **Bourgoignie, J., Hwang, K., Espinel, C., Klahr, S., and Bricker, N. S.,** A natriuretic factor in the serum of patients with chronic uremia, *J. Clin. Invest.*, 51, 1514, 1972.
54. **Kramer, H. J.,** Antinatriferic and natriuretic activities in human plasma following acute and chronic salt loading, in *Natriuretic Hormone,* Kramer, H. J. and Kruck, F., Eds., Springer-Verlag, New York, 1978, 24.
55. **Buckalew, V. M.,** Column chromatography of plasma antinatriferic activity, in *Natriuretic Hormones,* Kramer, H. J. and Kruck, F., Eds., Springer-Verlag, New York, 1978, 131.
56. **Gault, M. H., Vasdev, S. C., Longerich, L. L. et al.,** Plasma digitalis-like factor(s) increase with salt loading, *N. Engl. J. Med.*, 309, 1459, 1983.
57. **Vasdev, S., Longerich, L., Johnson, L., Brent, E., and Gault, M. H.,** Dehydroepiandrosterone sulfate as a digitalis like factor in plasma of healthy adults, *Res. Commun. Chem. Pathol. Pharmacol.*, 49, 387, 1985.
58. **Hamlyn, J. M., Levinson, P. D., Ringel, R., Levin, P. A., Hamilton, B. P., Blaustein, M. P., and Kowarski, A. A.,** Relationships among endogenous digitalis-like factors in essential hypertension, *Fed. Proc.*, 44, 2782, 1985.
59. **Valdes, R., Jr.,** Endogenous digoxin-immunoactive factor in human subjects, *Fed. Proc.*, 44, 2800, 1985.
60. **Izumo, H., Izumo, S., DeLuise, M., and Flier, J. S.,** Erythrocyte Na,K pump in uremia. Acute correction of a transport defect by hemodialysis, *J. Clin. Invest.*, 74, 581, 1984.
61. **Kramer, H. J.,** Natriuretic hormone, its possible role in fluid and electrolyte disturbances in chronic liver disease, *Postgrad. Med. J.*, 51, 532, 1975.
62. **Favre, H.,** Role of the natriuretic factor in the disorders of sodium balance, in *Advances in Nephrology,* Vol. 11, Hamburger, J., Crosnier, J., and Maxwell, M. H., Eds., Yearbook Medical Publishers, Chicago, IL
63. **Naccarato, R., Messa, P., Gregolin, C., and Zanon, G.,** Renal handling of sodium and water in early chronic liver disease, *Gastroenterology,* 81, 205, 1981.
64. **Nanji, A. A. and Greenway, D. C.,** Falsely raised plasma digoxin concentrations in liver disease, *Br. Med. J.*, 290, 432, 1985.
65. **Graves, S. W., Valdes, R., Jr., Brown, B., Knight, A. B., and Craig, H. R.,** Endogenous digoxin-immunoreactive substance in human pregnancies, *J. Clin. Endocrinol. Metab.*, 58, 748, 1984.
66. **Valdes, R., Jr., Graves, S. W., Brown, B. A., and Landt, M.,** Endogenous substance in newborn infants causing false positive digoxin measurements, *J. Pediatr.*, 102, 947, 1983.
67. **Gruber, K. A., Rudel, L. L., and Bullock, B. C.,** Increased circulating levels of an endogenous digoxin-like factor in hypertensive monkeys, *Hypertension,* 4, 348, 1982.
68. **Hennessy, J. F., Buckalew, V. M., Jr., Gruber, K. A., Ober, K. P., Bullock, B., Hannaert, P., and Garay, R.,** Ion transport characteristics in rhesus monkey erythrocytes: relationship to age and blood pressure, *Clin. Exp. Hypertension,* A6, 961, 1984.
69. **Gruber, K. A., Metzler, C. H., Robinson, T. E. J., Buggy, J., Bullock, B. C., and Lymangrover, J. R.,** Cardiovascular investigations of an endogenous digoxin-like factor, *Fed. Proc.*, 44, 2795, 1985.
70. **Schreiber, V., Kolbel, F., Stepan, J., Gregorova, I., and Pribyl, T.,** Digoxin-like immunoreactivity in the serum of rats with cardiac overload, *J. Mol. Cell. Cardiol.*, 13, 107, 1981.
71. **Kojima, I., Yoshihara, S., and Ogata, E.,** Involvement of endogenous digitalis-like substance in genesis of deoxycorticosterone-salt hypertension, *Life Sci.*, 30, 1775, 1982.
72. **Huang, C. T. and Smith, R. M.,** Lowering of blood pressure in chronic aortic coarctate hypertensive rats with anti-digoxin antiserum, *Life Sci.*, 35, 115, 1984.
73. **Kojima, I.,** Circulating digitalis-like substance is increased in DOCA-salt hypertension, *Biochem. Biophys. Res. Commun.*, 122, 129, 1984.
74. **Hamlyn, J. M., Ringel, R., Schaeffer, J., Levinson, P. D., Hamilton, B. P., Kowarski, A. A., and Blaustein, M. P.,** A circulating inhibitor of (Na + K)ATPase associated with essential hypertension, *Nature,* 300, 650, 1982.

75. **Liu, Z.-Q., Yao, R.-G., and Yang, D.-Y.,** Endogenous digoxin-like substance as an important factor in the development of hypertension in children, *Int. J. Cardiol.*, 29, 343, 1990.
76. **Takahashi, H., Matsusawa, M., Okabayashi, H., Suga, K., Ikegaki, I., Nishimura, M., and Yoshimura, M.,** Endogenous digitalislike substance in an adult population in Japan, *Am. J. Hypertension,* 1, 168S, 1988.
77. **Graves, S. W., Eder, J. P., Schryber, S. M., Sharma, K., Brena, A., Antman, K. H., and Peters, W. P.,** Endogenous digoxin-like immunoreactive factor and digitalis-like factor associated with the hypertension of patients receiving multiple alkylating agents as part of autologous bone marrow transplants, *Clin. Sci.*, 77, 501, 1989.
78. **Hillyard, S. D., Lu, E., and Gonick, H. C.,** Further characterization of the natriuretic factor derived from kidney tissue of volume-expanded rats, *Circ. Res.*, 38, 250, 1976.
79. **Raghaven, S. R. V. and Gonick, H. C.,** Partial purification and characterization of natriuretic factor from rat kidney, *Proc. Soc. Exp. Biol. Med.*, 164, 101, 1980.
80. **Haupert, G. T. and Sancho, J. M.,** Sodium transport inhibitor from bovine hypothalamus, *Proc. Natl. Acad. Sci. U.S.A.*, 76, 4658, 1979.
81. **Fishman, M. C.,** Endogenous digitalis-like activity in mammalian brain, *Proc. Natl. Acad. Sci. U.S.A.*, 76, 4661, 1979.
82. **Lichtstein, D. and Samuelov, S.,** Endogenous ''ouabain like'' activity in rat brain, *Biochem. Biophys. Res. Commun.*, 96, 1518, 1980.
83. **Akagawa, K., Hara, N., and Tsukada, Y.,** Partial purification and properties of the inhibitors of Na,K-ATPase and ouabain-binding in bovine central nervous system, *J. Neurochem.*, 42, 775, 1984.
84. **Morgan, K., Lewis, M. D., Spurlock, G., Collins, P. A., Foord, S. M., Southgate, K., Scanlon, M. F., and Mir, M. A.,** Characterization and partial purification of the sodium-potassium ATPase inhibitor released from cultured rat hypothalamic cells, *J. Biol. Chem.*, 260, 13595, 1985.
85. **Castaneda-Hernandez, G. and Godfraind, T.,** Effect of high sodium intake on tissue distribution of endogenous digitalis-like material in the rat, *Clin. Sci.*, 66, 225, 1984.
86. **Takahashi, H., Matsuzawa, M., Okabayashi, H., Suga, K., Ikegaki, I., Yoshimura, M., and Ijichi, H.,** Evidence for a digitalis-like substance in the hypothalamo-pituitary axis in rats, *J. Hypertension,* 4(Suppl. 6), S317, 1986.
87. **Takahashi, H., Matsusawa, M., Ikegaki, I., Suga, K., Nishimura, M., Yoshimura, M., Yamada, H., and Sano, Y.,** Digitalis-like substance is produced in the hypothalamus but not in the adrenal gland in rats, *J. Hypertension,* 6(Suppl. 4), S345, 1988.
88. **Bencsath, P., Szenasi, G., Ponec, J., Takacs, L., and Lichardus, B.,** Renal sodium excretion in acutely hypophysectomized rats with expanded extracellular fluid volume, in *Hormonal Regulation of Renal Sodium Excretion,* Lichardus, B., Schrier, R. W., and Ponec, J., Eds., Elsevier/North Holland, Amsterdam, 1980, 299.
89. **Yamada, H., Ihara, N., and Sano, Y.,** Morphological evidence of endogenous digitalis-like substance (EDLS) in the rat and macaque hypothalamus using digoxin-immunohistochemistry, *Endocrinol. Jpn.*, 34, 319, 1987.
90. **Ihara, N., Yuri, K., Yamada, H., and Sano, Y.,** Immunohistochemical studies on the distribution of endogenous digitalis-like substance (EDLS)-containing neurons in the rat hypothalamus, with special consideration on the possibility of their coexistence with posterior lobe hormones, *Arch. Histol. Cytol.*, 51, 35, 1988.
91. **Kim, R. S. and LaBella, F. S.,** Endogenous ligands and modulators of the digitalis receptor: some candidates, *Pharmacol. Ther.*, 14, 391, 1981.
92. **Templeton, J. F., Kumar, P. S., Bose, D., Smyth, D. D., Kim, R. S., and LaBella, F. S.,** Digitalis-like pregnanes. Cardiac and renal effects of a glycoside of 14B-hydroxyprogesterone, *Can. J. Physiol. Pharmacol.*, 66, 1420, 1988.
93. **Schreiber, V., Gregorova, I., Pribyl, T., and Stepan, J.,** Digitalis-like biological activity and immunoreactivity in chromatographic fractions of rabbit adrenal extract, *Endocrinol. Exp.*, 15, 299, 1981.

94. **Shilo, L., Dolev, S., Shapiro, M. S., and Shenkman, L.,** Endogenous digoxin-like material is of adrenal origin, *Isr. J. Med. Sci.*, 23, 294, 1987.
95. **Doris, P. A.,** Immunological evidence that the adrenal gland is a source of an endogenous digitalis-like factor, *Endocrinology,* 123, 240, 1988.
96. **Doris, P. A. and Stocco, D. M.,** An endogenous digitalis-like factor derived from the adrenal gland: studies of adrenal tissue from various sources, *Endocrinology,* 125, 2573, 1989.
97. **Halperin, J., Schaeffer, R., Galves, L., and Malave, S.,** Ouabain-like activity in human cerebrospinal fluid, *Proc. Natl. Acad. Sci. U.S.A.*, 80, 6101, 1983.
98. **Halperin, J. A., Riordan, J. F., and Tosteson, D. C.,** Characteristics of an inhibitor of the Na/K pump in human cerebrospinal fluid, *J. Biol. Chem.*, 263, 646, 1988.

Chapter 9

ATRIAL NATRIURETIC PEPTIDE, SODIUM TRANSPORT SYSTEMS, AND ESSENTIAL HYPERTENSION

Josep Closas, Jean R. Cusson, and Pierre Larochelle

TABLE OF CONTENTS

I. Introduction 184

II. Some Highlights in ANP Research (1981–1991) 184
  A. Discovery of ANP and First Investigations of its Production and Actions 184
  B. ANP and Human Subjects 185

III. Role of ANP in Essential Hypertension 185

IV. ANP and Sodium Transport Systems 187
  A. ANP Actions on Kidney Cells 187
  B. ANP Actions on Vascular Smooth Muscle Cells 188
  C. ANP Actions on Intestinal Cells 190
  D. Summary 190

V. ANP, Sodium Transport Systems, and Essential Hypertension 190

VI. Summary and Future Prospects 191

References 191

0-8493-5474-9/94/$0.00 + $.50

I. INTRODUCTION

Atrial natriuretic peptide (ANP) is one of the circulating hormones with blood pressure related biological actions which has been intensively studied in the last decade. The involvement of ANP in the pathophysiology of hypertensive disorders and its therapeutic potential as an antihypertensive agent have been explored in some detail. The purpose of this chapter is to review the available data on ANP and sodium transport systems. However, a brief overview on ANP and a more specific discussion of some aspects of the involvement of ANP in hypertensive disorders are initially presented. The current knowledge on ANP has been the subject of several excellent reviews to which the reader is referred.[1-3]

II. SOME HIGHLIGHTS IN ANP RESEARCH (1981–1991)

A. DISCOVERY OF ANP AND FIRST INVESTIGATIONS OF ITS PRODUCTION AND ACTIONS

Adolfo de Bold performed the critical experiment of injecting cardiac extracts in rats.[4] He showed the diuretic and hypotensive actions of the atrial extracts which contained specific granules that had been discovered 35 years earlier.[5] Soon, numerous investigators throughout the world explored this exciting research area. The 28-amino acid structure of ANP was elucidated.[6,7] The importance of atrial stretch as a stimulus for ANP secretion from the heart into the bloodstream was suggested[8] and clearly demonstrated[9] experimentally. The development of the radioimmunoassay for ANP was significant,[10] and subsequently, several molecular forms of ANP were found in blood.[11,12] The importance of the disulfide bound for the biological activity of ANP was demonstrated.[13] Early on, it became apparent that ANP had multiple actions on several target organs. For example, ANP can reduce blood pressure through a variety of mechanisms: a reduction in cardiac output and/or heart rate,[14] a reduction in plasma volume,[15] and a reduction in peripheral resistances.[16] The renal effects of ANP are also quite complex. ANP produces marked diuresis and natriuresis[4] through direct glomerular changes,[17,18] but also without changes in glomerular filtration rate.[19] Additionally, evidence exists for direct tubular actions of ANP,[1-3] and ANP also causes the suppression of aldosterone production.[20]

ANP is a peptidic hormone that interacts with specific membrane receptors.[1-3] Relaxation of arterial smooth muscle, the inhibition of aldosterone production, and the glomerular actions of ANP can be linked to specific receptor sites.[1-3] The degradation of ANP is also linked to specific "clearance" receptors.[21] Interaction between ANP and the receptor coupled to guanylate cyclase leads to guanosine 3′,5′-cyclic monophosphate (cGMP) production.[22] cGMP is thought to be the second messenger of ANP. ANP dose dependently stimulates cGMP production[23,24] and the measurement of cGMP in plasma and urine can serve as a useful marker of the biological activity of ANP.[23] Ultimately, several actions of ANP are linked to alterations in membrane sodium transport. This is discussed in detail below.

TABLE 1
Plasma ANP Levels in Untreated Essential Hypertension in Studies With Available Data on Age and Blood Pressure

Hypertensive patients				Normotensive controls				
N	Age (years)	MAP (mmHg)	ANP (pmol/l)	N	Age (years)	MAP (mmHg)	ANP (pmol/l)	Ref.
44	47	115	4	48	45	90	4	37
32	55	122	13	61	52	97	11	38
62	51	117	9	38	20–50	100	12	39
35	45	107	19	20	46	85	13	40
20	22–68	113	66[a]	9	20–71	93	25	41
43	53	127	16[a]	17	48	102	10	42
22	46	125	15[a]	22	45	87	12	43

Note: Data are rounded averages; range and standard deviations are omitted for simplicity.

[a] Plasma ANP significantly elevated in hypertensives vs. controls in the study.

B. ANP AND HUMAN SUBJECTS

The importance of atrial stretch in the production and secretion of ANP was also shown in humans through a variety of physiological maneuvers,[24-28] and in direct relationship with intracardiac pressure.[29] With regard to ANP actions, Richards et al.[30] were the first to intravenously administer ANP to healthy volunteers, and they were able to reproduce the ANP effects found by de Bold et al.[4] The renal effects of ANP were also carefully examined, but their complexity remains a challenge.[31,32] The dose-dependent cGMP production following ANP[33,34] was confirmed in humans, and the pharmacokinetic parameters of ANP[33] were determined. More recently, the effects of the inhibition of ANP degradation by inhibitors of an endopeptidase has received more attention. These oral agents produce a modest natriuresis.[35,36]

III. ROLE OF ANP IN ESSENTIAL HYPERTENSION

Essential hypertension remains a disorder of unknown etiology but for which evidence exists of several abnormalities of blood pressure-related systems and hormones. When ANP actions were uncovered, it soon became clear that essential hypertension could theoretically be a state of lack of ANP or resistance to ANP actions. Several groups investigated those hypotheses, but no convincing evidence has been found for either.

Measurement of plasma concentrations of ANP provided controversial data,[37-43] as shown in Table 1. Plasma ANP levels are often similar in mild to moderate untreated essential hypertension and in aged-matched normotensive controls, although they are reported to be elevated in patients with more severe hypertension.

Considering the elevation in intracardiac pressures in hypertensives[44] and that ANP secretion is correlated with intracardiac pressures,[29] it was somewhat surprising

TABLE 2
Effects of Head-Out Water Immersion

	Time (min.)	Normotensive controls	Essential hypertensives
Mean arterial pressure	Pre (0)	87 ± 3	108 ± 4
(mmHg)	Post (120)	76 ± 4[a]	96 ± 2[a]
Plasma C-terminal	Pre (0)	6.0 ± 1.3	6.1 ± 0.9
ANP levels (pmol/l)	Post (120)	16.3 ± 3.0[a]	13.2 ± 2.5[a,b]

Results: X ± SEM.

[a] $p < 0.01$, postimmersion vs. baseline values.
[b] $p = 0.13$ vs. values in normotensive controls.

to find normal plasma ANP levels in essential hypertension. However, no data yet clearly indicates a lack of ANP secretion in essential hypertension even following adoption of the supine posture and the increase in sodium intake or head-out thermoneutral water immersion.

In a recently completed investigation at the Institut de Recherches Cliniques de Montréal, the effect of head-out thermoneutral water immersion (HOI) on plasma concentrations of ANP were compared between 14 untreated essential hypertensives and 13 aged-matched normotensive controls. The subjects were studied on a 200 mmol/d sodium intake and a 2-h HOI test was compared to a 2-h "dry" test, both performed in the seated position. Each test was preceded and followed by 1-h rest periods, also in the seated position and out of the bath. As shown in Table 2, there was a nonsignificant trend for a smaller increase in plasma ANP levels following HOI in the hypertensive patients.

Thus, it still remains unclear whether some abnormalities exist with regards to ANP production and essential hypertension. No specific antagonist of ANP, such as monoclonal antibodies, have been administered to human subjects with hypertension, to see whether ANP played a role in blood pressure control in these subjects.

On the other hand, synthetic ANP was intravenously administered to hypertensive patients in several studies. Infusion of high doses or prolonged infusions of ANP reduces blood pressure in hypertensives.[45-47] This suggests that ANP could be used as an antihypertensive agent. Additionally, it could support the idea that hypertensives are relatively deficient in ANP production. Furthermore, ANP also produced more diuresis and natriuresis in hypertensives than in controls,[34] even at low infusion rates,[45,48] as shown in Table 3.

The fact that hypertensives are somewhat hyperresponsive to ANP infusion would also be in keeping with the hypothesis that ANP production is deficient in hypertensives, assuming an up-regulation phenomenon. Alternatively, an increase response in hypertension could be a nonspecific effect. Blood pressure is often reduced in proportion with baseline blood pressure with many antihypertensive drugs, and the elevation in blood pressure (and renal perfusion pressure) could in

TABLE 3
ANP-Induced Natriuresis in Essential Hypertension

	Exogenous ANP or vehicle	Subjects	n	Natriuretic response[a]	
Study 1[34]	Stepped infusion	Controls	7	V:	108 ± 22
	3 × 30 min period			ANP:	477 ± 104[b]
	4, 8, 16 pmol/kg/min	Patients	5	V:	201 ± 34[c]
	Controlled vehicle infusion			ANP:	1003 ± 11[b,c]
Study 2[48]	3-h constant infusion	Controls	6	ANP:	344 ± 50
	7 pmol/kg/min			ANP:	500 ± 61[c]
	No vehicle study	Patients	5		
Study 3[45]	12 h constant infusion	Controls	6	V:	242 ± 28
	0.5 pmol/kg/min			ANP:	221 ± 26
	Controlled vehicle infusion	Patients	6	V:	206 ± 30
				ANP:	290 ± 42[b,c]

Note: V, vehicle and ANP, a trial natriuretic peptide.

[a] Excretion rate in μmol/min (X ± SEM); study 1: during last 30-min period; study 2: average of 3-h period; study 3: average of 12-h period.
[b] $p < 0.05$: ANP vs. V.
[c] $p < 0.05$: Patients vs. controls.

itself act synergistically with ANP to produce an "exaggerated" natriuretic response.

IV. ANP AND SODIUM TRANSPORT SYSTEMS

Since the description was coined that ANP lacks an inhibitory effect on Na^+,K^+-ATPase[49,50] in order to establish the differences with the natriuretic hormone (ouabain-like factor), many efforts have been made to elucidate the cellular mechanism of action of ANP. However, early experiences[51,52] failed to find any effect of synthetic ANP on sodium transport systems (Na^+,K^+ pump, Na^+,K^+,Cl^- cotransport, and Na^+,Li^+ countertransport) in human red cells, peritoneal mouse macrophages, and cultured vascular smooth muscle and endothelial cells from the aorta. In this part of the chapter we summarize some investigations of the effect of ANP on cation membrane transport systems, mainly in the kidney, vascular, and intestinal cells.

A. ANP ACTIONS ON KIDNEY CELLS

As mentioned previously, the renal effects of ANP are basically of two types. First, ANP acts at the glomerular site to increase the glomerular filtration rate by raising the glomerular hydraulic pressure, and ANP also augments the glomerular permeability coefficient by the relaxation of mesangial cells.[53] The second type of ANP effects on the kidney are localized at the cellular level, directly affecting ionic transport. This is substantiated by the existence of ANP receptors in the medullary collecting duct,[54] cGMP accumulation after the exposition to ANP,[55] and the decrease in sodium uptake.

In the inner medullary collecting duct (IMCD), two cation transport systems exist: sodium enters the cell from the lumen through amiloride-sensitive sodium channels at the apical pole. The sodium is then pumped from the cytoplasm to the basolateral side by the Na^+,K^+-ATPase.[56,57]

The early demonstration that administration of cardiac atrial extract inhibited net sodium reabsorption in the IMCD,[58] was confirmed by Zeidel et al.[59] in fresh suspensions of highly purified rabbit IMCD cells, where the authors monitored the activity of cellular Na^+,K^+-ATPase and sodium entry by measuring ouabain-sensitive oxygen consumption. The findings indicated that ANP directly inhibits Na^+,K^+-ATPase-mediated O_2 consumption in IMCD, compatible with inhibition of sodium entry. In addition, it has been also demonstrated that sodium enters IMCD cells via conductive, amiloride-sensitive sodium channels which are regulated by ANP.[60] These results are in accordance with the finding that atriopeptin II directly inhibited Na^+ transport in renal epithelial cells LLC-PK_1 through an amiloride-sensitive conductive sodium transport pathway,[61] and without effect on the Na^+/H^+ exchanger. These actions are mediated by the second messenger cGMP, with the subsequent activation of protein kinase C (PKC).[62] On the other hand, Rocha and Kudo[57,63] showed in microperfused IMCD isolated from rat kidneys the existence of Na^+,K^+,Cl^- cotransport stimulated by ANP, that generates Na^+ and Cl^- secretion. It has been also observed a direct effect of ANP on NaCl transport that inhibited the lumen-to-bath flux of Na^+ and Cl^-. The addition of cGMP reproduced ANP actions, suggesting that cGMP is the second messenger of ANP in the IMCD.

In summary, ANP seems to regulate Na^+ and Cl^- excretion in IMCD by two mechanisms. One is the inhibition of sodium entry into the IMCD cells, affecting the Na^+,K^+-ATPase and amiloride-sensitive sodium transport. ANP also stimulates Na^+ and Cl^- secretion by the Na^+,K^+,Cl^- cotransport pathway.

Although it has been shown that the proximal tubule lacks ANP biologic receptors and particulate guanylate cyclase and does not generate cGMP in response to ANP,[53] Hammond et al.[64] found that synthetic ANP decreased tubular Na^+ reabsorption linked to reabsorption of HCO_3 in proximal tubules. These ANP effects were associated with the inhibition of Na^+,H^+ exchange in luminal brush border membranes (BBM). Recently, the same laboratory reported that the ANP-mediated inhibition on the rate of Na^+,H^+ exchange across renal BBM can be produced indirectly by enhancing intrarenal generation of dopamine, which in turn inhibits Na^+,H^+ exchange, or by a direct mechanism that potentiates the inhibitory action of dopamine on Na^+,H^+ exchange.[65] Finally, Moran et al.[66] demonstrated in cultured opossum kidney cells (similar to the epithelial cells of the proximal tubule) that ANP inhibited the activity of the Na^+,H^+ exchange, and generated cGMP as the second messenger.

B. ANP ACTIONS ON VASCULAR SMOOTH MUSCLE CELLS

In a series of experiments, O'Donnell et al.[67-70] described the effects of rat atriopeptin III (APIII) on primary cell cultures derived from rat thoracic aorta. They showed that rat APIII stimulated Na^+,K^+,Cl^- cotransport of vascular smooth muscle (VSM) cells in a concentration-dependent manner. By contrast, rat APIII had no effect on the two other transport systems known to be present in VSM cells (Na^+,H^+ exchange and Na^+,K^+-ATPase). These effects of ANP were also dependent upon the ability of the hormone to elevate intracellular cGMP levels. Finally, a clear correlation between biological activity of ANP and its ability to stimulate Na^+,K^+,Cl^- cotransport and to elevate intracellular cGMP levels was found. The authors hypothesize that the ANP vasodilatory effect can be related to the cotransport stimulation, leading to a decreased intracellular sodium concentration, and this in turn causes a decrease in intracellular calcium (Blaustein hypothesis) and vasorelaxation.

More conflicting results were reported regarding the effect of ANP on Na^+,K^+,Cl^- cotransport in bovine endothelial cells. While Fujita et al.[71] reported that ANP selectively activates the Na^+,K^+,Cl^- cotransporter in the aforementioned cells, the findings of O'Donnell[72] indicated that ANP reduces this cotransporter. One possible explanation for this difference may be the distinct transporter inhibitor used in the experiments.

In order to study the interaction between ANP and Na^+,K^+-ATPase, Sybertz and Desiderio[73] stated that the vasorelaxant effect of ANP was dependent on the activation state of the Na^+,K^+-ATPase. In fact, in rabbit aortic rings precontracted with norepinephrine, ANP induced a relaxation that was abolished by ouabain and a K^+-free medium, well-known conditions that inhibited Na^+,K^+-ATPase. These data suggested that ANP induces relaxation in rabbit VSM by an ouabain- and a K^+-sensitive mechanism, presumably Na^+,K^+-ATPase. Similar results were obtained by Sato et al.[74] on rat aortic rings. Their findings seem to indicate that the vasodilating effect of ANP is at least partially mediated by the activation of electrogenic Na^+,K^+-ATPase. Auguet et al.[75] also reported that inhibition of Na^+ pump activity by incubation with either ouabain or K^+-free medium inhibited the vasorelaxant action of ANP on isolated rabbit aorta. These authors as well as Garay et al.[76] hypothesized that the vasorelaxant effect of ANP could be explained by calcium sequestration in internal cellular stores, probably mediated by a cGMP-dependent protein kinase.

This interaction between ANP and the Na^+,K^+-ATPase also has been demonstrated in rat brain: ANP decreased the release of Na^+,K^+-ATPase inhibitor from incubated rat brain tissue after injection of the hormone.[77]

In vivo studies carried out in dogs by Chintala and Jandhyala[78] expanded the evidence that the vasorelaxant action of ANP was related to the activation of Na^+,K^+-ATPase. In those experiments, ANP infusion significantly depressed vascular responses to noradrenaline. However, the subsequent infusion of ouabain together with ANP reversed and restored the vascular reactivity to the control levels. This antagonism of ouabain on vasorelaxant effects of ANP does not preclude, however, the ability of ANP to enhance cGMP formation in the arterial smooth muscle, and it could be related to the mechanisms affecting calcium fluxes across the cell membrane, and not at the second messenger level.[79]

C. ANP ACTIONS ON INTESTINAL CELLS

Recent studies suggest that ANP may affect electrolyte transport in the intestinal tract. A direct inhibitory effect of APIII on Na^+,K^+,Cl^- cotransport has been demonstrated in marine teleost intestine,[80,81] also mediated by cGMP. Concerning the effects of ANP on mammalian intestine, Semrad et al.[82] found that ANP inhibited the amiloride-sensitive Na^+,H^+ exchange in isolated chicken enterocytes by stimulating increases in intracellular calcium activity. The data suggest that this event is initiated by an ANP-stimulated increase in cGMP concentration which, in turn, appears to increase calcium. Also in mammals, it has been suggested that ANP elicits Cl^- secretion in rat distal colon by a calcium-mediated neurogenic mechanism.[83] APIII and brain natriuretic peptide significantly increased the serosal-to-mucosal Cl^- flux in porcine distal colon epithelium and reduced net chloride absorption. These results indicate that natriuretic peptides stimulate K^+ and Cl^- secretion across the porcine distal colon epithelium by a direct regulation of transport properties of the epithelium.[84]

D. SUMMARY

ANP and its second messenger cGMP exert a diuretic and natriuretic effect on the inner medullary collecting duct. ANP inhibits Na^+ entry conductance and also stimulates Na^+ and Cl^- secretion through the Na^+,K^+,Cl^- cotransport system. In the proximal tubule ANP probably inhibits the Na^+,H^+ exchange. In cultured VSM cells ANP also stimulates the Na^+,K^+,Cl^- cotransport, and this may be the first step for its vasodilatory action. Some degree of activation of Na^+,K^+-ATPase also seems to be a prerequisite for this action. Finally, the secretion of Cl^- and Na^+ in the intestine can participate in the regulation of the homeostasis of sodium and water.

V. ANP, SODIUM TRANSPORT SYSTEMS, AND ESSENTIAL HYPERTENSION

Data on ANP and sodium transport systems in essential hypertension are limited at this time. Experiments conducted in borderline human hypertensives demonstrated that in normal plasma renin activity (PRA) hypertensives, ANP may modulate the release of plasma Na^+,K^+-ATPase inhibitor after the extracellular volume expansion. However, borderline hypertensive subjects with low PRA levels showed a rise in blood pressure and a peripheral vasoconstriction, probably due to a predominant hemodynamic role of Na^+,K^+-ATPase over the ANP release.[85] In a preliminary report, De la Sierra et al.[86] studied the kinetic parameters of ionic transport systems in 26 hypertensive patients in relation to plasma levels of vasoactive hormones and echocardiographic data. Despite that the differences were not significant, they found higher levels of ANP and blood pressure among patients with regulatory abnormalities of intraerythrocyte Na^+ or Ca^{2+}, when they were compared to those hypertensives having an abnormally high entry of Na^+ into cells or those without detectable defects of sodium transport.

VI. SUMMARY AND FUTURE PROSPECTS

ANP is a circulating peptidic hormone that interacts with specific receptors on cells of many target organs. Production of cGMP is the postreceptor event that has been best characterized. There is now a growing body of evidence that ANP can alter several sodium transport systems. ANP is not an inhibitor of Na^+,K^+-ATPase. ANP stimulates Na^+,K^+,Cl^- cotransport and inhibits Na^+,H^+ exchange. These mechanisms can partly explain the physiological and pharmacological effects of ANP on the kidney (natriuresis) and on blood vessels (vasodilation).

In essential hypertension, some evidence suggests that ANP secretion is relatively deficient. A reduced ANP availability could alter sodium transport systems and cause sodium retention and vasoconstriction, hallmarks of essential hypertension. Only limited data have been published on these aspects of ANP. Future studies should evaluate the closeness of the relationships between the ability to secrete ANP, sodium transport abnormalities, and characteristics of the pressure-natriuresis curve in essential hypertension.

REFERENCES

1. **Cernacek, P., Crawhall, J. C., and Levy, M.,** Atrial natriuretic peptide: blood levels in human disease and their measurement, *Clin. Biochem.*, 1988; 21:5–17.
2. **Needleman, P., Blaine, E. H., Greenwald, J. E., Michener, M. L., Saper, C. B., Stockmann, P. T., and Tolunay, H. E.,** The biochemical pharmacology of atrial peptides, *Annu. Rev. Pharmacol. Toxicol.*, 1989; 29:23–54.
3. **Goetz, K. L.,** Physiology and pathophysiology of atrial peptides, *Am. J. Physiol.*, 1988; 254: E1–E15.
4. **De Bold, A. J., Borenstein, H. B., Veress, A. T., and Sonnenberg, H.,** A rapid and potent natriuretic response to intravenous injection of atrial myocardial extract in rats, *Life Sci.*, 1981; 28:89–94.
5. **Kisch, B.,** Electron microscopy of the atrium of the heart, *Exp. Med. Surg.*, 1956; 14:99–112.
6. **Kangawa, K. and Matsuo, H.,** Purification and complete amino acid sequence of α-human natriuretic polypeptide (α-h-ANF), *Biochem. Biophys. Res. Commun.*, 1984; 118:131–139.
7. **Thibault, G., Garcia, R., Cantin, M., Genest, J., Lazure, C., Seidah, N. G., and Chretien, M.,** Primary structure of a high Mr form of rat atrial natriuretic factor, *FEBS Lett.*, 1984; 167:352–356.
8. **Lang, R. E., Tholken, H., Ganten, D., Luft, F. C., Ruskoaho, H., and Unger, T.,** Atrial natriuretic factor -- a circulating hormone stimulated by volume loading, *Nature*, 1985; 314: 264–266.
9. **Edwards, B. S., Zimmerman, R. S., Schwab, T. R., Heublein, D. M., and Burnett, J. C.,** Atrial stretch, not pressure, is the principal determinant controlling the acute release of atrial natriuretic factor, *Circ. Res.*, 1988; 62:191–195.
10. **Gutkowska, J., Bourassa, M., Roy, D., Thibault, G., Garcia, R., Cantin, M., and Genest, J.,** Immunoreactive atrial natriuretic factor (IR-ANF) in human plasma, *Biochem. Biophys. Res. Commun.*, 1985; 128:1350–1357.
11. **Myata, A., Kangawa, K., Toshimore, T., Hatoh, T., and Matsuo, H.,** Molecular forms of atrial natriuretic polypeptides in mammalian tissues and plasma, *Biochem. Biophys. Res. Commun.*, 1985; 129:248–255.

12. **Thibault, G.,** Atrial natriuretic factor: its circulating forms and prohormone processing, in *Atrial Natriuretic Peptides,* Samson, W. K. and Quirion, R., Eds., CRC Press, Boca Raton, FL, 1990: 33–40.
13. **Genest, J. and Cantin, M.,** The atrial natriuretic factor: its physiology and biochemistry. X. Structure-activity relationships, *Rev. Physiol. Pharmacol.,* 1988; 110:85–89.
14. **Ackermann, U., Irizawa, T. G., Milojevic, S., and Sonnenberg, H.,** Cardiovascular effects of atrial extracts in anesthetized rats, *Can. J. Physiol. Pharmacol.,* 1984; 62:819–826.
15. **Cody, R. J., Atlas, S. A., Laragh, J. H., Kubo, S. H., Covit, A. B., Ryman, K. S., Shaknovich, A., Pondolfino, K., Clark, M., Camargo, M. J. F., Scarborough, R. M., and Lewicki, J. A.,** Atrial natriuretic factor in normal subjects and heart failure patients — plasma levels and renal, hormonal, and hemodynamic responses to peptide infusion, *J. Clin. Invest.,* 1986; 78:1362–1374.
16. **Fugita, T., Ito, Y., Noda, H., Sato, Y., Ando, K., Kangawa, K., and Matsuo, H.,** Vasodilatory actions of α-human atrial natriuretic peptide and high Ca^{+2} effects in normal man, *J. Clin. Invest.,* 1987; 80:832–840.
17. **Burnett, J. C., Jr., Granger, J. P., and Opgenorth, T. J.,** Effects of synthetic atrial natriuretic factor on renal function and renin release, *Am. J. Physiol.,* 1984; 247:F863–F866.
18. **Murray, R. D., Itoh, S., Inagami, T., Misono, K., Seto, S., Scicli, A. G., and Canetero, O. A.,** Effects of synthetic atrial natriuretic factor in the isolated perfused rat kidney, *Am. J. Physiol.,* 1985; 249:F603–F609.
19. **Bourgoignie, J. J., Gavellas, G., and Hwang, K. H.,** Renal effects of atrial natriuretic factor in primate, *Am. J. Physiol.,* 1986; 251:F1049–1054.
20. **Chartier, L., Schiffrin, E., Thibault, G., and Garcia, R.,** Atrial natriuretic factor inhibits the stimulation of aldosterone secretion by angiotensin II, ACTH and potassium in vitro and angiotensin II-induced steroidogenesis in vivo, *Endocrinology,* 1984; 115:2026–2028.
21. **Jamison, R. L., Canaan-Kuhl, S., and Pratt, R.,** The natriuretic peptides and their receptors, *Am. J. Kidney Dis.,* 1992; 20:519–530.
22. **Hamet, P., Tremblay, J., Thibault, G., Garcia, R., Cantin, M., and Genest, J.,** Effect of atrial natriuretic factor on metabolism of cGMP, *Endocrinology,* 1983; 112:289.
23. **Hamet, P., Tremblay, J., Pang, S. C., Skuherska, R., Schiffrin, E. L., Garcia, R., Cantin, M., Genest, J., Palmour, R., Ervin, F. R., Martin, S., and Goldwater, R.,** Cyclic GMP as mediator and biological marker of atrial natriuretic factor, *J. Hypertension,* 1986; 4(Suppl. 2):S49–S56.
24. **Sagnella, G. A., Shore, A. C., Markandu, N. D., and MacGregor, G. A.,** Effects of changes in dietary sodium intake and saline infusion on immunoreactive atrial natriuretic peptide in human plasma, *Lancet,* 1985; II:1208–1210.
25. **Larose, P., Meloche, S., du Souich, P., De Lean, A., and Ong, H.,** Radioimmunoassay of atrial natriuretic factor: human plasma levels, *Biochem. Biophys. Res. Commun.,* 1985; 130: 553–558.
26. **Ogihara, T., Shima, J., Hara, H., Tabuchi, Y., Hashizume, K., Nagano, M., Katahira, K., Kangawa, K., Matsuo, H., and Kumahara, Y.,** Significant increase in plasma immunoreactive atrial natriuretic polypeptide concentration during head-out water immersion, *Life Sci.,* 1986; 38:2413–2418.
27. **Shenker, Y., Sider, R. S., Ostafin, E. A., and Grekin, R. J.,** Plasma levels of immunoreactive atrial natriuretic factor in healthy subjects and in patients with edema, *J. Clin. Invest.,* 1985; 76:1684–1687.
28. **Cusson, J. R., Gutkowska, J., Rey, E., Michon, N., Boucher, M., and Larochelle, P.,** Plasma concentration of atrial natriuretic factor in normal pregnancy, *N. Engl. J. Med.,* 1985; 313:1230–1231.
29. **Hirata, Y., Nozaki, A., Toda, I., Murakawa, Y., Sugimoto, T., Matsuoka, H., Ishii, M., Miyata, A., Kangawa, K., and Matsuo, H.,** Plasma concentration of atrial natriuretic polypeptide in patients with atrial tachycardia, *Jpn. Heart J.,* 1987; 28:53–61.

30. **Richards, A. M., Ikram, H., Yandle, T. G., Nicholls, M. G., Webster, M. W. I., and Espiner, E. A.,** Renal, haemodynamic, and hormonal effects of human alpha atrial natriuretic peptide in healthy volunteers, *Lancet,* 1985; 1:545–549.
31. **Weidmann, P., Hasler, L., Gnadinger, M. P., Lang, R. E., Uehlinger, D. E., Shaw, S., and Rascher, W.,** Blood levels and renal effects of atrial natriuretic peptide in normal man, *J. Clin. Invest.,* 1986; 77:734–742.
32. **Brown, J. and Corr, L.,** Renal mechanisms of human α-atrial natriuretic peptide in man, *J. Physiol.,* 1987; 387:31–46.
33. **Cusson, J. R., DuSouich, P., Hamet, P., Schiffrin, E. L., Kuchel, O., Tremblay, J., Cantin, M., Genest, J., and Larochelle, P.,** Effects and pharmacokinetics of bolus injections of atrial natriuretic factor in normal volunteers, *J. Cardiovasc. Pharmacol.,* 1988; 11:635–642.
34. **Cusson, J. R., Hamet, P., Gutkowska, J., Kuchel, O., Genest, J., Cantin, M., and Larochelle, P.,** Effects of atrial natriuretic factor on natriuresis and cGMP in patients with essential hypertension, *J. Hypertension,* 1987; 5:435–443.
35. **Sybertz, E. J., Chiu, P. J. S., Vemulapalli, S., Watkins, R., Haslanger, M. F.,** Atrial natriuretic factor-potentiating and antihypertensive activity of SCH 34826. An orally active neutral metalloendopeptidase inhibitor, *Hypertension,* 1990; 15:152–161.
36. **Richards, A. M., Wittert, G., Espiner, E. A., Yandle, T. G., Frampton, C., and Ikram, H.,** Prolonged inhibition of endopeptidase 24.11 in normal man: renal, endocrine and haemodynamic effects, *J. Hypertension,* 1991; 9:955–962.
37. **Larochelle, P., Cusson, J. R., Gutkowska, J., Schiffrin, E. L., Hamet, P., Kuchel, O., Genest, J., and Cantin, M.,** Plasma atrial natriuretic factor concentrations in essential and renovascular hypertension, *Br. Med. J.,* 1987; 294:1249–1252.
38. **Nakaoka, H., Imataka, K., Amano, M., Fujii, J., Ishibashi, M., and Yamaji, T.,** Plasma levels of atrial natriuretic factor in patients with congestive heart failure, *N. Engl. J. Med.,* 1985; 313:892–893.
39. **Zachariah, P. K., Burnett, J. C., Jr., Ritter, S. G., and Strong, C. G.,** Atrial natriuretic peptide in human essential hypertension, *Mayo Clin. Proc.,* 1987; 62:782–786.
40. **Schiffrin, E. L., St.-Louis, J., and Essiambre, R.,** Platelet binding sites and plasma concentration of atrial natriuretic peptide in patients with essential hypertension, *J. Hypertension,* 1988; 6:565–572.
41. **Wambach, G., Gotz, S., Suckau, G., Bonner, G., and Kaufmann, W.,** Plasma levels of atrial natriuretic peptide are raised in essential hypertension during low and high sodium intake, *Klin. Wochenschr.,* 1987; 65:232–237.
42. **Kohno, M., Yasunari, K., Matsuara, T., Murakawa, K., and Takeda, T.,** Circulating atrial natriuretic polypeptide in essential hypertension, *Am. Heart J.,* 1986; 113:1160–1163.
43. **Montorsi, P., Tonolo, G., Polonia, J., Hepburn, D., and Richards, M. A.,** Correlates of plasma atrial natriuretic factor in health and hypertension, *Hypertension,* 1987; 10:570–576.
44. **London, G. M., Safar, M. E., Safar, A. L., and Simon, A. C.,** Blood pressure in the "low pressure system" and cardiac performance in essential hypertension, *J. Hypertension,* 1985; 3:337–342.
45. **Cusson, J. R., Thibault, G., Cantin, M., and Larochelle, P.,** Prolonged low dose infusion of atrial natriuretic factor in essential hypertension, *Clin. Exp. Hypertension,* (A) 1990; 12: 111–135.
46. **Ishii, M., Sugimoto, T., Matsuoka, H., Hirata, Y., Ishimitsu, T., Fukui, K., Kangawa, K., and Matsuo, H.,** The haemodynamic, renal and endocrine effects of α-human atrial natriuretic polypeptide in normotensive people and patients with essential hypertension, *J. Hypertension,* 1986; 4(Suppl. 6):S542–S545.
47. **Janssen, W. M. T., De Zeeuw, D., van der Hem, K., and De Jong, P. E.,** Antihypertensive effect of a 5-day infusion of atrial natriuretic factor in humans, *Hypertension,* 1989; 13: 640–646.
48. **Cusson, J. R., Thibault, G., Kuchel, O., Hamet, P., Cantin, M., and Larochelle, P.,** Cardiovascular, renal and endocrine responses to low doses of atrial natriuretic factor in mild essential hypertension, *J. Hum. Hypertension,* 1989; 3:89–96.

49. **Thibault, G., Garcia, R., Cantin, M., and Genest, J.,** Atrial natriuretic factor. Characterization and partial purification, *Hypertension,* 1983; 5(Suppl. 1):I75–I80.
50. **Pamnani, M. B., Clough, D. L., Chen, J. S., Link, W. T., and Haddy, F. J.,** Effects of rat atrial extract on sodium transport and blood pressure in the rat, *Proc. Soc. Exp. Biol. Med.,* 1984; 176:123–131.
51. **Hernando, N., Caramelo, C., Tejedor, A., Fernández-Cruz, A., and López-Novoa, J. M.,** Lack of effect of synthetic atrial natriuretic factor on rubidium uptake by human erythrocytes, *Biochem. Biophys. Res. Commun.,* 1985; 130:1066–1071.
52. **Garay, R., Hannaert, P., Rodrigue, F. et al.** Involvement of cytosolic free calcium in the action mechanism of atrial natriuretic factor (ANF), *Reg. Peptides,* 1985; (Suppl. 4):97–100.
53. **Cogan, M. G.,** Renal effects of atrial natriuretic factor, *Annu. Rev. Physiol.,* 1990; 52: 699–708.
54. **Bianchi, C., Gutkowska, J., Garcia, R., Thibault, G., Genest, J., and Cantin, M.,** Localization of ^{125}I-atrial natriuretic factor (ANF)-binding sites in rat renal medulla. A light and electron microscope autoradiographic study, *J. Histochem. Cytochem.,* 1987; 35:149–153.
55. **Ishikawa, S., Saito, T., Okada, K., Kuzuya, T., Kangawa, K., and Matsuo, H.,** Atrial natriuretic factor increases cyclic GMP and inhibits cyclic AMP in rat renal papillary collecting tubule cells in culture, *Biochem. Biophys. Res. Commun.,* 1985; 130:1147–1153.
56. **Zeidel, M. L.,** Renal actions of atrial natriuretic peptide: regulation of collecting duct sodium and water transport, *Annu. Rev. Physiol.,* 1990; 52:747–759.
57. **Rocha, A. S. and Kudo, L. H.,** Factors governing sodium and chloride transport across the inner medullary collecting duct, *Kidney Int.,* 1990; 38:654–667.
58. **Sonnenberg, H., Cupples, W. A., DeBold, A. J., and Veress, A. T.,** Intrarenal localization of the natriuretic effects of cardiac atrial extract, *Can. J. Physiol. Pharmacol.,* 1982; 60: 1149–1152.
59. **Zeidel, M. L., Seifter, J. L., Lear, S., Brenner, B. M., and Silva, P.,** Atrial peptides inhibit oxygen consumption in kidney medullary collecting duct cells, *Am. J. Physiol.,* 1986; 251: F379–F383.
60. **Zeidel, M. L., Kikeri, D., Silva, P., Burrowes, M., and Brenner, B. M.,** Atrial natriuretic peptides inhibit conductive sodium uptake by rabbit inner medullary collecting duct cells, *J. Clin. Invest.,* 1988; 82:1067–1074.
61. **Cantiello, H. F. and Ausiello, D. A.,** Atrial natriuretic factor and cGMP inhibit amiloride-sensitive Na^+ transport in the cultured renal epithelial cell line, LLC-PK_1, *Biochem. Biophys. Res. Commun.,* 1986; 134:852–860.
62. **Mohrmann, M., Cantiello, H. F., and Ausiello, D. A.,** Inhibition of epithelial Na^+ transport by atriopeptin, protein kinase c, and pertussis toxin, *Am. J. Physiol.,* 253; 1987:F372–F376.
63. **Rocha, A. S. and Kudo, L. H.,** Atrial peptide and cGMP effects on NaCl transport in inner medullary collecting duct, *Am. J. Physiol.,* 1990; 259:258–268.
64. **Hammond, T. G., Yusufi, A. N. K., Knox, F. G., and Dousa, T. P.,** Administration of atrial natriuretic factor inhibits sodium-coupled transport in proximal tubules, *J. Clin. Invest.,* 1985; 75:1983–1989.
65. **Winaver, J., Burnett, J. C., Tyce, G. M., and Dousa, T. P.,** ANP inhibits Na^+-H^+ antiport in proximal tubular brush border membrane: role of dopamine, *Kidney Int.,* 1990; 38: 1133–1140.
66. **Moran, A., Montrose, M. H., and Murer, H.,** Regulation of Na^+-H^+ exchange in cultured opossum kidney cells by parathyroid hormone, atrial natriuretic peptide and cyclic nucleotides, *Biochim. Biophys. Acta,* 1988; 969:48–56.
67. **O'Donnell, M. E. and Owen, N. E.,** Atrial natriuretic factor stimulates Na/K/Cl cotransport in vascular smooth muscle cells, *Proc. Natl. Acad. Sci. U.S.A.,* 1986; 83:6132–6136.
68. **O'Donnell, M. E. and Owen, M. E.,** Role of cyclic GMP in atrial natriuretic factor stimulation of Na^+,K^+,Cl^- cotransport in vascular smooth muscle cells, *J. Biol. Chem.,* 1986; 261: 15461–15466.

69. **O'Donnell, M. E., Bush, E. N., Holleman, W., and Owen, N. E.,** Biolocally active atrial natriuretic peptides selectively activate Na/K/Cl cotransport in vascular smooth muscle cells, *J. Pharmacol. Exp. Ther.,* 1987; 243:822–828.
70. **Owen, N. E., Bush, E. N., Holleman, W., and O'Donnell, M. E.,** Effect of atrial natriuretic factor on Na^+-K^+-Cl^- cotransport of vascular smooth muscle cells, *Hypertension,* 1987; 10 (Suppl. I):I-128–I-130.
71. **Fujita, T., Hagiwara, H., Ohuchi, S., Kozuka, M., Ishido, M., and Hirose, S.,** Stimulation of Na-K-Cl cotransport in cultured vascular endothelial cells by atrial natriuretic peptide, *Biochem. Biophys. Res. Commun.,* 1989; 159:734–740.
72. **O'Donnell, M. E.,** Regulation of Na-K-Cl cotransport in endothelial cells by atrial natriuretic factor, *Am. J. Physiol.,* 1989; 257:C36–C44.
73. **Sybertz, E. J. and Desiderio, E. M.,** The role of Na^+-K^+-ATPase in the vasorelaxant actions of synthetic atrial natriuretic factor, *Arch. Int. Pharmacodyn. Ther.,* 1985; 278:142–149.
74. **Sato, K., Murakami, K., Nishimura, K., Ito, K., Kangawa, K., and Matsuo, H.,** Possible involvement of sodium pump in the relaxation of rat aorta induced by α-human atrial natriuretic polypeptide, *Jpn. J. Physiol.,* 1988; 38:187–198.
75. **Auguet, M., Delaflotte, S., Garay, R., Cantin, M., Clostre, F., and Braquet, P.,** Effects of sodium pump inhibition on the relaxation induced by synthetic atrial natriuretic factor (ANF) and sodium nitroprusside, *Reg. Peptides,* 1985; (Suppl. 4):107–109.
76. **Garay, R., Hannaert, P., Rodrigue, F. et al.,** Atrial natriuretic factor inhibits Ca^{2+}-dependent K^+ fluxes in cultured vascular smooth muscle cells, *J. Hypertension,* 1985; 3(Suppl. 3): S297–S298.
77. **Crabos, M., Ausiello, D. A., Haupert, G. T., and Cantiello, H. F.,** Atrial natriuretic peptide regulates release of Na^+-K^+-ATPase inhibitor from rat brain, *Am. J. Physiol.,* 1988; 254: F912–F917.
78. **Chintala, M. S. and Jandhyala, B. S.,** Interaction between atrial natriuretic factor and ouabain: vascular reactivity to noradrenaline in pentobarbital anaesthetized dogs, *Clin. Exp. Pharmacol. Physiol.,* 1988; 15:591–599.
79. **Hegde, S. S., DeFeo, M. L., and Jandhyala, B. S.,** Effects of atrial natriuretic factor on cyclic GMP content in the rat aortic smooth muscle: studies on the role of membrane Na^+-K^+-ATPase, *Clin. Exp. Pharmacol. Physiol.,* 1989; 16:623–629.
80. **O'Grady, S. M., Field, M., Nash, N. T., and Rao, M. C.,** Atrial natriuretic factor inhibits Na-K-Cl cotransport in teleost intestine, *Am. J. Physiol.,* 1985; 249:C531–C534.
81. **O'Grady, S. M.,** Cyclic nucleotide-mediated effects of ANF and VIP on flounder intestinal ion transport, *Am. J. Physiol.,* 1989; 256:C142–C146.
82. **Semrad, C. E., Cragoe, E. J., and Chang, E. B.,** Inhibition of Na/H exchange in avian intestine by atrial natriuretic factor, *J. Clin. Invest.,* 1990; 86:585–591.
83. **Moriarty, K. J., Higgs, N. B., Lees, M., Tonge, A., Wardle, T. D., and Warhurst, G.,** Influence of atrial natriuretic peptide on mammalian large intestine, *Gastroenterology,* 1990; 98:647–653.
84. **Traynor, T. R. and O'Grady, S. M.,** Brain natriuretic peptide stimulates K and Cl secretion across porcine distal colon epithelium, *Am. J. Physiol.,* 1991; 260:C750–C755.
85. **Borghi, C., Boschi, S., Costa, F. V., and Ambrosioni E.,** Atrial natriuretic factor modulates the plasma levels of a Na^+/K^+ATPase inhibitor in volume expanded borderline hypertensives, *Am. J. Hypertension,* 1991; 4:618–622.
86. **De la Sierra, A., Coca, A., Paré, J. C. et al.,** Clinical profile of essential hypertensives based on ion-transport abnormalities: preliminary results, *J. Hypertension,* 9(Suppl. 6), 5308, 1991.

Chapter 10

VASCULAR MUSCLE CALCIUM CHANNELS IN HYPERTENSION

Nancy J. Rusch and Kent Hermsmeyer

TABLE OF CONTENTS

I. Introduction 198

II. Voltage-Dependent Calcium Channels (VDCC) in Vascular Muscle Membranes 198
- A. Background 198
- B. Evidence for Different VDCC Subtypes 199
- C. Intrinsic Regulation of Vascular T- and L-Type VDCCs by Arterial Membrane Potential 203

III. Evidence for Abnormal VDCC Current in Vascular Muscle Membranes in Hypertension 207
- A. Background 207
- B. Functional Implications of Enhanced Arterial VDCC Current in Hypertension 208
- C. VDCC Currents in Vascular and Cardiac Myocytes in Genetic and Experimental Hypertension 212

IV. Mechanisms Regulating VDCCs in Arterial Muscle Membranes in Hypertension 214
- A. Pressure-Induced Membrane Depolarization 214
- B. Neurotransmission 215
- C. Endothelium and Paracrine Factors 218

V. Summary 219

Acknowledgments 220

References 220

0-8493-5474-9/94/$0.00 + $.50

I. INTRODUCTION

The presence of an increased peripheral vascular resistance in hypertension attests to the role of arterial smooth muscle in the pathogenesis of high blood pressure. The comprehensive basis for this enhanced vascular resistance likely includes both structural remodeling and functional alterations of the arterial wall.[1-5] With respect to the latter, the role of the calcium ion in the etiology of hypertension has received particular attention and has been the focus of comprehensive reviews.[6-9] The concept that an elevated level of cytosolic free Ca^{2+} is coupled to augmented arterial contraction in hypertension has been advanced as a hypothesis to explain the increased vascular resistance characteristic of this disease.[10-14]

Not surprisingly, defects in multiple cellular processes regulating Ca^{2+} homeostasis have been reported in arterial muscle. Of these, an augmented Ca^{2+} influx through voltage-dependent calcium channels (VDCC) is an attractive hypothesis to consider. Comparison of radiolabeled ^{45}Ca flux between arterial muscle from normo- and hypertensive models provides evidence for altered Ca^{2+} influx through arterial membrane VDCCs exposed to high levels of blood pressure.[8] More recently, direct measurement of VDCC currents by patch-clamp methods has suggested a genetic and pressure-induced basis for VDCC alteration in vascular and cardiac muscle membranes in hypertension.[15-18] Thus, with the advent of new methodologies for the measurement of VDCC function, it may be pertinent to reexamine the evidence for altered voltage-dependent Ca^{2+} influx in vascular muscle membranes in hypertension. We also discuss neurotransmitters and paracrine modulators as candidates for differences in VDCC current between arteries from normo- and hypertensive animals.

This chapter focuses first on the characteristics of VDCC subtypes in vascular muscle membranes and their modulation by arterial membrane potential. Consequently, it explores the hypothesis that an altered distribution, function, or regulation of arterial VDCCs are implicated in the pathogenesis and maintenance of high blood pressure.

II. VOLTAGE-DEPENDENT CALCIUM CHANNELS (VDCC) IN VASCULAR MUSCLE MEMBRANES

A. BACKGROUND

Membrane VDCCs in many cell types regulate Ca^{2+} influx and intracellular signaling processes.[19] In vascular muscle, intracellular free Ca^{2+} levels and contraction are among the mechanisms triggered by VDCCs. The ionic transitions through these Ca^{2+}-selective pathways recently have been characterized at the single cell and single-channel levels by application of patch-clamp techniques.[19,20] Calcium influx through VDCCs also has been determined by radiolabeled ^{45}Ca flux studies in vascular tissue.[8] Observations from flux experiments were compared with electromechanical coupling studies in arterial segments to provide initial insight into the likely electrical and pharmacological properties of arterial membrane VDCCs.[21] For example, it was noted that arterial membrane depolarization electropositive to −50 mV was associated with sustained contraction in rat caudal and rabbit pulmonary arteries.[22,23] Similar depolarization-induced contractions were seen in cat and rabbit basilar arteries at membrane potentials positive to −60 to −50 mV.[24,25] The observation that these depolarization-induced contractions were inhibited by organic Ca^{2+} channel blockers[8,25-29] suggested that an enhanced open state probability of VDCCs was critical for activator Ca^{2+} to sustain vascular muscle contraction.

The application of patch-clamp techniques has enabled the identification of two apparently distinct VDCC subtypes in a variety of vascular muscle preparations.[30-36] These two VDCC subtypes, termed the transient-type (T-type) and long-lasting type (L-type) channels, continue to be characterized in different vascular muscle cell types according to their biophysical, voltage-dependent, and pharmacological properties. Furthermore, molecular biology techniques may soon shed light on the regulation of VDCC subtypes at the molecular level.[37,38] The recent cloning and functional expression of the α-subunit of the L-type VDCC from rat aortic membranes promises that the relationship between VDCC structure and function may be clarified in the near future.[39,40] This section is a review of some of the recent progress in the electrophysiological characterization of T- and L-type VDCCs in vascular muscle. Summarizing the properties of these channels and their modulation by membrane potential in arteries from normotensive animals is a necessary prerequisite for evaluation of possible VDCC alterations in hypertension.

B. EVIDENCE FOR DIFFERENT VDCC SUBTYPES

Initial reports of voltage-dependent Ca^{2+} channel currents in vascular muscle membranes suggested that two distinct Ca^{2+} channel subtypes contribute to macroscopic Ca^{2+} influx.[30-36,41,42] First, low-amplitude depolarizations from membrane potentials more negative than −60 mV elicited an inward Ca^{2+} current component which rapidly inactivated within tens of milliseconds. The amplitude and kinetics of this low-threshold current were unaffected by the exchange of external Ca^{2+} with Ba^{2+} as the charge carrier, and showed insensitivity to organic Ca^{2+} channel blockers at negative membrane potentials. Due to the brief time course of Ca^{2+} influx through this low-threshold channel (Figure 1), this Ca^{2+} channel was designated the transient-type, or T-type VDCC. Analysis of the voltage-dependent activation and steady-state inactivation of the T-type VDCC suggested that this channel was available to conduct Ca^{2+} current between resting potentials negative to −45 mV and command potentials of −30 mV (Figure 2). This estimated "window current" (Figure 2, shaded area) from about −45 to −30 mV was indicated by the overlap of activation and inactivation curves in recordings using 10 m*M* Ba^{2+} or Ca^{2+} as the charge carrier.

Second, in whole-cell recordings from the same vascular muscle, membrane depolarization to potentials positive to −40 mV elicited a high-threshold activated Ca^{2+} current component, which inactivated slowly during maintained depolariza-

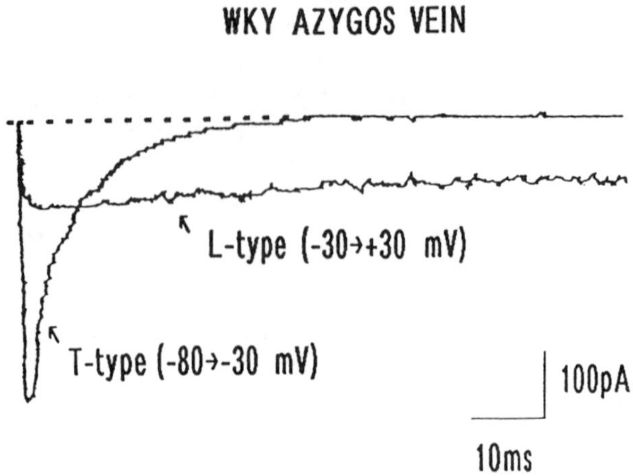

FIGURE 1. Whole-cell VDCC currents in a WKY rat azygos venous muscle cell. The T-type current was measured during an 80-ms depolarizing pulse from −80 to −30 mV, while the L-type current was recorded during depolarization from −30 to +30 mV. Comparison between T- and L-type currents illustrates the different voltage thresholds and kinetics of the two VDCC subtypes.

tion.[30-36,42] This channel preferentially conducted external Ba^{2+} for Ca^{2+}, and was blocked by organic Ca^{2+} channel blockers, showing particular sensitivity to dihydropyridine inhibition.[19,32,42,43] Based on its slow rate of channel inactivation (compared to the T-type VDCC) during maintained depolarization in whole-cell recordings (Figure 1), this high-threshold channel was termed the long-lasting, or L-type VDCC. In relation to the T-type VDCC, voltage-dependent activation and steady-state inactivation of L-type VDCCs occurred at more positive membrane potentials (Figure 2). The window current from −35 to −10 mV (Figure 2, shaded area) characterizes this high-threshold VDCC subtype, and highlights why L-type VDCCs carry Ca^{2+} current at more depolarized membrane potentials.

The presence of two distinct VDCC subtypes in vascular muscle membranes subsequently was confirmed by single-channel patch-clamp methods. Single-channel Ca^{2+} currents showing two different unitary amplitudes in high Ca^{2+}- or Ba^{2+}-containing solution were recorded in the same membrane patch under identical voltage and chemical gradients.[32,33,36,44] The low-threshold channel showed a unitary conductance of approximately 10 pS (Figure 3A), and voltage-dependent activation and steady-state inactivation at more negative membrane potentials. The single-channel kinetics of this VDCC subtype showed rapid inactivation after patch depolarization. This reflected, at the single-channel level, the brief time course of the whole-cell T-type current observed during small depolarizing pulses from negative membrane potentials (Figures 3B, C). A higher threshold single-channel current, showing a unitary conductance of about 25 pS, was revealed in the same membrane patches at more depolarized patch potentials (Figures 3A, B). This high-threshold VDCC showed persistent open states during maintained voltage steps to depolarized membrane potentials, and modulation of its open state probability by dihydropyr-

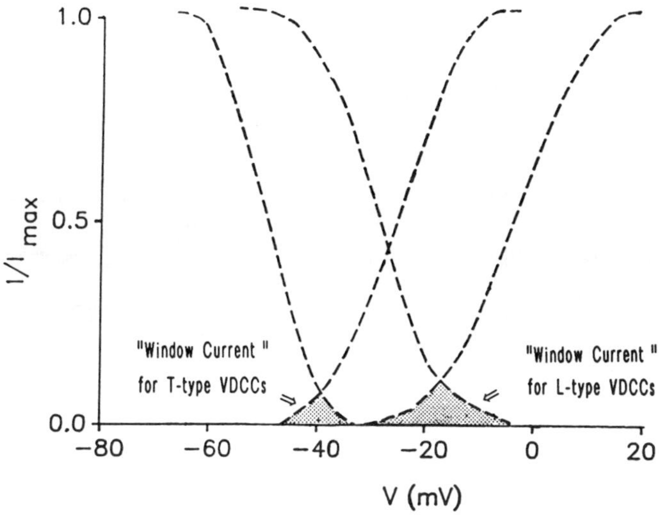

FIGURE 2. Plots of estimated voltage-activation relationships (dashed lines with positive slope) and voltage-inactivation relationships (dashed line with negative slope) for T- and L-type VDCCs. The respective overlap of activation and inactivation curves (shaded areas) show "window currents" for T- and L-type VDCCs, suggesting the voltage range compatible with steady-state channel activity. The "window current" for L-type VDCCs is at more depolarized potentials than for T-type VDCCs.

idine agonists and antagonists.[32,36] Thus, the single-channel kinetics and pharmacological characteristics of this channel were compatible with the recognized properties of the macroscopic L-type VDCC (Figures 1 and 3C).[33,36] Finally, summing of single-channel T- and L-type VDCC unitary currents identified during repeated voltage-clamp depolarizations produced the familiar integrated time course of the whole-cell VDCC currents. The comparison of T- and L-type whole-cell currents with integrated multiple single-channel records showed close correlation of single-channel events with macroscopic Ca^{2+} currents (Figure 3C).[33,36]

Accordingly, patch-clamp evidence based on kinetic, permeability, and pharmacological studies suggests that T- and L-type VDCCs are structurally distinct Ca^{2+}-conducting pathways which coexist in vascular muscle membranes. The detected density of these VDCC subtypes varies greatly between single cells from the same vascular muscle preparation and, not surprisingly, between membranes from different vascular muscle cell types. For example, the ratio of L- to T-type VDCC current amplitudes (L:T ratio) averaged 1:6 in rat azygos venous cells, one of the lowest ratios ever recorded. However, in some cells from this same vascular muscle type, the predominant T-type current could not be detected.[15,30] In contrast, guinea pig coronary arterial membranes showed an average L:T ratio of 10:1, with L-type current predominating.[44] Furthermore, the L:T ratio varied 30-fold between guinea pig mesenteric arterial cells,[35] and large ranges of L- to T-type current ratios also have been reported in rabbit ear artery[33] and rat tail artery.[34] In the latter two reports, the authors cautioned that the quality of the cells after enzymatic isolation appeared

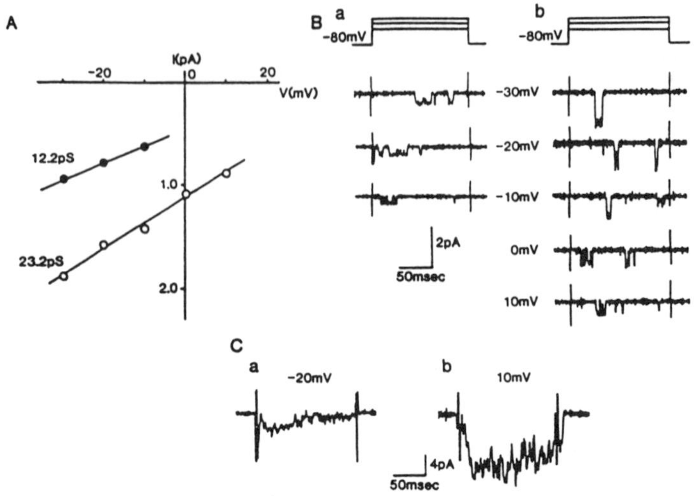

FIGURE 3. Two types of unitary current observed in smooth muscle cells of the rabbit basilar artery. The pipette was filled with 100 m*M* $BaCl_2$ solution, and the bath was superfused with high-K^+ solution containing 4 m*M* EGTA. The membrane was maintained at -80 mV, and a depolarizing pulse was applied to the membrane patch. (A) Relation between amplitude of the unitary Ba^{2+} current (I) and the patch membrane potential (V), with conductances defined by the slopes. (B) Sample tracings of the unitary Ba^{2+} current of two different amplitudes. (C) Summated unitary Ba^{2+} current with 50 nonblank tracings evoked by repetitive depolarizing pulses to -20 mV (a) and to $+10$ mV (b) (150 ms in duration, 15-s interval). (From Oike, M. et al., *Circ. Res.*, 67, 993, 1990. With permission.)

to influence the amplitude of macroscopic VDCC currents, pointing out the caveat that exposure to enzymatic dissociation may influence estimations of VDCC current density. However, high quality recordings of VDCC currents of long duration argue for a physiological basis for L:T ratio heterogeneity between different vascular cell types.

With this in mind, it has been estimated that a single vascular muscle cell membrane may express between 200 to 2000 VDCCs.[20,32,43] Virtually all patch-clamp reports in vascular membranes have demonstrated the presence of L-type channels, suggesting that arterial and venous muscle membranes may ubiquitously express this VDCC subtype. For example, in venous muscle membranes, both T- and L-type VDCCs have been detected in rat azygous,[30] rat portal,[41] and dog saphenous vein cells.[32] Similarly, both VDCC subtypes have been reported in many arterial muscle membranes, including rat aorta,[45,46] rabbit ear artery,[33] guinea pig mesenteric,[35] guinea pig coronary,[44] and rabbit basilar artery.[36] However, the T-type VDCC has been identified less consistently in membranes from arterial muscle. For example, single-channel recordings in rabbit cerebral, mesenteric, and coronary arterial membranes have revealed only L-type VDCCs, implying that T-type VDCCs may not be universally expressed in vascular muscle membranes.[47,48] Furthermore, the fact that L-type VDCCs may show multiple conductance levels in membranes of some cell types confounds the process of identifying particular VDCC subtypes according to their characteristic single-channel current amplitudes.[49] Reports of uncharacteristic voltage-dependent Ca^{2+} channel subtypes,[48,50-52] structurally and functionally distinct isoforms of VDCCs in different tissues,[39,53,54] and ligand-operated, nonselective ion channels in arterial membranes[55] suggest that the heterogeneity of vascular Ca^{2+}-conducting channels likely is underestimated at this time.

In this respect, the molecular isolation and characterization of Ca^{2+} channels in vascular muscle membranes would greatly expedite clarification of VDCC subtypes. However, the lack of specific radioligands for the T-type VDCC has impeded its isolation and characterization at the molecular level. Patch-clamp confirmation of the existence of the T-type VDCC in membranes from a single vascular muscle type also has been hampered by the lack of selective high-affinity pharmacological blockers for this channel. In contrast, the pharmacological sensitivity of the L-type VDCC to dihydropyridines has facilitated its electrophysiological and molecular isolation.[38] Recent reports indicate that the α-subunit of the vascular L-type VDCC in rat aortic muscle, which confers voltage sensitivity to the channel, is 96% homologous with the α-subunit of the L-type VDCC isolated from cardiac muscle membranes in rabbit, but may be an alternately spliced form.[39] As indicated by these authors, channel isolation combined with electrophysiological characterization likely will provide more definitive information on the diversity and single-channel properties of VDCCs in vascular muscle membranes.

C. INTRINSIC REGULATION OF VASCULAR T- AND L-TYPE VDCCs BY ARTERIAL MEMBRANE POTENTIAL

The level of membrane potential is the fundamental controller of VDCC open state probability in cell membranes. In arterial muscle, alterations in membrane potential regulate Ca^{2+} influx through VDCCs and consequently modulate vascular muscle cell excitability. Thus, in order to understand how *in situ* arterial membrane potential controls VDCC-dependent Ca^{2+} influx, and ultimately regulates vascular contraction to influence blood pressure, it is critical to: (1) define the physiological range of membrane potentials in arterial muscle *in situ,* and (2) characterize the voltage-dependent properties of the VDCC subtypes within this defined physiological voltage range. This statement appears simplistic from a theoretical perspective; however, the technical difficulties of obtaining membrane potentials from *in situ* arterial muscle cells and of resolving Ca^{2+} currents through VDCCs exposed to physiological ionic gradients are substantial. Although recent reports have begun to clarify the relationship between arterial membrane potential and VDCC behavior, it is apparent that an adequate understanding of this relationship awaits further careful investigation.

In considering the chronological progression of recent evidence coupling membrane potential to arterial VDCC function, it is important to realize that in the last decade we have redefined the accepted range of values for "physiological membrane potential" in arterial muscle. Initially, intracellular measurements by microelectrodes of vascular muscle membrane potentials usually were obtained in secured

TABLE 1
Values for Resting Membrane Potential in Unpressurized Arteries from Normotensive Animals

Arterial type	Membrane potential (mV)	Ref.
Rabbit pulmonary	−52, −60	23, 56
Rabbit basilar	−57	25
Rabbit ear	−66	28
Rat caudal		
Sprague-Dawley	−52, −56	26, 57
Wistar	−58	58
WKY	−55	59
Dahl	−52	60
Rat middle cerebral	−63	61
Rat mesenteric	−52, −56	57, 62
Guinea pig mesenteric	−70	63
Cat basilar	−62	24
Cat pial	−52	24
Cat middle cerebral	−70	64
Cat mesenteric	−49	64
Cat coronary	−58	64
Monkey coronary	−40	65
Porcine coronary	−51	66

segments of arterial muscle. Under these conditions, resting membrane potentials more negative than −50 mV were reported in most preparations. A survey of membrane potential values determined in a wide range of species and arterial muscle types shows a range from −40 to −70 mV, with most values falling between −50 to −65 mV (Table 1).[23-28,56-66] In contrast to these potentials, initial patch-clamp measurements of membrane Ca^{2+} currents through vascular muscle VDCCs showed detected voltage thresholds for macroscopic T- and L-type VDCC opening of about −45 and −30 mV, respectively (Figure 2). Correlating these values with measurements of arterial membrane potential, it was proposed that arterial muscle cell depolarization from resting membrane potentials of between −50 to −65 mV would sequentially activate the low-threshold T-type VDCC and then the high-threshold L-type VDCC. Maximum depolarization by norepinephrine or other vasoconstrictor agonists has been estimated between −30 and −15 mV in rat caudal artery,[27,58,59] at −33 mV in rabbit main pulmonary and cat basilar arteries,[24,67] and at −25 and −22 mV in cat middle cerebral and rabbit basilar arteries.[24,64] These levels of membrane potential are within the voltage range for steady-state L-type VDCC activation. Thus, it may be expected that an initial voltage-dependent opening of T-type VDCCs would permit a transient Ca^{2+} influx into the arterial muscle cell, followed by maintained Ca^{2+} influx through L-type VDCCs at more depolarized membrane potentials. The latter scenario implies activation of both T- and L-type VDCC subtypes during depolarization of arterial muscle from resting voltage levels.[15,30,31]

TABLE 2
Membrane Potential Values in Pressurized Arteries (Normotensive Animals)

Arterial type	Membrane potential (mV)		Ref.
Cat middle cerebral	−44	*(In vitro)*	75
Dog renal	−38, −38	*(In vitro)*	76, 78
Dog mesenteric	−47	*(In vitro)*	77
Rabbit cerebral	−37	*(In vitro)*	80
Rat saphenous	−39	*(In vitro)*	81
Frog tongue	−40	*(In situ)*	72
Rat mesenteric	−39, −43	*(In situ)*	73, 79
Rat gracilis	−37	*(In situ)*	79
Rat caudal (Wistar)	−38	*(In situ)*	74
Rat cremaster	−41	*(In situ)*	79
Guinea pig mesenteric	−39	*(In situ)*	73

Note: In vitro or *in situ* intraluminal pressures were between 80 to 120 mmHg.

However, resting membrane potentials in arterial muscle segments can be as much as 30 mV more negative than the detected threshold voltage for L-type VDCC activation defined by patch-clamp studies (Table 1, Figure 2). In the extreme, this may imply that L-type VDCCs are modulated by mechanisms other than membrane potential in resting arterial muscle. However, this implication seems unlikely because depolarization by vasoconstrictors in the intact system maintains membrane potential less negative than these resting potentials. Furthermore, selective blockers of L-type VDCCs reduce arterial vascular resistance in the intact circulation,[68] suggesting that L-type VDCCs are functional membrane pathways for activator Ca^{2+} influx under physiological conditions. Most importantly, the gap between resting membrane potential values and the threshold for L-type VDCC activation is resolved by imposing the physiological conditions of vascular distention on the successful measurement of intracellular membrane potential in "pressurized" arterial segments. Progressive pressurization of *in vitro* arterial segments (within the physiological range of distending pressures) results in depolarization of arterial muscle cells; the latter pressure-dependent depolarization may be dependent upon the presence of functional endothelium in some[69,70] but not all[71] vascular preparations. The key point is that most arterial segments pressurized to normal blood pressure values (80 to 120 mmHg) show membrane potentials between −37 and −47 mV (Table 2, *in vitro* values).[72-81] These transmembrane voltages are about 20 mV more depolarized than those reported previously in unpressurized arterial tissues (Table 1), and correspond to membrane potentials near the threshold for L-type VDCC steady-state opening in voltage-clamped arterial membranes. Interestingly, these "physiological membrane potentials" in arterial cells are near the maximal voltage-inactivation level reported for T-type VDCCs,[82] and thus would voltage-inactivate the low-threshold T-type channels. As such, T-type VDCCs likely contribute little to total Ca^{2+} influx in arterial muscle exposed to normal transmural pressures, unless hyperpolarization at least transiently occurs.

Critical to these statements, however, is the need to define the level of endogenous membrane potential in *in situ* pressurized arterial muscle, where VDCC activity depends on membrane potential levels influenced by integrated neural, endocrine, and physical factors. It is therefore very significant that membrane potential measurements in intact *in situ* arteries correspond closely to values obtained in pressurized *in vitro* arterial segments. Membrane potential values determined in arteries embedded in intact circulatory beds are between −43 and −37 mV at normal blood pressure levels of 80 to 120 mmHg (Table 2, *in situ* values). For example, arterial muscle cells of *in situ* mesenteric, gracilis, and cremaster arteries show membrane potential values of −43, −37, and −41 mV at normal blood pressure levels in the same rat strain.[79] The latter values concur with the level of membrane potential values in *in vitro* pressurized arteries, and thus further suggest that membrane potential fluctuations between about −45 and −20 mV may identify the physiological voltage range for functional arteries. Presumably, these values also represent the *in situ* voltages that regulate the potential-operated VDCC subtypes in intact arterial muscle membranes.

Thus, rapid progress in vascular microelectrode research has permitted estimates, at least tentatively, of levels of "physiological membrane potential" in arterial muscle. The challenge is now for patch-clamp electrophysiologists to further characterize the properties of T- and L-type VDCCs and their modulation within this range of functionally relevant transmembrane voltages. This has been, and remains, difficult to accomplish using prevailing patch-clamp recording techniques. Customarily, to permit adequate patch-clamp resolution of low amplitude VDCC currents, high external Ca^{2+} or Ba^{2+} concentrations (10 to 110 m*M*) resulting in artificially high divalent cation electrochemical gradients have been applied to enhance VDCC current amplitude. While this ionic manipulation has facilitated the study of Ca^{2+} current through these channels, high external cation concentrations shift the current-voltage relationship for VDCC activation and inactivation to more positive membrane potentials. For example, L-type VDCCs in rabbit cerebral arterial membranes appear to have similar open state probabilities at −5 mV in 80 m*M* Ba^{2+} as at −40 mV with 10 m*M* Ba^{2+} in the external solution.[48] This suggests that increased divalent cation gradients may shift the voltage regulation of the L-type VDCC by as much as 35 mV in the depolarizing direction. As a result, the majority of patch-clamp measurements of Ca^{2+} current through arterial VDCCs may have been shifted by at least 10 mV in the positive direction. If this is correct, VDCCs studied in normal Ca^{2+} gradients would likely show significant open state probabilities at more negative transmembrane voltages, and thus be optimally poised to be sensitive indicators of changes in membrane potential within the physiological voltage range. Another technical challenge in recording VDCC currents is that attempts to study these channels under physiological conditions are hampered by the short mean open time of this channel in cell-attached membrane patches of arterial muscle. The latter has led to the use of organic Ca^{2+} channel agonists (i.e., Bay K 8644) to increase L-type VDCC open times and enhance the ease of single-channel recording.[36,44,51,83] Thus, the low amplitude and short open times of VDCCs have required recording of Ca^{2+} currents under circumstances designed for optimal event detection, rather than for optimal physiological characterization. This has minimized the opportunity to predict what the intrinsic open state probability and voltage-dependent properties of VDCCs would be in vascular muscle membranes *in situ* at physiological membrane potentials.

Regardless, growing patch-clamp evidence suggests that the open state probability of L-type VDCCs in arterial membranes is modulated by physiological transmembrane voltages. For example, by using external solution minimally enhanced with 10 m*M* Ba^{2+}, single L-type VDCC currents have been recorded in cell-attached membrane patches of guinea pig coronary arterial cells during prolonged voltage-clamp at membrane potentials of −40 and −50 mV. Few T-type VDCC unitary currents were detected at these voltages in these same patches, implying again that T-type VDCCs may be voltage-inactivated at physiological membrane potentials. However, the same authors have suggested that T-type VDCCs may be available for activation following arterial muscle hyperpolarization by vasodilatory agonists.[82] Thus, a physiological role for the low-threshold T-type VDCC subtype should not be discounted. Despite this addendum, the time course of $[Ca]_i$ changes during pharmacological interventions strongly implicate L-type VDCCs as the predominate membrane pathway for voltage-dependent Ca^{2+} influx in arterial muscle. For example, arterial pressure-induced contraction, sometimes referred to as "myogenic activation", is inhibited profoundly by pharmacological block of L-type VDCCs.[70,84] This implies that pressure-activated "myogenic" tone likely depends on Ca^{2+} influx through L-type VDCC subtypes. However, this apparent dependence of pressure-induced arterial contraction on Ca^{2+} influx through L-type VDCCs has not been reported in all blood vessel types.[71,85] It is likely that within the wide variety of vascular muscle types, different subtypes of VDCCs exist. Until specific pharmacological blockers of the T-type VDCC, and perhaps other types and subtypes of VDCCs are available, investigation of the functional role of VDCCs in arterial contraction will remain difficult.

III. EVIDENCE FOR ABNORMAL VDCC CURRENT IN VASCULAR MUSCLE MEMBRANES IN HYPERTENSION

A. BACKGROUND

Abnormal voltage-dependent Ca^{2+} influx has been implicated as a mechanism for vascular reactivity changes in hypertension. The experimental approach generally used to correlate abnormal VDCC function to vascular contractile changes has been to alter VDCC open state probability by pharmacological or membrane potential manipulation, and to compare changes in arterial contraction between normo- and hypertensive arterial muscle. These studies have provided important insight into the functional importance of VDCCs in regulating vascular tone in arterial muscle types from genetic and experimental rat models of hypertension. However, pinpointing VDCC current alterations as mechanisms for arterial reactivity changes has been difficult, as many other cellular processes also regulate cytosolic free Ca^{2+} concentration ($[Ca]_i$) and the level of arterial contraction.[86] Also, as reviewed recently,[87] the contractile amplitude in smooth muscle is not dependent solely on the level of $[Ca]_i$, but also is modulated by many other regulatory mechanisms. Thus, recent reports by some investigators[88,89] that the Ca^{2+} sensitivity of arterial muscle contractile proteins may be altered in hypertension suggest that electromechanical coupling events distal to membrane VDCCs also may modulate the abnormal arterial contraction.

With this caveat in mind, functional evidence is nevertheless growing that arterial VDCCs are a mechanism for increased Ca^{2+} influx in hypertension. In addition to reports of an increased arterial sensitivity to direct membrane depolarizing agents,[90-100] an enhanced VDCC response to neurohumoral agents also has been reported in arterial muscle cells from some models of hypertension.[101,102] However, the multifaceted effects of neurohumoral agents on VDCCs, particularly in light of possible contractile protein Ca^{2+} sensitivity variability, leave coupling of changes in agonist-induced contraction to Ca^{2+} channel mechanisms as a very perplexing puzzle. For example, α-adrenoceptor agonists reportedly modulate the open state probability of arterial VDCCs by changing vascular membrane potential,[29,103] by cytosolic mediation of the open state of the channel,[104] and by a direct membrane effect on channel gating.[105] In view of this complexity, the more focused approach of defining VDCC mechanisms by altering membrane voltage or by using VDCC-selective agonists or antagonists has been the most likely to provide interpretable results.

B. FUNCTIONAL IMPLICATIONS OF ENHANCED ARTERIAL VDCC CURRENT IN HYPERTENSION

Arterial muscle obtained from genetically hypertensive rats, but not normotensive controls, develops a Ca^{2+}-dependent active tone after the application of passive stretch. For example, basal tension in the carotid artery and aorta from adult spontaneously hypertensive rats (SHR) is reduced by lowering the level of Ca^{2+} in the external solution or after chelation of external Ca^{2+} by ethylene glycol-tetraacetic acid (EGTA).[90,91,97] In the same experiments, the Ca^{2+}-dependent development of active basal tone was not observed in similar arteries obtained from normotensive Wistar Kyoto rats (WKY). The latter suggests that in physiological Ca^{2+} concentrations, the arterial muscle membrane from adult SHR is more permeable to Ca^{2+} under basal conditions. Similar results have been reported in femoral artery from 6-week-old WKY and SHR.[92] In these preparations, Ca^{2+}-free solution relaxed only SHR arteries. Furthermore, nifedipine, a blocker of the L-type VDCC, also caused dose-dependent relaxation of SHR but not WKY arterial basal tone. This apparent increase in nifedipine-sensitive basal Ca^{2+} influx in arterial muscle from young SHR suggests that an enhanced L-type VDCC current may occur early in the development of hypertension. However, because arterial pressures in these 6-week-old WKY and SHR rats were determined to be different (WKY = 114 mmHg;

SHR = 134 mmHg), it is unclear from these data alone whether vascular Ca^{2+} permeability changes preceded or were a consequence of the elevated blood pressure.

Logically, the most likely mechanism for an elevated arterial membrane Ca^{2+} permeability in genetic hypertension may be a depolarized membrane potential. In the event that membrane potential is not altered, the alternative is that VDCCs in arterial muscle membranes from hypertensive animals function abnormally to permit a higher Ca^{2+} influx. This hypothesis is considered in the next section, as several theories exist, including a higher membrane density of VDCCs, a different voltage-sensitivity of these channels, or altered subtypes of VDCCs in hypertensive membranes. While the possibility that vascular muscle cells are more depolarized in arterial segments from hypertensive animals must be tested in many different blood vessels and models of hypertension to give a definitive answer, considerable evidence weighs against a difference in resting membrane potential as a universal finding.[27,57,59,60,62,106] For this mechanism to explain increased vascular muscle contraction, the expectation is that the open state probability of VDCCs is regulated by membrane voltage,[107] such that a more electropositive membrane potential in arterial cells from hypertensive animals would result in an elevated VDCC current. Because of the technical difficulty in accurately measuring the membrane potential of vascular muscle, no vascular reactivity studies have compared altered basal Ca^{2+} permeability between arteries from normo- and hypertensive rats along with membrane potential in the same preparation.

However, measurements of resting membrane potential obtained by other laboratories allow comparison of the evidence for arterial membrane depolarization in hypertension. Briefly, similar resting membrane potentials between −52 and −56 mV have been reported in caudal arterial segments from hypertensive rats, including SHR,[59] stroke-prone SHR,[106] Dahl salt-sensitive rats,[60] and deoxycorticosone- (DOCA) salt-sensitive rats.[27,57] These membrane potentials in arteries exposed to hypertension were the same as those recorded in similar arteries from age-matched normotensive control rats. Resting membrane potentials in WKY and SHR mesenteric arterial cells also are reported to be comparable, averaging −56 and −57 mV, respectively.[62] Likewise, the reported membrane potential of −52 mV in mesenteric arteries from DOCA-salt hypertensive rats was the same as values obtained in arteries of the Sprague-Dawley controls.[57] These data imply similar resting membrane potentials between arteries obtained from normotensive rats and genetic or experimental rat models of hypertension, and indicate that membrane depolarization is not a likely mechanism for enhanced arterial VDCC current in arterial segments obtained from hypertensive rats. One report indicates however, that depolarized resting membrane potentials exist in arterial muscle from SHR. In external solution containing 6 m*M* KCl, comparable membrane potentials of −55 and −53 mV were recorded in aortas from 6-week-old WKY and SHR, while disparate potentials of −58 and −50 mV were recorded in aortas from 12-week-old rats of the same strains.[99] The latter suggests that the depolarized membrane potential in SHR aortic cells was related to the development of high blood pressure. However, even this 8 mV difference in membrane potential (−58 mV in WKY compared to −50 mV in SHR) found in the 12-week-old rats was abolished when

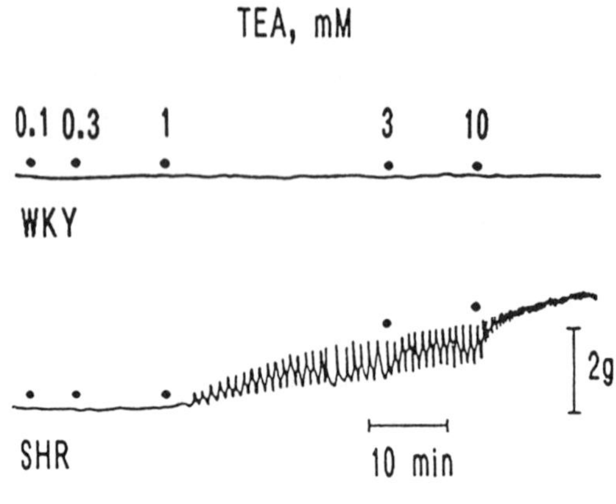

FIGURE 4. Exposure of rat aortic segments to increasing concentrations of TEA. Representative recordings show that application of TEA (0.1 to 10 m*M*) contracted SHR but not normotensive WKY aortas. (Adapted from Rusch, N. J. et al., *Hypertension,* 19, 301, 1992. With permission.)

the external K^+ concentration was lowered from 6 to 3 m*M*.[99] In view of this, it is difficult to contend that a distinct difference between WKY and SHR arterial membrane potentials exists within the physiological range of K^+ concentrations. In a separate study, rat aortic vascular muscle obtained 6 months after the induction of renal hypertension (2 kidney, 1 clip, 2K1C, model) showed a resting membrane potential of -50 mV as compared to -58 mV in control vascular muscle, indicating arterial depolarization in hypertension.[108] The latter suggestion is consistent with studies in which the L-type VDCC, dihydropyridine agonist Bay K 8644, contracted arterial preparations from SHR more readily than those from WKY.[92,94,96-98] This pharmacological effect may be secondary to a more electropositive resting membrane potential in the SHR arteries because dihydropyridines bind with higher affinity to the inactivated state of the L-type VDCC subtype.[31,51,109] Alternatively, the differential contractile effect of Bay K 8644 may indicate an altered ion channel protein in SHR arteries because dihydropyridines bind specifically to the α_1-subunit of L-type VDCCs in arterial muscle.[39] Thus, while it is possible that a depolarized resting membrane potential in arterial muscle may enhance VDCC current in certain, narrowly defined situations in hypertension, experimental data correlating membrane depolarization with enhanced basal tone in the same vascular preparation will be required to give credence to this possibility.

Elevated VDCC current also has been postulated to augment contractile reactivity during arterial excitation.[92-100] Thus, stroke-prone SHR carotid artery and SHR aorta show an enhanced contractile sensitivity to tetraethylammonium- (TEA) induced depolarization as compared to WKY arteries (Figure 4), and this difference can be abolished by pharmacological blockers of the L-type VDCC.[95,100] Similarly, an enhanced Ca^{2+}-dependent contractile sensitivity to TEA has been reported in rat aortas exposed to high arterial pressure after interrenal aortic coarctation.[100] These data imply that membrane excitation can unmask an underlying Ca^{2+}-dependent excitability in arteries from hypertensive rats, which likely is mediated by L-type VDCCs. Femoral and carotid arteries from SHR also contract with greater sensitivity to KCl-induced depolarization.[93,97] In the latter, the KCl concentration for half-maximal contraction (ED_{50}) was 25 m*M* in SHR as compared to 37 m*M* in WKY. Similarly, in isolated rat caudal arterial cells, the ED_{50} values for KCl-induced contraction were 30 m*M* in SHR compared to 38 m*M* in WKY.[96] However, in the mesenteric circulation, KCl dose-response curves reportedly are comparable between small (100 to 200 μm) WKY and SHR resistance arteries,[110] whereas larger SHR mesenteric arteries show an enhanced sensitivity to KCl.[94] In the same preparation, estimates of KCl-induced Ca^{2+} influx ^{45}Ca transport studies show no difference between WKY and SHR.[8] Thus, while functional evidence exists for abnormal VDCC current in vascular muscle in hypertension, determining the mechanism and distribution of VDCC abnormalities will likely require direct measurement of VDCC currents in membranes of a variety of blood vessels.

One notable clue to the hypertension puzzle is that VDCC abnormalities are only one facet of a generalized increase in vascular muscle membrane permeability. Multiple types of arterial muscle from genetic and experimental rat models of hypertension show concurrent increases in transmembrane permeability to Na^+, K^+, and Cl^-, as well as the Ca^{2+} ion.[111-114] These findings have prompted the suggestion that changes in transmembrane ionic flux in hypertension, including increased Ca^{2+} entry, are the manifestation of a universal membrane defect.[115] The molecular identity of this membrane defect remains unidentified. However, some investigators contend that a decreased binding of Ca^{2+} to the arterial sarcolemma in hypertension induces membrane instability and a generalized increase in transmembrane ionic flux.[116,117] This hypothesis is supported by measurements showing fewer Ca^{2+} binding sites in arterial muscle membranes in hypertension,[118] as well as reports that increases in $[Ca]_o$ normalize the enhanced ionic flux and functional abnormalities in arteries from genetic and renal hypertensive rats.[116,117,119] Furthermore, it has been reported that the fluidity of vascular membranes is reduced in hypertension,[120] and a decreased membrane fluidity may increase dihydropyridine-sensitive Ca^{2+} influx in arterial muscle.[121] The latter suggests that changes in membrane composition may regulate VDCC function in hypertension.[122] However, cause and effect are still a clouded issue, as VDCC abnormalities could conceivably lead to permeability and even membrane fluidity changes through inositol triphosphate, phospholipase C, protein kinase and other crucial signaling mechanisms that are dependent on subsarcolemmal Ca^{2+} levels.[5,123,124]

Finally, findings of increased VDCC activity in arteries isolated from hypertensive rats correspond with reports of abnormal VDCC function in intact vascular beds. In the renal vasculature of SHR, diameters of the resistance vessels in SHR are 18 to 35% smaller than in WKY, and this difference is eliminated by low calcium media.[125] Because the microcirculation is dependent on VDCC current both for tone and refilling of intracellular Ca^{2+} stores,[126] this observation suggests that elevated Ca^{2+}-dependent vascular tone, rather than structural changes, may account for the smaller microvascular diameter in SHR. Similarly, verapamil but not the nonspecific dilator nitroprusside, is more effective in dilating the forearm vasculature of hypertensive than normotensive human subjects.[127,128] This points to abnormal L-type VDCC behavior as a mechanism for enhanced vascular resistance in human hypertension. In the integrated system, organic Ca^{2+} channel blockers of L-type VDCCs cause more hypotension in SHR, renal, DOCA, and Dahl salt-sensitive hypertensive rats than in normotensive rats.[129-135] Clinically approved L-type VDCC blockers also reduce blood pressure more in hypertensive than in normotensive human subjects.[136-141] Collectively, these data provide a compelling argument that abnormal VDCC function in arterial muscle membranes may be related to the increased vascular tone observed in animal and human hypertension.

C. VDCC CURRENTS IN VASCULAR AND CARDIAC MYOCYTES IN GENETIC AND EXPERIMENTAL HYPERTENSION

Despite indications that changes in arterial reactivity in hypertension may reflect abnormal L-type VDCC function, few patch-clamp studies have compared VDCC current between cardiovascular membranes from normo- and hypertensive animals. Nevertheless, initial comparisons between WKY and SHR have suggested that L-type VDCC current may be altered in vascular muscle from genetically hypertensive rats.[15,16] Experiments in azygos vein cells from 1- to 3-day-old WKY and SHR, free from changes caused by hemodynamic rather than genetic factors, suggest that the amplitude of total whole-cell VDCC current is similar between WKY and SHR venous membranes. However, the relative contributions of T- and L-type current to total membrane current were different between the two strains (Figure 5A), with L-type current accounting for 33 and 62% of total VDCC current in WKY and SHR, respectively. The L:T ratio was variable among cells from the same rat strain, but averaged only 0.9 in WKY compared to 2.9 in SHR cells (Figure 5B). Because the vascular muscle in this study was obtained in neonatal rats from the low-pressure venous side of the circulation, it was suggested that the augmented L-type VDCC current was genetically determined rather than induced by elevated blood pressure. The close correspondence between physiological membrane potentials and the voltage domain of L-type VDCC window current, as outlined earlier in this chapter, fits well with the hypothesis that increased L-type VDCC current could be the key to the sustained vascular contraction seen in hypertension.[15]

Reported increases in the peak amplitude of whole-cell L-type current, however, do not indicate which single-channel mechanism(s) contribute to this augmentation. Changes in whole-cell L-type current imply a change in the membrane density, unitary amplitude, and/or open state probability of L-type VDCCs in hypertension because total current (I) is the product of (n)(i)(p) [n = channel number, i = single-channel current amplitude, p = open state probability]. In this respect, comparisons of L-type VDCC current density (whole-cell current amplitude normalized to membrane area) between vascular membranes from normo- and hypertensive animals, as well as humans, are an important goal of future research. Single-channel characterization of the biophysical and pharmacological properties of unitary L-type VDCC currents, as well as molecular investigation of possible channel

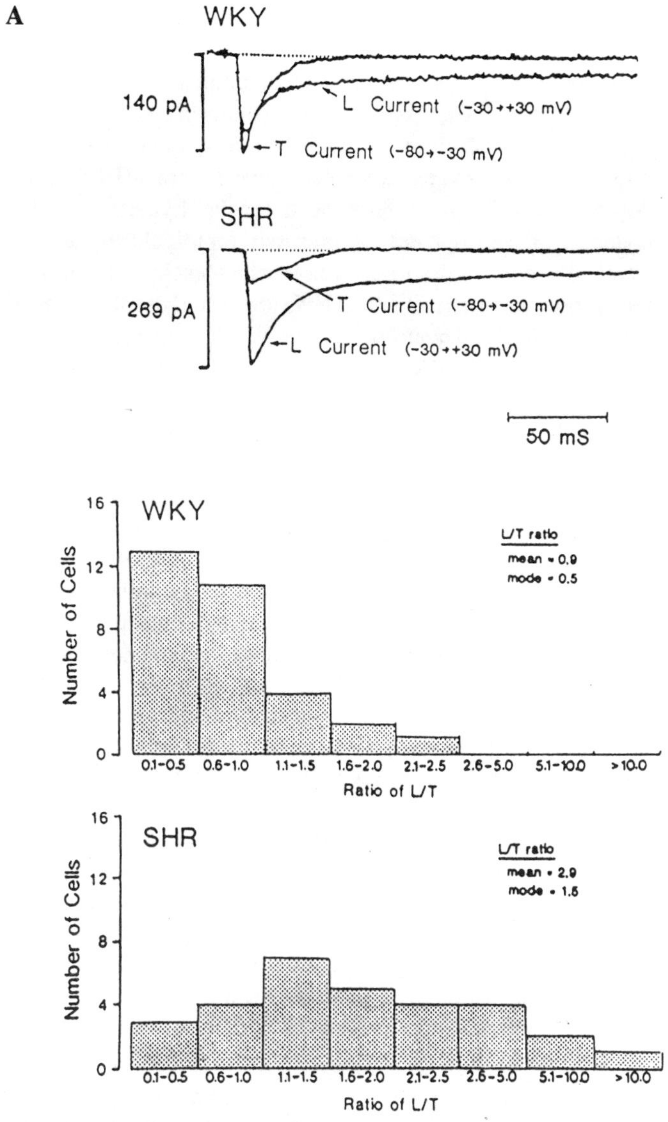

FIGURE 5. (A) Whole-cell calcium currents in WKY (upper tracings) and SHR (lower tracings) azygos venous muscle cells. The T-type (T) current was measured during a 300-ms depolarizing pulse from −80 to −30 mV, while the L-type (L) current was recorded during depolarization from −30 to +30 mV. The WKY cell showed predominantly T-type current (peak T- and L-type current, 140 and 112 pA, respectively), while the SHR cell showed more L-type current (peak T- and L-type current, 90 and 269 pS, respectively). (B) Graph showing the frequency distribution of the ratio of L-type to T-type (L/T) calcium current for 30 WKY and 30 SHR azygos venous cells. WKY cells had a lower L/T ratio (mean, 0.9; mode, 0.5). SHR cells had a higher L/T ratio (mean, 2.9; mode, 1.5). Note that scale changes on the abscissa. (Adapted from Rusch, N. J. and Hermsmeyer, K., *Circ. Res.*, 63, 997, 1988. With permission.)

structural alterations, also will add critical data to clarify the nature of VDCC alterations in hypertension.

Encouraging progress from a related field comes from reports that cardiac muscle cells show L-type VDCC density changes during normal development and under pathophysiological conditions. Patch-clamp characterization of whole-cell VDCC currents in cardiac myocytes suggests that L-type VDCC density changes during development, and in pressure-induced cardiac hypertrophy. In rabbit ventricular myocytes, L-type current density increases rapidly during development from fetal to neonatal to adult maturation, without changes in voltage-dependent activation or inactivation properties.[142,143] These data suggest that ventricular membranes accumulate a higher density of L-type VDCCs during development, while the intrinsic nature of this VDCC subtype is not altered. Furthermore, pressure-induced hypertrophy of feline ventricular cells delays inactivation of the slow component of whole-cell L-type VDCC current, thus possibly prolonging the action potential and contractile pattern of these myocytes. In the same cells, however, peak L-type VDCC current was similar between normal and hypertrophied ventricular cells;[17] however, macroscopic L-type currents in hypertrophied rat myocytes (Goldblatt renovascular hypertension) revealed an increased current density and a similar slower inactivation of whole-cell current.[18] Myocardial hypertrophy also is associated with changes in at least two types of K^+ currents,[144] suggesting that even in a single muscle cell membrane, multiple ionic channels can be affected by exposure to high blood pressure.

IV. MECHANISMS REGULATING VDCCs IN ARTERIAL MUSCLE MEMBRANES IN HYPERTENSION

A. PRESSURE-INDUCED MEMBRANE DEPOLARIZATION

As reviewed earlier, arterial muscle shows pressure-dependent depolarization, resulting in resting membrane potential levels in pressurized arterial muscle within the transmembrane voltage range associated with steady-state L-type VDCC activation (Table 2; Figure 2). In hypertension, it is likely that this process of pressure-dependent depolarization is enhanced, as transmural pressure rises during the course of this disease. For example, in pressurized canine ileum arteries, a normal transmural pressure of 100 mmHg was associated with a resting membrane potential of −47 mV, whereas membrane potential was −39 mV during additional pressurization to 160 mmHg.[77] Similarly, membrane potential was reduced from −38 to −33 mV by pressurization of dog renal arteries from 100 to 140 mmHg.[78] In *in situ* rat caudal artery, membrane potential showed rapid change from −37 to −31 mV during blood pressure fluctuation from about 130 to 150 mmHg. These authors noted that the gain of the depolarization-pressure relationship was much steeper at higher than at normal blood pressures.[74] Finally, comparison of pressure-induced depolarization between WKY and SHR cerebral arteries indicates that at transmural pressures between 40 to 160 mmHg, SHR cerebral arteries depolarize more than their normotensive counterparts. For example, at a transmural pressure of

140 mmHg, WKY cerebral arteries showed resting membrane potentials of −43 mV, whereas comparable SHR arteries were further depolarized to about −33 mV.[84] Collectively, these data suggest that in hypertension, the membrane depolarizing effects of elevated blood pressure will redefine the pressure-depolarization relationship in arterial muscle, and that arterial membranes from genetically hypertensive animals may be more sensitive to this effect.

This augmented pressure-induced depolarization in hypertension is a likely mechanism for the increased L-type VDCC activity postulated to occur in *in situ* arteries of hypertensive animals and humans. As reviewed earlier,[145] the resting membrane potential of the arterial cell regulates the amplitude of steady-state VDCC current and sets the physiological "holding potential" from which depolarization-induced increases in VDCC current occur. In hypertension, enhanced arterial depolarization may be obligatorily coupled to promoting Ca^{2+} influx through L-type VDCCs, by optimally accessing the voltage range for window current. The more electropositive membrane potentials in arteries exposed to high transmural pressure would virtually eliminate any possibility for contribution of T-type VDCCs to voltage-dependent Ca^{2+} influx. If this analysis is correct, T-type VDCCs would play little role in regulating arterial contraction in hypertension except during a hyperpolarizing circumstance such as release of endothelium-derived hyperpolarizing factors.[108,146-149] In this regard, the strong correlation of spontaneous contractions with genetic hypertension[116] suggests that T-type VDCCs, thought to provide a pacemaker function,[15,30] may be important under certain circumstances.

Despite the apparent predominance of the L-type VDCCs as pathways for Ca^{2+} influx in arterial muscle in hypertension, other Ca^{2+}-conducting pathways may be activated by stretch of the arterial membranes. Many recent studies have been directed at elucidating the identity of "stretch-activated channels" (SACs) in membranes from vascular muscle and other cell types.[71,85,150] Recent evidence from patch-clamp studies on porcine coronary arteries suggest that SACs likely represent mechanosensitive cation channels, permeable to Na^+ and K^+, as well as Ca^{2+}, during mechanical stimulation of the vascular muscle membrane.[150] While the role of SACs in pressure-induced activation of arterial muscle is unclear, it is possible they serve a dual role in enhancing $[Ca]_i$ during arterial pressurization, both by providing a pathway for Ca^{2+} influx and also by enhancing the open state probability of L-type VDCCs by causing membrane depolarization. Further, it should be noted that preliminary evidence suggests that current through L-type VDCCs is not modulated directly by membrane stretch. Whole-cell recordings of L-type VDCC current indicate that L-type current amplitude in single arterial cells is not altered during mechanical perturbation of the membrane,[150] suggesting that mechanisms other than the direct mechanical effects of stretch must be invoked to produce abnormal VDCC currents in hypertension.

B. NEUROTRANSMISSION

Although patch-clamp experiments on isolated arterial cells and cell membranes have clarified the voltage-dependent properties of VDCC subtypes, the final open state probability of these channels *in situ* will be influenced by numerous endogenous modulators. Of these, it may be particularly important to appraise modulation of VDCC activity by the sympathetic nervous system because an enhanced noradrenergic output to blood vessels likely contributes to arterial excitability in many models of hypertension.[21] Although sympathetic activation involves the release of multiple transmitter types, the actions of norepinephrine on vascular muscle VDCCs has received the most attention in recent electrophysiology experiments.

Whole-cell patch-clamp recordings have suggested that norepinephrine has opposing effects on T- and L-type VDCCs. In rat portal vein, norepinephrine (1 μM) increased the amplitude of T-type current by 41%, but partially blocked L-type current.[104] Norepinephrine-induced block of L-type VDCCs also was reported in rabbit ear artery.[105] This block of L-type VDCCs may be explained as one inhibitory aspect of norepinephrine action that is exaggerated by the nonphysiological conditions of whole-cell recording;[151] in particular, that norepinephrine-induced rises in $[Ca]_i$ result in sequential Ca^{2+} inactivation of L-type VDCCs. In smooth muscle cells, release of Ca^{2+} from intracellular stores inhibits voltage-dependent Ca^{2+} entry by acting at the cytosolic mouth of the calcium channel.[152] The $[Ca]_i$ required for half-maximal inactivation of L-type current in vascular muscle may be as low as 100 nM, suggesting that $[Ca]_i$ may be a powerful, physiological regulator of L-type VDCC current in vascular muscle.[153] It is interesting that whole-cell L-type VDCC current in SHR vascular muscle appears more sensitive to Ca^{2+} inactivation than WKY, as evidenced by the more pronounced block of SHR L-type current amplitude by rises in $[Ca]_i$.[16] Paradoxically, it is possible that Ca^{2+} inactivation in functional vascular muscle cells is deficient because L-type current appears to be augmented despite local Ca^{2+} increases in the subsarcolemmal space.[12] The latter implies that these Ca^{2+} "hotspots" do not have access to the inactivation site on the L-type VDCC, or perhaps that the Ca^{2+} inactivation process is abnormal in more obscure aspects.

However, in contrast to norepinephrine-induced Ca^{2+} inactivation of L-type current in whole-cell recordings, single-channel, cell-attached recordings of arterial VDCC currents suggest that the predominant effect of norepinephrine on L-type VDCCs is a depolarization-mediated increase in open state probability. In rabbit ear artery, norepinephrine (0.5 to 2.5 μM) activates single L-type VDCCs by membrane depolarization, and also by a mediation pathway independent of voltage but dependent on cytosolic mediation.[103] Thus, in this arterial preparation, norepinephrine activation of L-type VDCCs may permit Ca^{2+} entry required for tonic arterial contraction. These findings would explain many previous reports that norepinephrine-induced contractions in arterial muscle are partially dependent on Ca^{2+} influx through L-type VDCCs, and are of particular interest because norepinephrine-induced contractions in SHR arteries may be abnormally dependent on Ca^{2+} entry.[101] They further provide a possible mechanism by which an enhanced sympathetic output (increased neuronal release of norepinephrine) in hypertension would increase the open state probability of L-type VDCCs, and promote an elevated arterial tone.

The latter concept has been suggested implicitly by studies comparing resting membrane potentials of *in situ* mesenteric arteries in WKY and SHR rats. In these

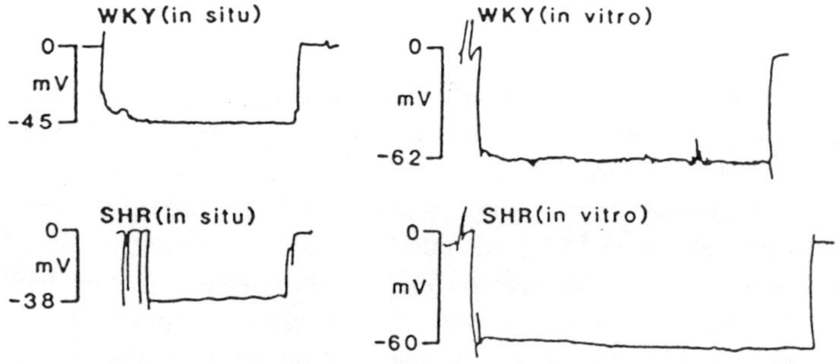

FIGURE 6. Intracellular recording of membrane potential in normotensive WKY (upper traces) and in SHR (lower traces) mesenteric arterial cells. Measurements were made in cells from intact arteries in anesthetized rats (*in situ;* traces on left) or in pinned segments of similar arterial muscle (*in vitro;* traces on right). Note the more electropositive membrane potential of *in situ* compared to *in vitro* preparations, and the further depolarization of SHR compared to WKY *in situ* mesenteric arterial cell. (From Rusch, N. J. and Stekiel, W. J., in *Cellular and Molecular Mechanisms in Hypertension,* Cox, R. H., Ed., Plenum Press, New York, 1991, 1. With permission.)

vessels exposed to endogenous neurogenic and humoral factors, membrane potential was −43 mV in WKY arteries compared to −38 mV in SHR arteries (Figure 6, left traces).[62,79,145] After local chemical denervation of sympathetic nerve endings by 6-hydroxydopamine, a comparable membrane potential of −45 mV was measured in the same *in situ* WKY and SHR arteries, suggesting that local sympathetic output depolarized SHR arteries more than their WKY counterparts (not shown). Membrane potentials of *in vitro* WKY and SHR arteries also were similar at −56 and −57 mV, respectively (Figure 6, right traces). The approximately 10 mV depolarization between membrane potentials of WKY and SHR in *in vitro* segments (−56 to −57 mV) and the value of −45 mV measured in denervated, pressurized *in situ* arteries from both rat strains likely reflects pressure-dependent depolarization of the arterial muscle in the *in situ* vessels. Thus, the integrated influences of transmural pressure and sympathetic output indicate that the sympathetic nervous system, in combination with pressure-induced depolarization, powerfully mediate arterial excitability in some *in situ* vascular beds. They further suggest an augmentation of this tonic excitatory influence in arterial muscle in hypertension. The exact neuroeffector mechanisms for the enhanced sympathetically mediated depolarization are unclear, but could involve augmented norepinephrine availability at the neuromuscular junction[21] or an enhanced sensitivity of arterial muscle to norepinephrine at elevated transmural pressures.[78] Regardless, it has been postulated that the amplified neuronally induced depolarization of *in situ* SHR arterial muscle may position membrane potential to optimally activate L-type VDCCs.[145] It could be contended that the final consequence in the integrated system would be an enhanced Ca^{2+} influx into arterial muscle cells and an increased arterial tone in hypertension.[15,22,103,145]

C. ENDOTHELIUM AND PARACRINE FACTORS

Restating the hypothesis, the more electropositive arterial membrane potential induced by elevated transmural pressure and sympathetic noradrenergic output in hypertension may augment VDCC activity of *in situ* arterial membranes. In the normal environment, these and other depolarizing stimuli may be buffered by factors released by the vascular endothelium, which can induce arterial hyperpolarization and concomitant relaxation.[146-149] The latter hyperpolarization appears to be due to activation of arterial K^+ channels by endothelium-derived factors because it is blocked by K^+ channel antagonists such as tetraethylammonium.[108] In view of this, it has been proposed that endothelium-mediated hyperpolarization may reduce the level of Ca^{2+} influx through vascular muscle VDCCs and thus regulate arterial tone.[108,149]

However, the level of endothelium-dependent relaxation appears to be reduced in hypertension. Arteries from renal,[108,154] Dahl salt-sensitive,[155] and genetically hypertensive rats[149] show attenuated endothelium-dependent dilations as compared to their normotensive counterparts. This attenuated relaxation correlates with the loss of endothelium-induced hyperpolarization of the arterial muscle, suggesting close electromechanical coupling of membrane potential and relaxation.[108,149] For example, in rat mesenteric arteries under basal conditions, acetylcholine elicits an endothelium-dependent hyperpolarization of 17 mV in WKY but only 8 mV in SHR. In the same vessels under conditions of depolarization with norepinephrine, acetylcholine-induced hyperpolarizations average 29 and 6 mV in WKY and SHR arterial muscle, respectively. This reduced acetylcholine-induced hyperpolarization in SHR was associated with a blunted relaxation response to endothelium-dependent dilating factors.[149] In another study comparing aortas from control and renal-hypertensive rats (2K, 1C), the hyperpolarization induced by carbacol in control vessels was 11 mV as compared to only 2 mV in aortas in 2K, 1C. This blunting of endothelium-dependent hyperpolarization in aortas from 2K, 1C was associated with a reduced endothelium-mediated relaxation.[108] These findings may be relevant to human hypertension because reduced endothelium-dependent dilations in forearm blood vessels of hypertensive patients also have been measured.[156] Thus, an inability of the endothelium to buffer arterial depolarization in hypertension may result in enhanced excitability of the arterial muscle cell and further voltage-activation of arterial VDCCs.[108,149]

In addition to regulation of VDCCs by membrane voltage alteration, evidence is growing that endothelium-derived constricting factors may enhance the open state probability of arterial L-type VDCCs independent of membrane potential changes. Patch-clamp reports suggest that endothelin, the potent vasoconstrictor peptide released by the vascular endothelium,[157] increases L-type VDCC current in multiple arterial muscle cell types. For example, the peak amplitude of whole-cell, dihydropyridine-sensitive Ca^{2+} channel current in porcine coronary arterial cells was enhanced twofold by external application of endothelin (10 n*M*).[158] In segments of the same vascular preparation, endothelin-induced contractions were partially blocked by dihydropyridine antagonists, suggesting an obligatory role of L-type VDCCs in endothelin-induced contractions. Endothelin also increased the frequency, but not the conductance or mean open time, of single-channel L-type currents in cell-attached patches of the same arterial cells.[159] The latter findings implicate involvement of an intracellular second messenger system in the endothelin-induced enhancement of L-type VDCC open state probability, at least in this arterial muscle cell type.

This recent evidence of endothelin-mediated regulation of arterial VDCCs conveys the important point that multiple endogenous modulators of VDCCs, in addition to membrane potential, are likely to determine the final open state probability of these channels in vascular muscle. In addition to endothelium-derived products, angiotensin II increases L-type VDCC current in rabbit aortic muscle cells.[160] Other circulating substances, such as platelet-derived growth factor (PDGF), may exert their effect on vascular smooth muscle by activation of L-type VDCCs.[102] In the latter case, a verapamil-sensitive increase in $[Ca]_i$ was greater in SHR than in WKY aortic muscle cells, prompting the suggestion that PDGF may produce a greater activity of Ca^{2+} channels in SHR vascular membranes. Thus, it may be reasonable to define the regulation of VDCCs of *in situ* arterial muscle as the integrated response of membrane potential and endogenous modulation. Changes in the summated influences of these determinants will determine the final open state probability of VDCCs in arterial muscle membranes in hypertension.

V. SUMMARY

The primary purpose of this chapter has been to examine the literature implicating VDCC abnormalities in arterial membranes in hypertension. Evidence is presented that two VDCC subtypes coexist in arterial muscle membranes, although their relative distribution in different arterial muscle types appears extremely variable. To judge from measurements of membrane potential in *in situ* arteries, the low-threshold, T-type VDCC subtype may be mainly voltage-inactivated in arterial muscle cells exposed to physiological levels of transmural pressure, and thus play only a minor role in regulating voltage-dependent Ca^{2+} influx under steady-state conditions. In contrast, evidence is presented that the open state probability of the L-type VDCC subtype may be closely coupled to *in situ* membrane potential, and thus poised as a sensitive pathway to regulate Ca^{2+} current during changes in transmembrane voltage. It is very likely that studies directed at correlating changes in arterial membrane potential with altered VDCC current and vascular reactivity responses will be helpful in clarifying the role of VDCCs in arterial excitation-contraction coupling.

There is abundant and increasing evidence from vascular reactivity studies to support the hypothesis that L-type VDCC current is augmented in arterial muscle membranes of genetically hypertensive rats. In addition, studies in both the intact animal and human circulation have implicated augmented L-type VDCC current as a mechanism of increased vascular resistance in hypertension. However, efforts at identifying the exact cellular events by which augmented arterial voltage-dependent

Ca^{2+} influx may occur in hypertension have just begun. Patch-clamp experiments in isolated arterial and cardiac cell membranes have provided initial evidence for altered density and kinetics of VDCCs, implicating genetic and pressure-induced mechanisms in these abnormalities. In addition, microelectrode measurements show a sympathetically mediated depolarization of *in situ* arteries, which may confer closer coupling between membrane potential and L-type VDCC activation in hypertension. However, the open state probability of arterial VDCCs at a given membrane potential is likely modulated further by such diverse influences as membrane composition, humoral substances, and endothelium-derived factors. The latter suggests that much careful investigation will be required to define VDCCs at the molecular level, and to predict their integrated responses to voltage, physical, and endogenous stimuli under physiological recording conditions.

ACKNOWLEDGMENTS

Supported by grants HL-HL40474 (to N. J. R.), PPG HL-29587 (to N. J. R.), HL-38645 (to K. H.), and HL-38537 (to K. H.) from the National Institutes of Health.

REFERENCES

1. **Folkow, B.,** Physiological aspects of primary hypertension, *Physiol. Rev.,* 1982; 62:347–504.
2. **Hermsmeyer, K.,** Altered arterial muscle ion transport mechanism in the spontaneously hypertensive rat, *J. Cardiovasc. Pharmacol.,* 1984; 6:S10–S15.
3. **Mulvany, M. J.,** The structure of the resistance vasculature in essential hypertension, *J. Hypertension,* 1987; 5:129–136.
4. **Hermsmeyer, K. and Erne, P.,** Cellular calcium regulation in hypertension, *Am. J. Hypertension,* 1989; 655–658.
5. **Hermsmeyer, K. and Erne, P.,** Subsarcolemmal increase in intracellular free calcium in vascular muscle cells from newborn spontaneously hypertensive rats, in *Cellular Aspects of Hypertension,* Bruschi, G. and Borghetti, A., Eds., Springer-Verlag, Berlin, 1991, 91–96.
6. **Aoki, K.,** Development of the calcium-membrane theory of hypertension, in *Membrane Abnormalities in Hypertension,* Kwan, C. Y., Ed., Boca Raton, FL, CRC Press, 1989, 79–114.
7. **Kwan, C. Y.,** Abnormalities of vascular muscle membranes with special reference to calcium handling, in *Membrane Abnormalities in Hypertension,* Kwan, C. Y., Ed., Boca Raton, FL, CRC Press, 1989, 115–144.
8. **Cauvin, C., Johns, A., Yamamoto, M. K. et al.,** Ca^{2+} movements in vascular smooth muscle and their alterations in hypertension, in *Membrane Abnormalities in Hypertension,* Kwan, C. Y., Ed., Boca Raton, FL, CRC Press, 1989, 145–179.
9. **Wadsworth, R. M.,** Calcium and vascular reactivity in aging and hypertension, *J. Hypertension,* 1990; 8:975–983.
10. **Sugiyama, T., Yoshizumi, M., Takaku, F. et al.,** The elevation of the cytoplasmic calcium ions in vascular smooth muscle cells in SHR: measurement of the free calcium ions in single living cells by laser microfluorospectrometry, *Biochem. Biophys. Res. Commun.,* 1986; 141: 340–345.

11. **Bohr, D. F. and Webb, R. C.,** Vascular smooth muscle in hypertension, *Annu. Rev. Pharmacol. Toxicol.,* 1988; 28:389–409.
12. **Erne, P. and Hermsmeyer, K.,** Intracellular vascular muscle Ca^{2+} modulation in genetic hypertension, *Hypertension,* 1989; 14:145–151.
13. **Sada, T., Koike, H., Ikeda, M. et al.,** Cytosolic free calcium of aorta of hypertensive rats, *Hypertension,* 1990; 16:245–251.
14. **Papageorgiou, P. and Morgan, K. G.,** Intracellular free Ca^{2+} is elevated in hypertrophic aortic muscle from hypertensive rats, *Am. J. Physiol.,* 1991; 260:H507–H515.
15. **Rusch, N. J. and Hermsmeyer, K.,** Calcium currents are altered in the vascular muscle cell membrane of spontaneously hypertensive rats, *Circ. Res.,* 1988; 63:997–1002.
16. **Hermsmeyer, K. and Rusch, N. J.,** Calcium channel alterations in genetic hypertension, *Hypertension,* 1989; 14:453–456.
17. **Kleiman, R. B. and Houser, S. R.,** Calcium currents in normal and hypertrophied isolated feline ventricular myocytes, *Am. J. Physiol.,* 1988; 255:H1434–H1442.
18. **Keung, E. C.,** Calcium current is increased in isolated adult myocytes from hypertrophied rat myocardium, *Circ. Res.,* 1989; 64:753–763.
19. **Bean, B. P.,** Pharmacology of calcium channels in cardiac muscle, vascular muscle and neurons, *Am. J. Hypertension,* 1991; 4:406S–411S.
20. **Tsien, R. W.,** Calcium channels: mechanism of selectivity, permeation, and block, *Annu. Rev. Biophys. Chem.,* 1987; 16:265–290.
21. **Stekiel, W. J.,** Electrophysiological mechanisms of force development by vascular smooth muscle membrane in hypertension, in *Blood Vessel Changes in Hypertension: Structure and Function,* Lee, E. M. K. W., Ed., Boca Raton, FL, CRC Press, 1989, 127–170.
22. **Hermsmeyer, K., Trapani, A., and Abel, P. W.,** Membrane potential-dependent tension in vascular muscle, in *Vasodilation,* Vanhoutte, P. M. and Leusen, I., Eds., New York, Raven Press, 1981, 273–284.
23. **Haeusler, G.,** Relationship between noradrenaline-induced depolarization and contraction in vascular smooth muscle, *Blood Vessels,* 1978; 15:46–54.
24. **Harder, D. R., Abel, P. W., and Hermsmeyer, K.,** Membrane electrical mechanism of basilar artery constriction and pial artery dilation by norepinephrine, *Circ. Res.,* 1981; 49:1237–1242.
25. **Harder, D. R.,** Membrane activation of smooth muscle from rabbit basilar artery by dopamine, *Pfluegers' Arch.,* 1981; 390:296–298.
26. **Hermsmeyer, K.,** Electrophysiology of vascular muscle, in *Microcirculation,* Vol. 3, Kaley, G. and Altura, B. M., Eds., Baltimore, University Park Press, 1980, 439–460.
27. **Hermsmeyer, K.,** Electrogenic ion pumps and other determinants of membrane potential in vascular muscle (the 1982 Bowditch Lecture), *Physiologist,* 1982; 25:454–465.
28. **Cheung, D. W. and McKay, M. J.,** The effects of Bay K 8644 and nifedipine on the neural response of the rabbit ear artery, *Br. J. Pharmacol.,* 1986; 88:363–368.
29. **Hermsmeyer, K. and Bian, K.,** Calcium channel hypothesis in hypertension, *J. Vasc. Med. Biol.,* 1991; 3:219–222.
30. **Sturek, M. and Hermsmeyer, K.,** Calcium and sodium channels in spontaneously contracting vascular muscle cells, *Science,* 1986; 233:475–477.
31. **Bean, B. P., Sturek, M., Puga, A. et al.,** Calcium channels in muscle cells isolated from rat mesenteric arteries: modulation by dihydropyridine drugs, *Circ. Res.,* 1986; 59:229–235.
32. **Yatani, A., Seidel, C. L., Allen, J. et al.,** Whole-cell and single channel calcium currents of isolated smooth muscle cells from saphenous vein, *Circ. Res.,* 1987; 60:523–533.
33. **Benham, C. D., Hess, P., and Tsien, R. W.,** Two types of calcium channels in single smooth muscle cells from rabbit ear artery studied with whole-cell and single-channel recordings, *Circ. Res.,* 1987; 61:I-10–I-16.
34. **Wang, R., Karpinski, E., and Pang, P. K. T.,** Two types of calcium channels in isolated smooth muscle cells from rat tail artery, *Am. J. Physiol.,* 1989; 256:H1361–H1368.
35. **Ohya, Y. and Sperelakis, N.,** ATP regulation of the slow calcium channels in vascular smooth muscle cells of guinea pig mesenteric artery, *Circ. Res.,* 1989; 64:145–154.

36. **Oike, M., Inoue, Y., Kitamura, K. et al.**, Dual action of FRC8653, a novel dihydropyridine derivative, on the Ba^{2+} current recorded from the rabbit basilar artery, *Circ. Res.*, 1990; 67: 993–1006.
37. **Lory, P., Varadi, G., and Schwartz, A.**, Molecular insights into regulation of L-type Ca channel function, *NIPS*, 1991; 6:277–281.
38. **Slish, D. F., Schultz, D., and Schwartz, A.**, Molecular biology of the calcium antagonist receptor, *Hypertension*, 1992; 19:19–24.
39. **Koch, W. J., Ellinor, P. T., and Schwartz, A.**, cDNA cloning of a dihydropyridine-sensitive calcium channel from rat aorta, *J. Biol. Chem.*, 1990; 265:17786–17791.
40. **Catterall, W. A. and Striessing, J.**, Receptor sites for Ca^{2+} channel antagonists, *TIPS*, 1992; 13:256–262.
41. **Loirand, G., Pacaud, P., Mironneau, C. et al.**, Evidence for two distinct calcium channels in rat vascular smooth muscle cells in short-term primary culture, *Pfluegers' Arch.*, 1986; 407:566–568.
42. **Hermsmeyer, K., Sturek, M., and Rusch, N. J.**, Nitrendipine inhibition of calcium current in rat vascular muscle cells, *J. Cardiovasc. Pharmacol.*, 1988b; 12:S100–S103.
43. **Worley, J. F., Deitmer, J. W., and Nelson, M. T.**, Single nisoldipine-sensitive calcium channels in smooth muscle cells isolated from rabbit mesenteric artery, *Proc. Natl. Acad. Sci. U.S.A.*, 1986; 83:5746–5750.
44. **Ganitkevich, V. Y. and Isenberg, G.**, Contribution of two types of calcium channels to membrane conductance of single myocytes from guinea-pig coronary artery, *J. Physiol.*, 1990; 426: 19–42.
45. **Akaike, N., Kanaide, H., Kuga, T. et al.**, Low-voltage-activated calcium current in rat aorta smooth muscle cells in primary culture, *J. Physiol.*, 1989; 416:141–160.
46. **Kuga, T., Sadoshima, J., Tomoike, H. et al.**, Actions of Ca^{2+} antagonists on two types of Ca^{2+} channels in rat aorta smooth muscle cells in primary culture, *Circ. Res.*, 1990; 67: 469–480.
47. **Matsuda, J. J., Volk, K. A., and Shibata, E. F.**, Calcium currents in isolated rabbit arterial smooth muscle myocytes, *J. Physiol.*, 1990; 427:657–680.
48. **Worley, J. F., Quayle, J. M., Standen, N. B. et al.**, Regulation of single calcium channels in cerebral arteries by voltage, serotonin and dihydropyridines, *Am. J. Physiol.*, 1991; 261: H1951–H1960.
49. **Kunze, D. L. and Ritchie, A. K.**, Multiple conductance levels of the dihydropyridine-sensitive calcium channel in GH_3 cells, *J. Membr. Biol.*, 1990; 118:171–178.
50. **Aaronson, P. I., Bolton, T. B., Lang, R. J. et al.**, Calcium currents in single isolated smooth muscle cells from the rabbit ear artery in normal-calcium and high-barium solutions, *J. Physiol.*, 1980; 405:57–75.
51. **Nelson, M. T. and Worley, J. F.**, Dihydropyridine inhibition of single calcium channels and contraction in rabbit mesenteric artery depends on voltage, *J. Physiol.*, 1989; 412:65–90.
52. **Simard, J. M.**, Calcium channel currents in isolated smooth muscle cells from the basilar artery of the guinea pig, *Pfluegers' Arch.*, 1991; 417:528–536.
53. **Chen, C. and Hess, P.**, Mechanism of gating of T-type calcium channels, *J. Gen. Physiol.*, 1990; 96:603–630.
54. **Nargeot, J., Dascal, N., and Lester, H. A.**, Heterologous expression of calcium channels, *J. Membr. Biol.*, 1992; 126:97–108.
55. **Benham, C. D. and Tsien, R. W.**, A novel receptor-operated Ca^{2+}-permeable channel activated by ATP in smooth muscle, *Nature*, 1987; 328:275–278.
56. **Su, C. and Bevan, J. A.**, Electrical and mechanical responses of pulmonary artery muscle to neural and chemical stimulation, *Bibl. Anat.*, 1966; 8:30–34.
57. **Longhurst, P. A., Rice, P. J., Taylor, D. A. et al.**, Sensitivity of caudal arteries and the mesenteric vascular bed to norepinephrine in DOCA-salt hypertension, *Hypertension*, 1988; 12:133–142.

58. **Neild, T. O. and Kotecha, N.,** Relation between membrane potential and contractile force in smooth muscle of the rat tail artery during stimulation by norepinephrine, 5-hydroxytryptamine and potassium, *Circ. Res.*, 1987; 60:791–795.
59. **Hermsmeyer, K.,** Electrogenesis of increased norepinephrine sensitivity of arterial vascular muscle in hypertension, *Circ. Res.*, 1976; 38:362–367.
60. **Abel, P. W., Trapani, A., Matsuki, N. et al.,** Unaltered membrane properties of arterial muscle in Dahl strain genetic hypertension, *Am. J. Physiol.*, 1981; 241:H224–H227.
61. **Hirst, G. D. S., Silverberg, G. D., and van Helden, D. F.,** The action potential and underlying ionic currents in proximal rat middle cerebral arteries, *J. Physiol.*, 1986; 371:289–304.
62. **Stekiel, W. J., Contney, S. J., and Lombard, J. H.,** Small vessel membrane potential, sympathetic input, and electrogenic pump rate in SHR, *Am. J. Physiol.*, 1986; 250:C547–C556.
63. **Kuriyama, H. and Suzuki, H.,** Adrenergic transmissions in the guinea-pig mesenteric artery and their cholinergic modulations, *J. Physiol.*, 1981; 317:383–396.
64. **Harder, D. R.,** Comparison of electrical properties of middle cerebral and mesenteric artery in cat, *Am. J. Physiol.*, 1980; 239:C23–C26.
65. **Mekata, F.,** The role of hyperpolarization in the relaxation of smooth muscle of the monkey coronary artery, *J. Physiol.*, 1986; 371:257–265.
66. **Ito, Y., Kitamura, K., and Kuriyama, H.,** Effects of acetylcholine and catecholamines on the smooth muscle cell of the porcine coronary artery, *J. Physiol.*, 1979; 294:595–611.
67. **Haeusler, G.,** Contraction, membrane potential and calcium fluxes in rabbit pulmonary arterial muscle, *Fed. Proc.*, 1983; 42:263–268.
68. **Fleckenstein, A.,** The practical significance of calcium antagonists in cardiovascular therapy, in *Calcium Antagonism in Heart and Smooth Muscle,* Wiley Interscience, New York, 1983, 306–310.
69. **Katusic, Z. S., Shepherd, J. T., and Vanhoutte, P. M.,** Endothelium-dependent contraction to stretch in canine basilar arteries, *Am. J. Physiol.*, 1987; 252:H671–H673.
70. **Rubanyi, G. M.,** Endothelium-dependent pressure-induced contraction of isolated canine carotid arteries, *Am. J. Physiol.*, 1988; 255:H783–H788.
71. **Laher, I. and Bevan, J. A.,** Stretch of vascular smooth muscle activates tone and $^{45}Ca^{2+}$ influx, *J. Hypertension,* 1989; 7:S17–S20.
72. **Funaki, S.,** Studies on membrane potentials of vascular smooth muscle with intracellular microelectrodes, *Proc. Jpn. Acad.*, 1958; 34:534–536.
73. **Steedman, W. M.,** Microelectrode studies on small mammalian arteries, *Bibl. Anat.*, 1966; 8:25–29.
74. **Bryant, H. J., Harder, D. R., Pamnani, M. B. et al.,** In vivo membrane potentials of smooth muscle cells in the caudal artery of the rat, *Am. J. Physiol.*, 1985; 249:C78–C83.
75. **Lombard, J. H., Smeda, J., Madden, J. A. et al.,** Effect of reduced oxygen availability upon myogenic depolarization and contraction of cat middle cerebral artery, *Circ. Res.*, 1986; 58: 565–569.
76. **Harder, D. R., Gilbert, R., and Lombard, J. H.,** Vascular muscle cell depolarization and activation in renal arteries on elevation of transmural pressure, *Am. J. Physiol.*, 1987; 253: F778–F781.
77. **Smeda, J. S. and Daniel, E. E.,** Elevations in arterial pressure induce the formation of spontaneous action potentials and alter neurotransmission in canine ileum arteries, *Circ. Res.*, 1988; 62:1104–1110.
78. **Lombard, J. H., Eskinder, H., Kauser, K. et al.,** Enhanced norepinephrine sensitivity in renal arteries at elevated transmural pressure, *Am. J. Physiol.*, 1990; 259:H29–H33.
79. **Stekiel, W. J., Contney, S. J., and Lombard, J. H.,** Sympathetic neural control of vascular muscle in reduced renal mass hypertension, *Hypertension,* 1991; 17:1185–1191.
80. **Brayden, J. E. and Nelson, M. T.,** Regulation of arterial tone by activation of calcium-dependent potassium channels, *Science,* 1992; 256:532–535.
81. **Berczi, V., Stekiel, W. J., Contney, S. J. et al.,** Pressure-induced activation of membrane K^+ current in rat saphenous artery, *Hypertension,* 1992; 19:725–729.

82. **Ganitkevich, V. Y. and Isenberg, G.,** Stimulation-induced potentiation of T-type Ca^{2+} channel currents in myocytes from guinea-pig coronary artery, *J. Physiol.*, 1991; 443:703–725.
83. **Huang, Y., Quayle, J. M., Worley, J. F. et al.,** External cadmium and internal calcium block of single calcium channels in smooth muscle cells from rabbit mesenteric artery, *Biophys. J.*, 1989; 56:1023–1028.
84. **Harder, D. R., Smeda, J., and Lombard, J. H.,** Enhanced myogenic depolarization in hypertensive cerebral arterial muscle, *Circ. Res.*, 1985; 57:319–322.
85. **Laher, I., Hwa, J. J., and Bevan, J. A.,** Calcium and vascular myogenic tone, *Ann. N.Y. Acad. Sci.*, 1988; 522:216–225.
86. **Ives, H. E.,** Ion transport defects and hypertension. Where is the link?, *Hypertension* 1989; 14:590–596.
87. **Stull, J. T., Gallagher, P. J., Herring, B. P. et al.,** Vascular smooth muscle contractile elements, *Hypertension,* 1991; 17:723–732.
88. **Rinaldi, G. J., Cattaneo, E. A., Mattiazzi, A. et al.,** Dissociation between calcium influx blockage and smooth muscle relaxation by nifedipine in spontaneously hypertensive rats, *Circ. Res.*, 1987; 60:367–374.
89. **Soloviev, A. I. and Bershtein, S. A.,** The contractile apparatus in vascular smooth muscle cells of spontaneously hypertensive rats possess increased calcium sensitivity: the possible role of protein kinase C, *J. Hypertension,* 1992; 10:131–136.
90. **Noon, J. P., Rice, P. J., and Baldessarini, R. J.,** Calcium leakage as a cause of high resting tension in vascular smooth muscle from the spontaneously hypertensive rat, *Proc. Natl. Acad. Sci. U.S.A.*, 1978; 75:1605–1607.
91. **Fitzpatrick, D. F. and Szentivanyi, A.,** The relationship between increased myogenic tone and hyporesponsiveness in vascular smooth muscle of spontaneously hypertensive rats, *Clin. Exp. Hypertension,* 1980; 2:1023–1037.
92. **Aoki, K. and Asano, M.,** Effects of Bay K 8644 and nifedipine on femoral arteries of spontaneously hypertensive rats, *Br. J. Pharmacol.*, 1986; 88:221–230.
93. **Aoki, K. and Asano, M.,** Increased responsiveness to calcium agonist BAY k 8644 and calcium antagonist nifedipine in femoral arteries of spontaneously hypertensive rats, *J. Cardiovasc. Pharmacol.*, 1987; 10:S62–S64.
94. **MacKay, M. J. and Cheung D. W.,** Increased reactivity in the mesenteric artery of spontaneously hypertensive rats to phorbol ester, *Biochem. Biophys. Res. Commun.*, 1987; 145: 1105–1111.
95. **Thompson, L. P., Bruner, C. A., Lamb, F. S., King, D. M., and Webb, R. C.,** Calcium influx and vascular reactivity in systemic hypertension, *Am. J. Cardiol.*, 1987; 59:29A–34A.
96. **Bolzon, B. J. and Cheung, D. W.,** Isolation and characterization of single vascular smooth muscle cells from spontaneously hypertensive rats, *Hypertension,* 1989; 14:137–144.
97. **Bruner, C. A. and Webb, R. C.,** Increased vascular reactivity to Bay K 8644 in genetic hypertension, *Pharmacology,* 1990: 41:24–35.
98. **Storm, D. S., Turla, M. B., Todd, K. M., and Webb, R. C.,** Calcium and contractile responses to phorbol esters and the calcium channel agonist, Bay K 8644, in arteries from hypertensive rats, *Am. J. Hypertension,* 1990; 3:245S–248S.
99. **Tomobe, Y., Ishikawa, T., Yanagisawa, M. et al.,** Mechanisms of altered sensitivity to endothelin 1 between aortic smooth muscle of spontaneously hypertensive and Wistar-Kyoto rats, *J. Pharmacol. Exp. Ther.*, 1991; 257:555–561.
100. **Rusch, N. J., De Lucena, R. G., Wooldridge, T. A. et al.,** A Ca^{2+}-dependent K^+ current is enhanced in arterial membranes of hypertensive rats, *Hypertension,* 1992; 19:301–307.
101. **Pederson, O. L., Mikkelsen, E., and Andersson, K. E.,** Effects of extracellular calcium on potassium and noradrenaline induced contractions in the aorta of spontaneously hypertensive rats — increased sensitivity to nifedipine, *Acta Pharmacol. Toxicol.*, 1978; 43:137–144.
102. **Bendhack, L. M., Sharma, R. V., and Bhalla, R. C.,** Altered signal transduction in vascular smooth muscle cells of spontaneously hypertensive rats, *Hypertension,* 1992; 19:II-142–II-148.

103. **Nelson, M. T., Standen, N. B., Brayden, J. E. et al.,** Noradrenaline contracts arteries by activating voltage-dependent calcium channels, *Nature,* 1988; 336:382–385.
104. **Pacaud, P., Loirand, G., Mironneau, C. et al.,** Opposing effects of noradrenaline on the two classes of voltage-dependent calcium channels of single vascular smooth muscle cells in short-term primary culture, *Pfluegers' Arch.,* 1987; 410:557–559.
105. **Droogmans, G., Declerck, I., and Casteels, R.,** Effect of adrenergic agonists on Ca^{2+}-channel currents in single vascular smooth muscle cells, *Pfluegers' Arch.,* 1987; 409:7–12.
106. **Lamb, F. S. and Webb, R. C.,** Regenerative electrical activity and arterial contraction in hypertensive rats, *Hypertension,* 1989; 13:70–76.
107. **Hosey, M. M. and Lazdunski, M.,** Calcium channels, molecular pharmacology, structure and regulation, *J. Membr. Biol.,* 1988; 104:81–105.
108. **Van de Voorde, J., Vanheel, B., and Leusen, I.,** Endothelium-dependent relaxation and hyperpolarization in aorta from control and renal hypertensive rats, *Circ. Res.,* 1992; 70:1–8.
109. **Chin, J. H.,** Differential sensitivity of calcium channels to dihydropyridines. The modulated receptor hypothesis, *Biochem. Pharmacol.,* 1986; 35:4115–4120.
110. **Mulvany, M. J. and Nyborg, N.,** An increased calcium sensitivity of mesenteric resistance vessels in young and adult spontaneously hypertensive rats, *Br. J. Pharmacol.,* 1980; 71: 585–596.
111. **Jones, A. W.,** Altered ion transport in vascular smooth muscle from spontaneously hypertensive rats, *Circ. Res.,* 1973; 33:563–572.
112. **Jones, A. W.,** Reactivity of ion fluxes in rat aorta during hypertension and circulatory control, *Fed. Proc.,* 1974; 33:133–137.
113. **Friedman, S. M. and Friedman, C. L.,** Cell permeability, sodium transport, and the hypertensive process in the rat, *Circ. Res.,* 1976; 39:433–441.
114. **Jones, A. W.,** Arterial tissue cations, in *Hypertension, Physiology and Treatment,* Genest, J., Kuchel, O., Hamet, P., and Cantin, M., Eds., New York, McGraw-Hill, 1983, 488–497.
115. **Kwan, C. Y.,** Dysfunction of calcium handling by smooth muscle in hypertension, *Can. J. Physiol. Pharmacol.,* 1985; 63:366–374.
116. **Bruner, C. A., Webb, R. C., and Bohr, D. F.,** Vascular reactivity and membrane stabilizing effect of calcium in spontaneously hypertensive rats, in *Calcium in Essential Hypertension,* Aoki, K. and Frohlich, E. D., Eds., San Diego, CA, Academic Press, 1989, 276–305.
117. **Bohr, D. F.,** Cell membrane in hypertension, *NIPS,* 1989; 4:85–88.
118. **Postnov, Y. V. and Orlox, S. N.,** Cell membrane alteration as a source of primary hypertension, *J. Hypertension,* 1984; 2:1–6.
119. **Rinaldi, G. and Bohr, D. F.,** Potassium-induced relaxation of arteries in hypertension: modulation by extracellular calcium, *Am. J. Physiol.,* 1989; 256:H707–H712.
120. **Bohr, D. F., Dominiczak, A. F., and Webb, R. C.,** Pathophysiology of the vasculature in hypertension, *Hypertension,* 1991; 18:III-69–III-75.
121. **Gleason, M. M., Medow, M. S., and Tulenko, T. N.,** Excess membrane cholesterol alters calcium movements, cytosolic calcium levels, and membrane fluidity in arterial smooth muscle cells, *Circ. Res.,* 1991; 69:216–227.
122. **Cox, R. H. and Tulenko, T. N.,** Altered excitation-contraction coupling in hypertension: role of plasma membrane phospholipids and ion channels, in *Regulation of Smooth Muscle Contraction,* Moreland, R. S., Ed., New York, Plenum Press, 1991, 273–290.
123. **Hermsmeyer, K.,** Calcium antagonist effects on vascular muscle membrane potentials and intracellular Ca^{2+}, in *Calcium in Biological Systems,* Rubin, R. P., Weiss, G., and Putney, J. W., Eds., New York, Plenum Press, 1985, 423–430.
124. **Hermsmeyer, K.,** Cellular calcium control in hypertension, *J. Cardiovasc. Pharmacol.,* 1988; 12:S8–S9.
125. **Gebremedhin, D., Fenoy, F. J., Harder, D. R. et al.,** Enhanced vascular tone in the renal vasculature of spontaneously hypertensive rats, *Hypertension,* 1990; 16:648–654.
126. **Hynes, M. R. and Duling, B. R.,** Ca^{2+} sensitivity of isolated arterioles from the hamster cheek pouch, *Am. J. Physiol.,* 1991; 260:H355–H361.

127. **Robinson, B. F., Dobbs, R. J., and Bayley, S.,** Response of forearm resistance vessels to verapamil and sodium nitroprusside in normotensive and hypertensive men: evidence for a functional abnormality of vascular smooth muscle in primary hypertension, *Clin. Sci.*, 1982; 63:33–42.
128. **Hulthen, U. L., Bolli, P., Amann, F. W. et al.,** Enhanced vasodilatation in essential hypertension by calcium channel blockade with verapamil, *Hypertension,* 1982; 4:26–31.
129. **Ishii, H., Itoh, K., and Nose, T.,** Different antihypertensive effects of nifedipine in conscious experimental hypertensive and normotensive rats, *Eur. J. Pharmacol.*, 1980; 64:21–29.
130. **Garthoff, S. and Kasda, S.,** Calcium antagonist nifedipine normalizes high blood pressure and prevents mortality in salt-loaded DS substrain of DAHL rats, *Eur. J. Pharmacol.*, 1981; 74:111–112.
131. **Kubo, T., Fujie, K., Yamashita, M. et al.,** Antihypertensive effects of nifedipine on conscious normotensive and hypertensive rats, *J. Pharm. Dyn.* 1981; 4:294–300.
132. **Thievant, P., Baranes, J., Le Hegarat, M. et al.,** Effects of diltiazem on renovascular-hypertensive and on normotensive rats, *Gen. Pharmacol.*, 1982; 13:165–167.
133. **Pedersen, O. L., Mikkelsen, E., and Jespersen, L. T.,** Treatment with verapamil reduces blood pressure and tends to normalize vascular responsiveness and ion transport in the spontaneously hypertensive rat, *J. Cardiovasc. Pharmacol.*, 1982; 4:S294–S297.
134. **Narita, H., Nagao, T., Yabana, H. et al.,** Hypotensive and diuretic actions of diltiazem in spontaneously hypertensive and Wistar Kyoto rats, *J. Pharmacol. Exp. Ther.*, 1983; 227: 472–477.
135. **Takata, Y. and Hutchinson, J. S.,** Exaggerated hypotensive responses to calcium antagonists in spontaneously hypertensive rats, *Clin. Exp. Hypertension,* 1983; A5:827–847.
136. **Pedersen, O. L., Christensen, N. J., and Ramsch, K. D.,** Comparison of acute effects of nifedipine in normotensive and hypertensive man, *J. Cardiovasc. Pharmacol.*, 1980; 2: 357–366.
137. **Maeda, K., Takasugi, T., Tsukano, Y. et al.,** Clinical study of the hypotensive effect of nifedipine and its relationship to severity of hypertension, *Int. J. Clin. Pharmacol. Ther.*, 1981; 19:47–55.
138. **Aoki, K., Kawaguchi, Y., Sato, K. et al.,** Clinical and pharmacological properties of calcium antagonists in essential hypertension in humans and spontaneously hypertensive rats, *J. Cardiovasc. Pharmacol.*, 1982; 4:S298–S302.
139. **Muiesan, G., Agabiti-Rosei, E., Castellano, M. et al.,** Antihypertensive and humoral effects of verapamil and nifedipine in essential hypertension, *J. Cardiovasc. Pharmacol.*, 1982; 4: S325–S329.
140. **Lewis, G. R. J.,** Long-term results with verapamil in essential hypertension and its influence on serum lipids, *Am. J. Cardiol.*, 1986; 57:35D–38D.
141. **Frishman, W., Charlap, S., Kimmel, B. et al.,** Twice daily administration of oral verapamil in the treatment of essential hypertension, *Arch. Intern. Med.*, 1986; 146:561–565.
142. **Osaka, T. and Joyner, R. W.,** Developmental changes in calcium currents of rabbit ventricular cells, *Circ. Res.*, 1991; 68:788–796.
143. **Huynh, T. V., Chen, F., Wetzel, G. T., Friedman, W. F., and Klitzner, T. S.,** Developmental changes in membrane Ca^{2+} and K^+ currents in fetal, neonatal, and adult rabbit ventricular myocytes, *Circ. Res.*, 1992; 70:508–515.
144. **Ten Eick, R. E., Whalley, D. W., and Rasmussen, H. H.,** Connections: heart disease, cellular electrophysiology, and ion channels, *FASEB J.*, 1992; 6:2568–2580.
145. **Rusch, N. J. and Stekiel, W. J.,** Ionic channels of vascular smooth muscle in hypertension, in *Cellular and Molecular Mechanisms in Hypertension,* Cox, R. H., Ed., New York, Plenum Press, 1991, 1–7.
146. **Komori, K., Lorenz, R. R., and Vanhoutte, P. M.,** Nitric oxide, ACh, and electrical and mechanical properties of canine arterial smooth muscle, *Am. J. Physiol.*, 1988; 255:H207–H212.
147. **Chen, G. and Suzuki, H.,** Calcium dependency of the endothelium-dependent hyperpolarization in smooth muscle cells of the rabbit carotid artery, *J. Physiol.*, 1990; 421:S21–S24.

148. **Tare, M., Parkington, H. C., Coleman, H. A. et al.,** Hyperpolarization and relaxation of arterial smooth muscle caused by nitric oxide derived from the endothelium, *Nature,* 1990; 346:69–71.
149. **Fujii, K., Tominaga, M., Ohmori, S. et al.,** Decreased endothelium-dependent hyperpolarization to acetylcholine in smooth muscle of the mesenteric artery of spontaneously hypertensive rats, *Circ. Res.,* 1992; 70:660–669.
150. **Davis, M. J., Donovitz, J. A., and Hood, J. D.,** Stretch-activated single-channel and whole-cell currents in vascular smooth muscle cells, *Am. J. Physiol.,* 1992; 262:C1083–C1088.
151. **Rusch, N. J. and Hermsmeyer, K.,** Measurement of whole-cell calcium current in voltage-clamped vascular muscle cells, *Mol. Cell. Biochem.,* 1988; 80:87–93.
152. **Komori, S. and Bolton, T. B.,** Inositol triphosphate releases stored calcium to block voltage-dependent calcium channels in single smooth muscle cells, *Pfluegers' Arch.,* 1991; 418: 437–441.
153. **Ohya, Y., Kitamura, K., and Kuriyama, H.,** Regulation of calcium current by intracellular calcium in smooth muscle cells of rabbit portal vein, *Circ. Res.,* 1988; 62:375–383.
154. **Bell, D. R. and Bohr, D. F.,** Endothelium in functional aortic changes of coarctation hypertension, *Am. J. Physiol.,* 1991; 260:H1187–H1193.
155. **Luscher, T. F., Raij, L., and Vanhoutte, P. M.,** Endothelium-dependent vascular responses in normotensive and hypertensive Dahl rats, *Hypertension,* 1987; 9:157–168.
156. **Panza, J. A., Quyyumi, A. A., and Brush, J. E.,** Abnormal endothelium-dependent vascular relaxation in patients with essential hypertension, *N. Engl. J. Med.,* 1990; 323:22–27.
157. **Yanigasawa, M., Kurihara, H., Kimura, S. et al.,** A novel potent vasoconstrictor peptide produced by vascular endothelial cells, *Nature,* 1988; 332:411–415.
158. **Goto, K., Kasuya, Y., Matsuki, N. et al.,** Endothelin activates the dihydropyridine-sensitive, voltage-dependent Ca^{2+} channel in vascular smooth muscle, *Proc. Natl. Acad. Sci. U.S.A.,* 1989; 86:3915–3918.
159. **Silberberg, S. D., Poder, T. C., and Lacerda, A. E.,** Endothelin increases single-channel calcium currents in coronary arterial smooth muscle cells, *FEBS Lett.,* 1989; 247:68–72.
160. **Bkaily, G., Peyrow, M., and Sculptoreanu, A. et al.,** Angiotensin II increases I_{Si} and blocks I_K in single aortic cell of rabbit, *Pfluegers' Arch.,* 1988; 412:448–450.

Chapter 11

ABNORMALITIES OF THE CALCIUM PUMP IN PRIMARY HYPERTENSION

Alejandro De la Sierra, Javier Sobrino, and Antonio Coca

TABLE OF CONTENTS

I. Introduction 230

II. The Ca^{2+}-Dependent ATPase (the Calcium Pump): Essential Aspects 230
- A. Structure and Function of the Calcium Pump 230
- B. Interaction of the Calcium Pump With Calmodulin 232
- C. Regulation of the Calcium Pump 233
- D. The Calcium Pump of the Sarcoplasmic Reticulum 234

III. Disorders of the Calcium Pump in Hypertension 234
- A. Alterations in Calcium Binding Capacity by Cell Membranes 234
- B. Abnormalities of the Calcium Pump in Experimental Hypertension 235
- C. Abnormalities of the Calcium Pump in Essential Hypertension 238

IV. Summary and Conclusions 242

References 242

0-8493-5474-9/94/$0.00+$.50

I. INTRODUCTION

The increase in vascular peripheral resistance that characterizes the established phase of essential hypertension depends mainly on the contractile tone of vascular smooth muscle cells. Progress in the knowledge of cell physiology has shown the central role of calcium in the regulation of the contractile tone.[1]

Contraction of the smooth muscle cells begins with the opening of voltage-operated and receptor-operated calcium channels, located in the cell membrane and in the sarcoplasmic reticulum. All this results in the increase of free cytosolic Ca^{2+} content. Calcium acts on the contractile proteins of the smooth muscle (actin and myosin) that change their spatial conformation, interacting with each other to cause the cell contraction.

The relaxation of the muscle cell is the direct consequence of the decrease in free cytosolic Ca^{2+} concentration. Cytosolic Ca^{2+} is carried out against its electrochemical gradient by means of different calcium transport systems that are capable of extruding calcium to the extracellular space, and intruding Ca^{2+} into the sarcoplasmic reticulum. By now, the existence of two distinct mechanisms capable of extruding Ca^{2+} outside the cell is known. On the one hand, a system of Na^+-Ca^{2+} exchange, specially developed in excitable cells such as those of myocardial muscle, couples the entry of three Na^+ molecules from outside with the extrusion of one molecule of Ca^{2+}. On the other hand, the Ca^{2+}-dependent ATPase uses the energy produced by ATP hydrolysis for the extrusion of calcium against its electrochemical gradient. This transport system is also responsible for the calcium sequestrum into the sarcoplasmic reticulum that causes the relaxation of the contractile cell.

Since the first observations by Postnov et al.,[2,3] showing a defect in the calcium binding capacity of the cell membranes from rats with primary hypertension and patients suffering from essential arterial hypertension, ongoing evidence suggests the existence of some disorder in the Ca^{2+}-dependent ATPase function in these cases. Although the essential nature of this abnormality is not well known, it seems plausible that it could be responsible, at least in part, for the increase of free cytosolic calcium exhibited by some essential hypertensive patients.[4,5] The aim of this chapter is to review the mechanism of action of the Ca^{2+}-dependent ATPase of the plasma membrane and the abnormalities that have been described in arterial hypertension.

II. THE Ca^{2+}-DEPENDENT ATPase (THE CALCIUM PUMP): ESSENTIAL ASPECTS

A. STRUCTURE AND FUNCTION OF THE CALCIUM PUMP

The Ca^{2+}-dependent ATPase is one of the seven or eight transport mechanisms existing in the cell membrane that move calcium from inside to outside the cell. Together with the Na^+-Ca^{2+} exchanger, it is the main mechanism for extruding calcium from cell cytoplasm and it is present in almost all cell membranes. In general, ATPase dominates in nonexcitable cells and the Na^+-Ca^{2+} exchanger dominates in excitable cells.[6] This is due to the fact that the latter cells require a high-capacity system of transport, even to the detriment of its affinity for calcium, such a condition exhibited by the Na^+-Ca^{2+} exchanger. On the contrary, Ca^{2+}-dependent ATPase presents a high affinity for Ca^{2+} and a lesser transport capacity. Therefore, the activity of the Ca^{2+}-dependent ATPase maintains the physiological low content of calcium inside the cell.

Several preliminary studies published in 1966 showing that erythrocytes were able to extrude Ca^{2+} by means of a specific ATPase promoted a large amount of further studies, mainly on red blood cells (RBC), in order to achieve the characterization of this enzyme. It is a classic E_1-E_2 ATPase with high affinity for free Ca^{2+} (<1 μM), which is inhibited specifically for low concentrations of vanadate ($K_{1/2}$ < 1 μM). Due to this high affinity it is qualified to continuously extrude Ca^{2+} from the cell. This is why it plays the most important role in the maintenance of the Ca^{2+} gradient between the cell cytosol and the extracellular medium.

The Ca^{2+}-dependent ATPase is a polypeptide of 138,000 Da in its monomeric shape, though it works as a functional dimer in the cell membrane.[8-10] The amount of this protein among the total membrane proteins is low, 0.1 to 0.2%, which constitutes in turn about 0.5% of the cell weight. In the presence of the regulating enzyme calmodulin, the properties of the erythrocyte ATPase, the best studied, are quite well known. The pump apparently transports the equivalent to passive influx of Ca^{2+}, which is about 50 μmol/(l cell h^{-1}) at an inner concentration of Ca^{2+} lower than 30 nmol/l cells.[11] If we take into account that the extracellular concentration of Ca^{2+} is approximately 1.3 mmol/l, it can be set up a gradient in opposition of 40,000. Thus, it can be asserted that a small amount of the pump capacity is normally used. If the concentration of intracellular calcium is saturated (10 μmol/l cells) the transport rate can reach 20 mmol/(l cells h^{-1}), corresponding to several thousands of units per minute. The affinity for calcium is high on the inside (lower than 1 μM) and low on the outside of the membrane (10 mM).[12]

This system hydrolyzes ATP at the same rate at which the calcium is transported (1 atom of calcium transported per molecule of ATP hydrolyzed).[13] Two specific sites in the ATPase are the locations for the fixation of ATP. The enzymatic site itself has an affinity constant of 2 to 3 μM. With this site alone the system operates at about one tenth of the rate at high ATP concentrations. In addition another regulating site for ATP has an affinity constant between 100 and 300 μM; its occupancy sets up the maximal rate.[14]

It is important to point out that the system requires the presence of Mg^{2+} ions to operate. The affinity constant for Mg^{2+} is 15 μM[15] inside the membrane, which should not be mistaken for the fact that the system transports this cation. In fact, the specificity of the pump for calcium is highly selective, allowing only Sr^{2+} and probably Pb^{2+} as the other divalent cations transported.[16]

It is quite certain that the system does not exchange Ca^{2+} for another cation, though initially an exchange by Na^+,K^+ or Mg^{2+} had been postulated. Ca^{2+} is not countertransported by any other anion.[17] Nevertheless, recent experimental evidence suggests that an exchange for protons takes place, i.e., that the mobile Ca^{2+} site returns in protonated form to the inner side of the membrane.[18] This

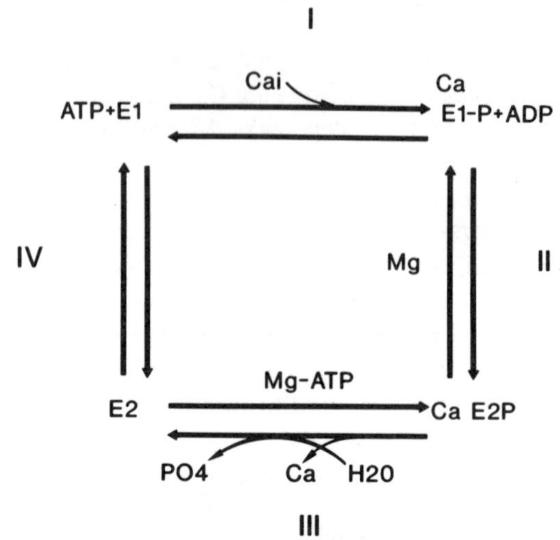

FIGURE 1. Reaction cycle of the Ca^{2+}-dependent ATPase. The cycle starts at the upper left-hand corner and runs in a clockwise direction. E_1 and E_2 designate two conformations of the protein, E_1-P and E_2-P are phosphorylated forms of the protein. Ca^{2+} is translocated across the membrane during reaction II. Reaction II requires Mg^{2+}, and reaction III, a high concentration of ATP.

suggestion is predicted on the fact that when the anion carrier is blocked with 4,4′-diisothiocyanatostilbene-2,2′-disulfonic acid (DIDS), those anions that pass through the membrane in undissociated form, such as acetate, stimulate calcium transport, whereas those that pass through it in ionized form, such as thyocianate, do not present this feature.

The reaction cycle of the calcium pump (Figure 1) is similar to other ATPases, such as the sodium pump. Essentially, the ATP hydrolysis phosphorylates the protein in the presence of calcium. The phosphorylated protein changes its configuration from E_1-P to E_2-P. Such a change is accelerated by the presence of Mg^{2+} ions.[19] During this configuration shift, Ca^{2+} is extruded outside. The protein dephosphorylates later and changes back into its initial configuration.

B. INTERACTION OF THE CALCIUM PUMP WITH CALMODULIN

An important feature of Ca^{2+}-dependent ATPase is its capacity to be stimulated by calmodulin,[20,21] an intracellular soluble protein with four metal binding sites, present in all cells, and responsible for the modulation of several actions in which Ca^{2+} acts as a second messenger. Calmodulin stimulates the calcium pump when several of its metal binding sites are occupied by Ca^{2+}. The interaction of Ca^{2+} with calmodulin determines the formation of a calmodulin-calcium pump complex, which results in an increase in the Ca^{2+} affinity of the transporter site of the pump by a factor of 30.[22] For some authors[23] the Ca^{2+}-dependent ATPase should have two configurations: a form associated with calmodulin and another form dissociated from this protein. The dissociated form would represent a low-affinity state in which maximum activity is achieved at a concentration of free calcium between 100 and 300 μM, presenting just one transporter site for calcium. On the contrary, in its form associated with calmodulin, the calcium pump turns into a high-affinity enzyme that reaches its maximum activity at free cytosolic calcium concentrations between 10 and 50 μM, and for which there are three sites for calcium.

The physiological role of the calcium pump regulation by calmodulin is somewhat unclear. Some authors believe that at the basal state Ca^{2+}-dependent ATPase would be dissociated from calmodulin. Then, the increase of intracellular calcium would be responsible for the association between calmodulin and the calcium pump. Consequently, intracellular calcium increases both the affinity for Ca^{2+} and the maximal rate through the intracellular calcium occupation of the specific locus of calmodulin. This would obtain the desired result, i.e., the restoration of the basal concentration of calcium. Once reached, calmodulin would dissociate again from the pump. This phenomenon has obvious regulating implications because calmodulin would serve as an activator capable of changing the enzyme from a state of low affinity for Ca^{2+} and low pumping rate to a state of diametrically opposite features. Nevertheless, other authors give little credit to this hypothesis[24] and suggest that at its basal state 98% of the calcium pump units would be linked to calmodulin. This means that the regulating role of this intracellular protein would be almost nil.

C. REGULATION OF THE CALCIUM PUMP

Disregarding the regulation of the calcium pump by calmodulin that acts as a negative feedback mechanism in the presence of increases of free cytosolic calcium, the functional characteristics of the ATPase of the plasma membrane depend largely on the lipidic environment in which it exists.[25] Phospholipids, either neutral or negatively charged, are absolutely required for the basal enzymatic activity.[26] However, if a neutral phospholipid such as phosphatidylcholine is used for the reconstitution of the Ca^{2+}-ATPase, the addition of other negatively charged phospholipids such as phosphatidylinositol-monophosphate and phosphatidylinositol-biphosphate can still additionally stimulate the ATPase activity.[27] Although it has not been proven that this regulation plays any physiological role, it seems possible that phosphatidylinositol-monophosphate could be a regulator of the Ca^{2+} transport by the pump of the cell membrane.

It has been reported that cyclic guanosine monophosphate (cGMP) exerts a stimulator effect on the plasmalemmal Ca^{2+} transport and that this effect is mediated through a direct phosphorylation of the enzyme.[28] Nevertheless, other authors[29] have proved that this phosphorylated enzyme does not possess the features of the calcium pump and is probably a myosin light-chain kinase. This cGMP-dependent kinase is capable of stimulating the calcium transport by the pump, probably through the formation of phosphatidylinositol-monophosphate. Therefore, cGMP-increasing agents such as endothelium-derived relaxing factor (EDRF), atrial natriuretic factor (ANF), and nitrocompounds may lower the free cytosolic calcium concentration through the indirect stimulation of the activity of the calcium pump.[29]

Other substances can modulate this enzyme activity, depending on the cellular model, in such a way that insulin can inhibit the calcium transport through ATPase in the adipocyte membranes;[30] 1,25-hydroxyvitamin D_3 can activate it in intestinal cells.[31] Oxytocin has inhibitory properties in myometrial cells, whereas thyroid hormones are stimulators in erythrocytes.[33] It was recently postulated that the toxic effect of cadmium can be caused by the inhibition of the calcium pump of the cell membrane.[34]

D. THE CALCIUM PUMP OF THE SARCOPLASMIC RETICULUM

The enzyme responsible for the reuptake of free cytosolic Ca^{2+} into the sarcoplasmic reticulum is an ATPase of a type similar to that of the plasmalemmal membrane. This ATPase interacts with Ca^{2+} with high affinity ($<0.5\ \mu M$) and the stoichiometry for ATP is 2:1. Because a large amount of this Ca^{2+}-ATPase is found in the membrane of the sarcoplasmic reticulum (>90% of the total membrane proteins in some skeletal muscles), it can quickly attract large amounts of cytosolic Ca^{2+} (from 20 to 40 nmol/g/s). The Ca^{2+}-dependent ATPase of the sarcoplasmic reticulum has been purified and is a polypeptide of 115,000 Da.[35] It can also be stimulated by calmodulin, but contrary to the ATPase of the cell membrane, where the stimulation is caused by the direct interaction of the activator with the pump, in the sarcoplasmic reticulum this activation is mediated by a calmodulin-dependent kinase. The regulation of the Ca^{2+}-dependent ATPase of the sarcoplasmic reticulum is carried out by phospholomban, a protein present both in the cardiac tissue and in the smooth or skeletal muscle.[36-38] Phospholomban acts through the phosphorylation mediated by several kinases, which depend either on cyclic adenosine monophosphate (cAMP), calmodulin, or cGMP.[38,39] Thus, similar to what happens with the cytoplasmic membrane calcium pump, those substances capable of stimulating G proteins and the phosphatidylinositol cycles such as ANF, EDRF, and beta-blockers can exert their relaxing effect.[29]

III. DISORDERS OF THE CALCIUM PUMP IN HYPERTENSION

A. ALTERATIONS IN CALCIUM BINDING CAPACITY BY CELL MEMBRANES

In 1979, Postnov et al.[3] showed that the erythrocyte membrane was characterized by a decrease in the Ca^{2+}-binding ability, both in patients suffering from essential hypertension and in spontaneously hypertensive rats (SHR). Further investigations carried out on erythrocyte membrane fractions enriched by right-side-out and inside-out vesicles (IOV) demonstrated that this defect affected only the inner surface of the plasma membrane.[40,41] This conclusion was confirmed by other studies using Ca^{2+} ionophores.[42]

The defect of the Ca^{2+}-binding ability in primary hypertension seems not to be limited to the erythrocyte membrane. Several studies carried out on SHR have proved the same disturbances in vascular smooth muscle cells,[40,43,44] cardiomyocytes,[40,45] plasma membranes of hepatocytes,[46] adipocytes,[47] and synaptosomes.[46] Scatchard analysis suggested that these disturbances may be caused by the decrease in the number of Ca^{2+}-binding sites rather than by the decrease of their affinity for calcium.[46]

Among the possible Ca^{2+}-binding membrane groups, it is necessary to consider carboxylic groups, such as glutamic and aspartic amino acids, as well as the negatively charged groups of acid phospholipids, such as phosphatidylinositol, phosphatidylserine and phosphatidylethanolamine.[48,49] In fact, 20% of the membranous calcium is linked to these phospholipids. Nevertheless, as for the lipidic composition of the erythrocyte membrane, no differences seem to exist between normotensive subjects or animals and essential hypertensive patients or SHR.[50]

Apart from Ca^{2+}-binding membrane groups, the cellular cytoplasm contains several substances that are able to bind divalent cations. However, under physiological conditions, most are characterized by calcium dissociation constant values which are two to three orders of magnitude larger than the range of possible changes in cytoplasmic calcium concentration. In this context, only highly selective fixation proteins such as troponins, parvalbumins, or calmodulin can play a certain regulating role.[50]

The studies carried out up to now have not disclosed differences in the cytoplasmic concentration, properties, and distribution of calmodulin between hyper- and normotensive patients.[51] However, as discussed later, a defect seems to exist in the stimulation by calmodulin of the calcium transport mediated by Ca^{2+}-dependent ATPase.

The failure to prove that the physicochemical properties of the cell membrane are responsible for the defect of fixation of calcium leads to the assumption that the disorder must be based on the active transport of this cation. If we take into account that the calcium pump of both the cell membrane and the sarcoplasmic reticulum is mainly responsible for the maintenance of the low free cytosolic calcium, it seems logical to hypothesize that a defect in this transport system may play a relevant role in primary hypertension.

B. ABNORMALITIES OF THE CALCIUM PUMP IN EXPERIMENTAL HYPERTENSION

The first studies of the active transport of Ca^{2+} were published in 1983 by the Postnov group.[53] The studies were carried out on preparations of erythrocyte membrane-forming vesicles in which the inner layer of the membrane was exposed to the extracellular medium, the so-called IOV. In these experiments, the authors demonstrated a decrease in the active transport of Ca^{2+} stimulated by calmodulin in SHR.[53] Although the rate of accumulation of calcium in basal conditions did not significantly differ between hyper- and normotensive rats, the addition of calmodulin to the extracellular medium caused a maximal stimulation of the active transport of Ca^{2+}, which was significantly higher in normotensive than in hypertensive rats (Figure 2). The authors suggested that the increase in the intracellular pool of Ca^{2+} observed in hypertension could be the consequence of a deficient stimulation, caused

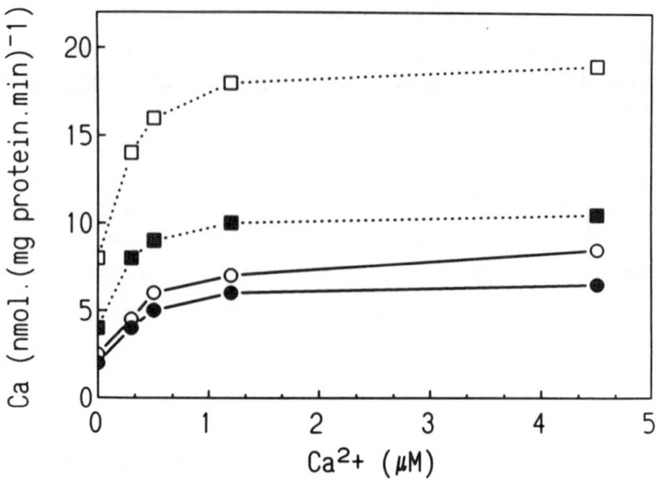

FIGURE 2. Dependence of the rate of Ca^{2+} accumulation by the IOV of the erythrocyte membranes as a function of free Ca^{2+} concentration in the incubation medium. Continuous lines represent the basal state and dotted lines represent Ca^{2+} transport after the addition of calmodulin (2 μg/ml). Empty circles and squares, WKY; filled circles and squares, SHR. (From Orlov, S. N. et al., *Pfluegers' Arch.*, 397, 54, 1983. With permission.)

either by a failure in the interaction of calmodulin molecules and the Ca^{2+}-dependent ATPase or by a disorder in the phospholipid medium of the membrane.

The same authors demonstrated similar results in other cellular patterns such as brain synaptosomes and myocardial cells of SHR.[54,55] However, in the latter work,[55] the basal activity of the Ca^{2+}-dependent ATPase in membranes without calmodulin appeared to be higher in hypertensive than in normotensive rats.

Other models of laboratory animals with hypertension of genetic origin seem to exhibit the same characteristics with respect to the Ca^{2+} transport. Thus, Vezzoli et al.[56] published the results of their investigations on the active transport of Ca^{2+} in preparations of erythrocyte membranes from Milan hypertensive rats. This strain is also characterized by the development of genetic hypertension, but differs from the classical SHR in the kinetics of its transport systems. The classical SHR present an inhibition of Na^+,K^+,Cl^- cotransport[57] and a tendency toward increased levels of intracellular Na^+ content when they are exposed to a saline overload. This increase of intracellular Na^+ could provoke a decrease in Ca^{2+} transport and an increase in free cytosolic Ca^{2+} through the inhibition of Na^+,Ca^{2+} countertransport in cells other than erythrocytes.[58] The Milan hypertensive rats have a hyperactive Na^+,K^+,Cl^- cotransport and lower intracellular Na^+ levels,[59] a fact that leads to disregard for this mechanism for the Ca^{2+} transport inhibition. In the sample of Milan hypertensive rats studied by Vezzoli et al.[56] the basal activity of the Ca^{2+}-dependent ATPase in the absence of calmodulin appeared slightly increased, though the differences with respect to normotensive rats were not statistically significant. On the contrary, the addition of calmodulin to the extracellular medium stimulated the active transport of Ca^{2+} in normotensives in a significantly higher fashion than in hypertensive rats. The kinetic analysis of this transport pathway showed a 30% decrease in the maximal rate in Milan hypertensive rats, with no differences in calcium affinity between both strains. Working on the same laboratory model, similar results were published later by Cirillo et al.[60] as well as by other authors[61] who studied the smooth muscle cell membrane of Dahl salt-sensitive rats in saline overload conditions.

The main criticism for these works is found in the use of preparations of membranes in an artificial medium. Although the studies carried out up to the present show almost opposing results, it is also true that the methodology used does not reflect the normal cellular physiology.[62] Theoretically, the proper conditions for measuring the calcium pump activity should be found in intact cells. As for the measurement of this activity in laboratory hypertension, two works must be taken into account.

Dagher et al.[63] developed a new method in 1987 for the study of the kinetic properties of the Ca^{2+}-dependent ATPase in intact RBC. The erythrocytes were exposed to the presence of the A23187 ionophore, which increases the passive permeability of the cell membrane for divalent cations and promotes the intracellular accumulation of Ca^{2+}. The addition of cobalt chloride to the medium immediately blocks all movements of calcium due to the A23187 ionophore, without affecting the active extrusion of calcium through the pump. The application of this methodology to the study of laboratory hypertension was not able to show significant differences in calcium affinity or maximal transport rate in SHR, as can be seen in Table 1.

Finally, Orlov et al.,[64] using a different technique in which erythrocytes are loaded with the calcium chelator Quin-2 and the ATPase is blocked by means of the addition of Na_3VO_4, could not observe significant differences in the basal activity of the calcium pump in two types of genetically hypertensive rats, the SHR and the Milan hypertensive rats. The addition of R24571, an inhibitor of calmodulin-mediated reactions, did not result in differences in the intracellular concentration of Ca^{2+}. These authors conclude that contrary to what happened in membrane preparations, calmodulin did not play a significant role in the calcium transport of intact cells. On the other hand, they also suggested that the increase of intracellular calcium in arterial hypertension could be caused by the increase of the passive influx of this ion. Oshima et al.,[65] after studying platelets of rats with primary hypertension, reached similar conclusions.

In summary, studies carried out on membrane preparations from SHR have established the existence of a defect in the interaction between calmodulin and the calcium pump. This abnormality determines a decrease in the extrusion of this cation. Nevertheless, investigations performed in intact cells, where the role that calmodulin plays in the activation of Ca^{2+}-dependent ATPase is not well defined, have not been able to reproduce the former results.

TABLE 1
Maximal Efflux Rate (V_{max}, in mmol/l cells h^{-1}) and Intracellular Ca^{2+} Concentration Required for Half-Maximal Stimulation ($K_{0.5}$, in μmol/l cells) in Normotensive Controls, Essential Hypertensives, WKR, and SHR

	V_{max}	$K_{0.5}$
Normotensive controls	16.9 ± 3.1	16.2 ± 7.9
WKR	25.1 ± 12.1	12.1 ± 4.9
Essential hypertensives	15.6 ± 6.6	21.0 ± 11.2[a]
SHR	30.0 ± 12.9	11.7 ± 5.3

[a] $p < 0.1$, when compared with normotensive controls.

From Dagher, G. et al., *Biochim. Biophys. Acta,* 903, 218, 1987. With permission.

C. ABNORMALITIES OF THE CALCIUM PUMP IN ESSENTIAL HYPERTENSION

Research on the activity of the Ca^{2+}-dependent ATPase in essential hypertension has paralleled that in experimental hypertension. The main difference is that almost all studies have been carried out in circulant cells for obvious reasons.

Again, the Postnov group[51,54] reported the decrease in calmodulin-stimulated Ca^{2+} transport in erythrocyte membranes of patients suffering from essential hypertension. The results were liable to oppose those found in SHR. In membrane preparations under calmodulin depletion, no differences were observed in the active transport of calcium, neither in the ATPase affinity for Ca^{2+}, nor in the maximal transport rate. On the contrary, the addition of calmodulin (2 μg/ml), independent of its origin, gave rise to an increase both in the affinity for Ca^{2+} and in the maximal rate. The increases were significantly higher in normotensive subjects than in essential hypertensives. Whereas in hypertensive patients the addition of calmodulin doubled the maximal transport rate and tripled the affinity for Ca^{2+}, both parameters were multiplied five times in preparations of erythrocyte membranes from normotensive subjects. The final conclusion was that a defect should occur in the interaction of calmodulin with the calcium pump in erythrocyte membrane.

These results were confirmed later by other authors. Olorunsogo et al.[66] corroborated that erythrocytes from essential hypertensive patients presented a stimulation of the active transport of Ca^{2+} representing 50% of the stimulation obtained in normotensive subjects. Similarly, Resinck et al.[67] found a decrease in the stimulation of the Ca^{2+} transport by calmodulin in platelets from patients with essential hypertension, though the basal activity of ATPase was increased in these patients.

In opposition to these results, Vincenzi et al.[68] found a decrease in the basal activity of the ATPase in their study of a group of 36 essential hypertensives. This basal activity is considered resistant to the inhibition via trifluoperazine, an inhibitor of the actions of calmodulin.[69] Conversely, in the absence of this inhibitor and considering these conditions are the maximal activity of ATPase, no differences were found between normo- and hypertensives.

In the first study in which intact RBC from SHR and essential hypertensive patients were used, Dagher et al.[63] concluded that no disturbances in the maximal transport rate nor in the affinity for Ca^{2+} of the erythrocyte Ca^{2+}-dependent ATPase existed in essential hypertensives. Nevertheless, more detailed analysis of these results revealed slight differences in the tendency of essential hypertensive patients to present lower affinity values for intracellular Ca^{2+} than those obtained in the normotensive population. In fact, the same authors suggested in the discussion of their results the possibility that a small subgroup of patients did present alterations in the Ca^{2+}-dependent ATPase.

In order to clarify the controversy regarding a possible disturbance of the calcium pump in essential hypertension, we carried out a kinetic study of this transport system in intact erythrocytes from 22 essential hypertensive patients and 20 normotensive healthy subjects.[70] We developed a new technique using Sr^{2+} as a calcium analog for the Ca^{2+} pump.[71-75] The intracellular concentrations of Sr^{2+} and Ca^{2+} were modified using the A23187 ionophore in a Ringer isotonic solution.[76,77] For each subject studied, 8 to 12 aliquots of cells containing different intracellular Sr^{2+} and Ca^{2+} concentrations were prepared. The first four to six were prepared with increasing concentrations of Sr^{2+} (0.2 to 3 mmol/l cell) and the following four to six were prepared with increasing concentrations of Ca^{2+} (0.1 to 2 mmol/l cell) and a fixed concentration of Sr^{2+} equivalent to the maximum reached in the previous concentrations. For the measurement of the Sr^{2+} efflux, the aliquots were suspended in the same Ringer medium with the addition of $MgCl_2$ 1 mmol/l, necessary for the correct function of the Ca^{2+} pump, and were incubated at 37°C for 15 min under continuous agitation.

For each subject studied, Sr^{2+} efflux was plotted against the total intracellular Sr^{2+} concentration (Figure 3, left). As previously described for internal Ca^{2+},[78] the stimulation of the Sr^{2+} efflux via increases in the intracellular Sr^{2+} concentration is clearly sigmoid, and in this part of the curve it is possible to calculate the apparent dissociation constant for Sr^{2+} and the maximal efflux rate. The increases of the intracellular Ca^{2+} concentration cause a competitive inhibition of the Sr^{2+} efflux (Figure 3, right) from which a valuation of the apparent dissociation constant for total internal Ca^{2+} can be drawn.

In previous experiments we observed that the Sr^{2+} efflux exhibited the properties of a flux mediated by the calcium pump because it was inhibited by La^{3+}, ATP depletion, and intracellular Ca^{2+}. The substitution of extracellular Na^+ did not modify this efflux.

The results of this study showed significant differences in the kinetic parameters of the erythrocyte calcium pump between hyper- and normotensives. As seen in Table 2, the values of the apparent dissociation constants for intracellular Ca^{2+} and Sr^{2+} as well as the maximal efflux rate were clearly increased in essential hypertensives.

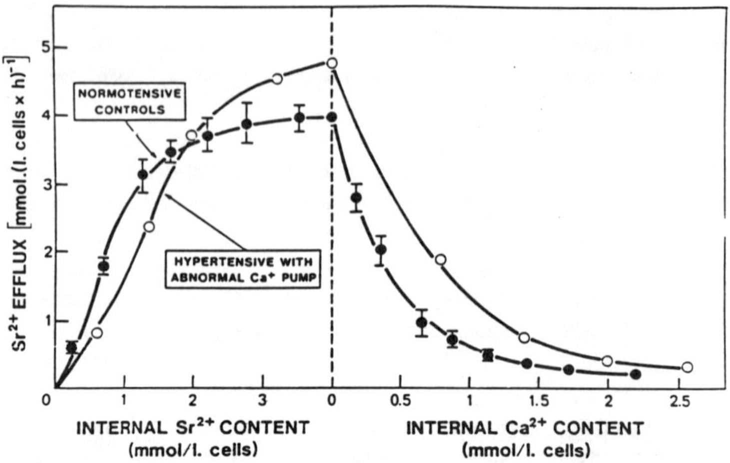

FIGURE 3. Stimulation of Sr^{2+} efflux by increases in total Sr^{2+} content (left side) and inhibition by increases in total internal Ca^{2+} (right side). A hypertensive patient with abnormal Ca^{2+} pump kinetics is represented against mean ± SEM values of 20 normotensive controls, showing: the Sr^{2+}-stimulation curve displaced to the right (increased K_{Sr}), increased V_{max} of Sr^{2+} efflux, and the Ca^{2+}-inhibition curve (right side) displaced to the right (increased K_{Ca}). (From De la Sierra, A. et al., *J. Hypertension,* 8, 285, 1990. With permission.)

TABLE 2
Kinetic Parameters of Erythrocyte Ca^{2+}-Dependent ATPase in Essential Hypertensive Patients and Normotensive Controls

	Normotensive controls (N = 20)	Essential hypertensives (N = 22)
V_{max}	5.0 ± 0.2	5.7 ± 0.4
K_{Sr}	394 ± 23	480 ± 61
K_{Ca}	55 ± 3	73 ± 7[a]

Note: V_{max}, maximal efflux rate of Sr^{2+}; K_{Sr}, apparent dissociation constant for intracellular Sr^{2+}; K_{Ca}, apparent dissociation constant for total intracellular Ca^{2+}.

[a] $p = 0.042$.

From De la Sierra, A., Hannaert, P., Ollivier, J. P., Senn, N., and Garay, R., *J. Hypertension,* 1990; 8:285–293. With permission.

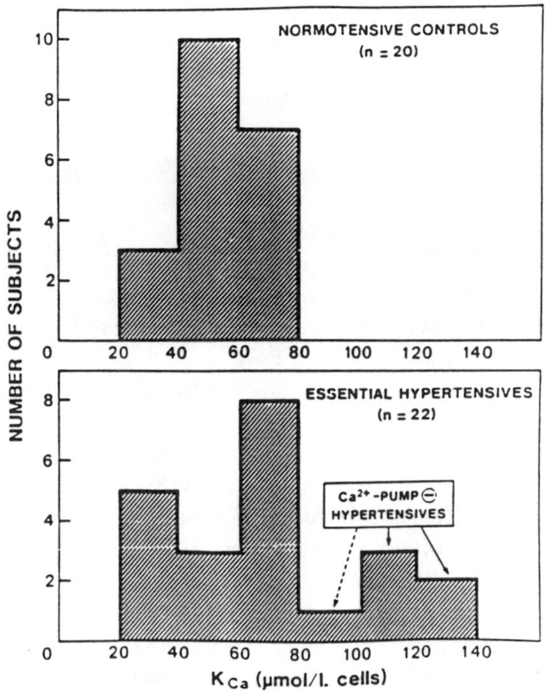

FIGURE 4. Individual values of the apparent dissociation constant for internal Ca^{2+} (K_{Ca}) in normo- and hypertensive subjects. With the 95% confidence limit of the normotensive population (87 μmol/l cells) as a cutoff point, six hypertensive patients had an increased K_{Ca}. (From De la Sierra, A. et al., *J. Hypertension,* 8, 285, 1990. With permission.)

Figure 4 shows the individual values of the apparent dissociation constant for intracellular Ca^{2+} in all the subjects studied. It can be observed that this parameter presents a bimodal distribution in essential hypertensives. Thus, using the confidence interval of 95% as the higher normal limit, a subgroup of six hypertensive patients showed values clearly above this upper normal limit (86 ± 7 μmol/l cell).

These results confirmed the observations of Dagher et al.,[63] that primary and essential hypertension are not associated with a unique disturbance of the erythrocyte calcium pump. Conversely, the population of essential hypertensives is heterogeneous with respect to this transport system. Whereas most (75%) exhibit an activity similar to that of the normotensive population, a small subset [25%, Ca^{2+} pump (−) hypertensives] presents an alteration of this pump characterized by a lower affinity for intracellular calcium. The increase in the maximal efflux rate in these patients can be explained as a compensatory mechanism of the affinity defect. Analogous with what happens with the Na^+,K^+-ATPase,[79] the Ca^{2+}-dependent ATPase-mediated efflux can be found to be normal, increased, or decreased under basal conditions and dependent on the intracellular concentration of Ca^{2+}. However, these subjects with an affinity defect for Ca^{2+} can present a decrease in the capacity for intracellular Ca^{2+} regulation when the latter exceeds the basal values.

As a result of this investigation, we postulated that this defect in the stimulation of the active transport of Ca^{2+} may cause, at the level of the vascular smooth muscle cells, a difficulty in the extrusion of the exceeding free cytosolic Ca^{2+} that takes place after the opening of the calcium channels when cellular contraction takes place. The final result would be the increase of the free cytosolic Ca^{2+} and consequently the increase in the tone of this cell and in the vascular peripheral resistances.

IV. SUMMARY AND CONCLUSIONS

In recent years, evidence has been convincing that some disturbances in the regulation of cell calcium concentration may play an important role in the pathogenesis of essential hypertension. In vascular smooth muscle cells, one of the main mechanisms implicated in this regulation is the Ca^{2+}-dependent ATPase of the plasma membrane. The calcium pump is a membrane protein capable of extruding Ca^{2+} from cells against its electrochemical gradient, using the energy produced by ATP hydrolysis. Ca^{2+}-dependent ATPase is regulated by calmodulin, a cytoplasmic protein, and by the phospholipidic composition of the plasma membrane, especially by phosphatidylinositol metabolites.

Studies carried out in patients and animal models with primary hypertension have demonstrated some abnormalities in the calcium pump performance. These abnormalities involve the net Ca^{2+} movements dependent on the Ca^{2+}-ATPase as well as the interaction of the Ca^{2+} pump with calmodulin. Most authors have concluded that the calcium transport capacity of the Ca^{2+}-dependent ATPase is decreased in primary hypertension. This defect in myocardial cells and vascular smooth muscle cells could be responsible for the increase in the cytosolic free calcium concentration, and thus, for the increase in total peripheral resistances that characterize the established phase of essential hypertension.

REFERENCES

1. **Rasmussen, H.,** The calcium messenger system, *N. Engl. J. Med.*, 1986; 314: 1094–1101.
2. **Postnov, Y. V., Orlov, S. N., Shevchenko, A., and Alder, A. M.,** Altered sodium permeability, calcium binding and Na,K, ATPase activity in red blood cell membrane in essential hypertension, *Pfluegers' Arch.*, 1977; 371: 268–269.
3. **Postnov, Y. V., Orlov, S. N., and Pokudin, N. I.,** Decrease of calcium binding by the red blood cell membrane in spontaneously hypertensive rats and in essential hypertension, *Pfluegers' Arch.*, 1979; 379: 191–195.
4. **Erne, P., Bolli, P., Burgisser, E., and Buhler, F. R.,** Correlation of platelet calcium with blood pressure. Effect of the antihypertensive therapy, *N. Engl. J. Med.*, 1984; 310: 1084–1088.
5. **Bruschi, G., Bruschi, M. E., Caroppo, M., Orlandini, G., Spaggiari, M., and Cavatorta, A.,** Cytoplasmic free [Ca^{2+}] is increased in the platelets of spontaneously hypertensive rats and essential hypertensive patients, *Clin. Sci.*, 1985; 68: 179–184.

6. **Blaustein, M. P. and Nelson, M. T.,** Sodium-calcium exchange: its role in the regulation of cell calcium, in *Membrane Transport of Calcium,* Carafoli, E., Ed., London, Academic Press, 1982; 217–236.
7. **Schatzmann, H. J.,** ATP dependent Ca^{2+} extrusion from human red cells, *Experientia,* 1966; 22: 364–365.
8. **Minocherhomjee, A. M., Beauregard, G., Potier, M., and Roufogalis, B. D.,** The molecular weight of the Ca^{2+}-transport ATPase of the human red blood cell determined by radiation inactivation, *Biochem. Biophys. Res. Commun.,* 1983; 116: 895–900.
9. **Cavieres, J. D.,** Calmodulin and the target size of the (Ca^{2+} + Mg^{2+})-ATPase of human red cell ghosts, *Biochim. Biophys. Acta,* 1984; 771: 241–246.
10. **Hymel, L., Nielsen, M., and Gietzen, K.,** Target size of human erythrocyte membrane Ca^{2+}-ATPase and Mg^{2+}-ATPase activities in the presence and absence of calmodulin, *Biochim. Biophys. Acta,* 1985; 815: 461–467.
11. **Lew, V. L., Tsien, R. Y., Miner, C., and Bookchin, R. M.,** Physiological (Ca_i^{2+}) level and pump-leak in intact red cells measured using incorporated Ca chelator, *Nature,* 1982; 298: 478–481.
12. **Kratje, R. B., Garrahan, P. J., and Rega, A. F.,** Two modes of inhibition of the Ca^{2+} pump in red cells by Ca^{2+}, *Biochim. Biophys. Acta,* 1985; 816: 365–378.
13. **Schatzmann, H. J.,** The red cell calcium pump, *Annu. Rev. Physiol.,* 1983; 45: 303–312.
14. **Richards, D. F., Rega, A. F., and Garrahan, P. J.,** Two classes of site for ATP in the Ca^{2+}-ATPase from human red cell membranes, *Biochim. Biophys. Acta,* 1978; 511: 194–211.
15. **Schatzmann, H. J.,** The plasma membrane calcium pump of erythrocytes and other animal cells, in *Membrane Transport of Calcium,* Carafoli, E., Ed., London, Academic Press, 1982; 41–108.
16. **Simons, T. J. B.,** Active transport of lead by human red cells, *FEBS Lett.,* 1984; 172: 250–254.
17. **Rossi, J. P. F. C. and Schatzmann, H. J.,** Is the red cell calcium pump electrogenic?, *J. Physiol.,* 1982; 327: 1–15.
18. **Smallwood, J. I., Waisman, D. M., Lafreniere, D., and Rasmussen, H.,** Evidence that erythrocyte calcium pump catalyzes a Ca^{2+}:nH^+ exchange, *J. Biol. Chem.,* 1983; 258: 11092–11097.
19. **Garrahan, P. J. and Rega, A. F.,** Activation of partial reactions of the Ca^{2+}-ATPase from human red cells by Mg^{2+} and ATP, *Biochim. Biophys. Acta,* 1978; 513: 59–65.
20. **Gopinath, R. M. and Vincenzi, F. F.,** Phosphodiesterase protein activator mimics red blood cell cytoplasmic activator of (Ca^{2+} + Mg^{2+})-ATPase, *Biochem. Biophys. Res. Commun.,* 1977; 77: 1203–1209.
21. **Jarrett, H. W. and Penniston, J. T.,** Partial purification of the (Ca^{2+} + Mg^{2+})-ATPase activator from human erythrocytes. Its similarity to the activator of 3′:5′-cyclic nucleotide phosphodiesterase, *Biochem. Biophys. Res. Commun.,* 1977; 77: 1210–1216.
22. **Foder, B. and Scharff, O.,** Decrease of apparent calmodulin affinity of erythrocyte (Ca^{2+} + Mg^{2+})-ATPase at low Ca^{2+} concentration, *Biochim. Biophys. Acta,* 1981; 649: 367–376.
23. **Scharff, O.,** Ca^{2+} activation of membrane-bound (Ca^{2+} + Mg^{2+})-dependent ATPase from human erythrocytes prepared in the presence or absence of Ca^{2+}, *Biochim. Biophys. Acta,* 1976; 443: 206–218.
24. **Vincenzi, F.,** Regulation of a plasma membrane calcium pump: a speculative model, *Ann. N.Y. Acad. Sci.,* 1978; 307: 229–231.
25. **Missiaen, L., Vrolix, M., Raeymaekers, L., and Casteels, R.,** Regulation of the Ca^{2+}-transport ATPases of smooth-muscle cells, *Adv. Prot. Phosphatases,* 1989; 5: 239–260.
26. **Wuytack, F., De Schutter, G., and Casteels, R.,** Purification of (Ca^{2+} + Mg^{2+})-ATPase from smooth muscle by calmodulin affinity chromatography, *FEBS Lett.,* 1981; 129: 297–300.
27. **Vrolix, M., Raeymaekers, L., Wuytack, F., Hofmann, F., and Casteels, R.,** Cyclic GMP-dependent protein kinase stimulates the plasmalemmal Ca^{2+} pump of smooth muscle via phosporilation of phosphatidilinositol, *Biochem. J.,* 1988; 255: 855–863.

28. **Furakawa, K. I. and Nakamura, H.,** Characterization of the (Ca^{2+}, Mg^{2+})-ATPase purified by calmodulin affinity chromatography from bovine aortic smooth muscle, *J. Biochem.*, 1987; 101: 287–290.
29. **Eggermont, J. A., Raeymaekers, L., and Casteels, R.,** Ca^{2+}-transport by smooth muscle membranes and its regulation, *Biomed. Biochim. Acta*, 1989; 48: S370–S381.
30. **Pershadsing, H. A. and McDonald, J. M.,** Direct addition of insulin inhibits a high affinity Ca^{2+}-ATPase in isolated adipocyte plasma membranes, *Nature*, 1979; 281: 495–497.
31. **Ghijsen, W. E. and Van Os, C. H.,** 1α,25-Dihydroxy-vitamin D-3 regulates ATP-dependent calcium transport in basolateral plasma membranes of rat enterocytes, *Biochim. Biophys. Acta*, 1982; 689: 170–172.
32. **Soloft, M. S. and Sweet, P.,** Oxytocin inhibition of (Ca^{2+} + Mg^{2+})-ATPase activity in rat myometral plasma membranes, *J. Biol. Chem.*, 1982; 257: 10687–10693.
33. **Davis, P. J. and Blas, S. D.,** In vitro stimulation of human red blood cell Ca^{2+} ATPase by thyroid hormone, *Biochem. Biophys. Res. Commun.*, 1981; 99: 1073–1080.
34. **Verbost, P. M., Flick, G., Lock, R. A. C., and Wendelaar Bonga, S. E.,** Cadmium inhibits plasma membrane calcium transport, *J. Membr. Biol.*, 1988; 102: 97–104.
35. **McLennan, D. H.,** Purification and properties of an adenosine triphosphatase from sarcoplasmic reticulum, *J. Biol. Chem.*, 1970; 245: 4508–4518.
36. **Kirchberger, M. A. and Tada, M.,** Effects of adenosine 3′:5′-monophosphate-dependent protein kinase on sarcoplasmic reticulum isolated from cardiac and slow and fast contracting skeletal muscles, *J. Biol. Chem.*, 1976; 251: 725–729.
37. **Eggermont, J. A., Vrolix, M., Raeymaekers, L., Wuytack, F., and Casteels, R.,** Phosphorylation of the sarcoplasmic reticulum and sarcolemma, *Circ. Res.*, 1988; 62: 266–278.
38. **Raeymaekers, L. and Jones, R. L.,** Evidences for the presence of phospholomban in the endoplasmic reticulum of smooth muscle, *Biochim. Biophys. Acta*, 1986; 882: 258–265.
39. **Raeymaekers, L., Hofmann, F., and Casteels, R.,** Cyclic GMP-dependent protein kinase phosphorylates phospholomban in isolated sarcoplasmic reticulum form cardiac and smooth muscle, *Biochem. J.*, 1988; 252: 269–273.
40. **Orlov, S. N. and Postnov, Y. V.,** Calcium accumulation and calcium binding by the cell membrane of cardiomyocytes and smooth muscle of aorta in spontaneously hypertensive rats, *Clin. Sci.*, 1980; 59(Suppl.): 207s–209s.
41. **Postnov, Y. V. and Orlov, S. N.,** Alteration on membrane control over intracellular calcium in essential hypertension and spontaneously hypertensive rats, in *Intracellular Electrolytes and Arterial Hypertension*, Zumkley, H. and Losse, H., Eds., Stuttgart, George Thieme Verlag, 1980; 144–151.
42. **Devinck, M. A., Pernollet, M. G., Nunez, A., and Meyer, P.,** Analysis of calcium handling in erythrocyte membranes of genetically hypertensive rats, *Hypertension*, 1981; 3: 397–403.
43. **Wei, J. W., Janis, R. A., and Daniel, E. E.,** Studies of subcellular fraction from mesenteric arteries of spontaneously hypertensive rats: alteration in both calcium uptake and enzyme activities, *Blood Vessels*, 1976; 13: 293–308.
44. **Wei, J. W., Janis, R. A., and Daniel, E. E.,** Alterations in calcium transport and binding by the plasma membranes of mesenteric arteries from spontaneously hypertensive rats, *Blood Vessels*, 1977; 14: 55–64.
45. **Pernollet, M. G., Devinck, M. A., and Meyer, P.,** Abnormal calcium handling by isolated cardiac plasma membranes from spontaneously hypertensive rats, *Clin. Sci.*, 1981; 61: 453–462.
46. **Devinck, M. A., Pernollet, M. G., Nunez, A. M., and Meyer, P.,** Calcium binding alteration in plasma membrane from various tissues of spontaneously hypertensives rats, *Clin. Exp. Hypertension*, 1981; 3: 797–808.
47. **Postnov, Y. V. and Orlov, S. N.,** Evidence of altered calcium accumulation and calcium binding by the membranes of adipocytes in spontaneously hypertensive rats, *Pfluegers' Arch.*, 1980; 385: 85–89.

48. **Forstner, J. and Manery, P.,** Calcium binding by human erythrocyte membranes, *Biochem. J.,* 1971; 124: 563–571.
49. **Forstner, J. and Manery, P.,** Calcium binding by human erythrocyte membranes. Significance of carboxyl, amino and thiol groups, *Biochem. J.,* 1971; 125: 343–352.
50. **Postnov, Y. V. and Orlov, S. N.,** Ion transport across plasma membrane in primary hypertension, *Physiol. Rev.,* 1985; 65: 904–945.
51. **Postnov, Y. V., Orlov, S. N., Reznikova, M. B., Rjazhsky, G. G., and Pokudin, N. I.,** Calmodulin distribution and Ca^{2+} transport in the erythrocytes of patients with essential hypertension, *Clin. Sci.,* 1984; 66: 459–463.
52. **Orlov, S. N. and Postnov, Y. V.,** Ca^{2+} binding and membrane fluidity in essential and renal hypertension, *Clin. Sci.,* 1982; 63: 281–284.
53. **Orlov, S. N., Pokudin, N. I., and Postnov, Y. V.,** Calmodulin-dependent Ca^{2+} transport in erythrocytes of spontaneously hypertensive rats, *Pfluegers' Arch.,* 1983; 397: 54–56.
54. **Postnov, Y. V. and Orlov, S. N.,** Calmodulin-dependent Ca^{2+} transport across plasma membranes in primary hypertension, *J. Hypertension,* 1983; 1(Suppl. 2): 9–10.
55. **Cirillo, M., David-Dufilho, M., and Devinck, M. A.,** Altered active sodium and calcium transport by heart sarcolemmal membranes from young spontaneously hypertensive rats: modulation by calmodulin, *J. Hypertension,* 1984; 2(Suppl. 3): 485–487.
56. **Vezzoli, G., Elli, A. A., Tripodi, G., Bianchi, G., and Carafoli, E.,** Calcium ATPase in erythrocytes of spontaneously hypertensive rats of the Milan strain, *J. Hypertension,* 1985; 3: 645–648.
57. **Garay, R., Rosati, C., and Meyer, P.,** Na^+ transport in primary hypertension, *Ann. N.Y. Acad. Sci.,* 1986; 488: 187–195.
58. **Blaustein, M. P.,** Sodium ions, calcium ions, blood pressure regulation, and hypertension: a reassessment and a hypothesis, *Am. J. Physiol.,* 1977; 232: C165–C173.
59. **Bianchi, G., Ferrari, P., Trizio, D. et al.,** Red blood cell abnormalities and spontaneous hypertension in the rat, *Hypertension,* 1985; 7: 319–325.
60. **Cirillo, M., Galletti, F., Corrado, M. F., and Strazzullo, P.,** Disturbances of renal and erythrocyte calcium handling in rats of the Milan hypertensive strain, *J. Hypertension,* 1986; 4: 443–449.
61. **Kwan, C. Y., Triggle, C. R., Grover, A. K., and Daniel, E. E.,** Subcellular membrane properties in vascular and non-vascular smooth muscles of Dahl hypertensive rats, *J. Hypertension,* 1986; 4: 49–55.
62. **Garay, R. P. and Garrahan, P. J.,** The interaction of adenosintriphosphate and inorganic phosphate with the sodium pump in red cells, *J. Physiol.,* 1975; 249: 51–67.
63. **Dagher, G., Amar, M., and Khefif, A.,** Red blood cells Ca^{2+} pump is not altered in essential hypertension of humans and Kyoto rats, *Biochim. Biophys. Acta,* 1987; 903: 218–228.
64. **Orlov, S. N., Pokudin, N. I., and Postnov, Y. V.,** Calcium transport in erythrocytes of rats with spontaneous hypertension, *J. Hypertension,* 1988; 6: 829–837.
65. **Oshima, T., Young, E. W., Bukoski, R. D., and McCarron, D. A.,** Abnormal calcium handling by platelets of spontaneously hypertensive rats, *Hypertension,* 1990; 15: 606–611.
66. **Olorunsogo, O. O., Okudolo, B. E., Lawal, S. O. A., and Falase, A. O.,** Erythrocyte Ca^{2+}-pumping of hypertensive humans: reduced stimulation by calmodulin, *Biosci. Rep.,* 1985; 5: 525–531.
67. **Resinck, T. J., Tkachuk, V. A., Erne, P., and Bühler, F. R.,** Platelet membrane calmodulin-stimulated calcium-adenosine triphosphatase. Altered activity in essential hypertension, *Hypertension,* 1986; 8: 159–166.
68. **Vincenzi, F. F., Morris, C. D., Kinsel, L. B., Kenny, M., and McCarron, D. A.,** Decreased calcium pump adenosine triphosphatase in red blood cells of hypertensive subjects, *Hypertension,* 1986; 8: 1058–1066.
69. **Vincenzi, F. F.,** The pharmacology of calmodulin antagonism: a reappraisal, in *Calmodulin and Intracellular Ca^{2+} Receptors,* Kakiuchi, S., Hidaka, H., and Means, A., Eds., New York, Plenum Medical, 1982; 1–17.

70. **De la Sierra, A., Hannaert, P., Ollivier, J. P., Senn, N., and Garay, R.,** Kinetic study of the Ca^{2+} pump in erythrocytes from essential hypertensive patients, *J. Hypertension,* 1990; 8: 285–293.
71. **Schatzmann, H. J. and Vincenzi, F. F.,** Calcium movements across the membrane of human red cells, *J. Physiol.,* 1969; 201: 369–395.
72. **Olson, E. J. and Cazort, R. J.,** Active calcium and strontium transport in human erythrocyte ghosts, *J. Gen. Physiol.,* 1969; 53: 311–322.
73. **Schatzmann, H. J.,** Active calcium transport and Ca^{2+}-activated ATPase in human red cells, in *Current Topics in Membrane and Transport,* Bronner, F. and Kleinzeller, A., Eds., New York, Academic Press, 1975; 125–168.
74. **Quist, E. E. and Roufogalis, B. D.,** Determination of the stoichiometry of the calcium pump in human erythrocytes using lanthanum as a selective inhibitor, *FEBS Lett.,* 1975; 50: 135–139.
75. **Pfleger, H. and Wolf, H. U.,** Activation of membrane-bound high-affinity calcium ion-sensitive adenosine triphosphatase of human erythrocytes by bivalent metal ions, *Biochem. J.,* 1975; 147: 359–361.
76. **Ferreira, H. G. and Lew, V. L.,** Use of ionophore A23187 to measure cytoplasmic Ca buffering and activation of the Ca pump by internal Ca, *Nature,* 1976; 259: 47–49.
77. **Lew, V. L. and García-Sancho, J.,** Use of the ionophore A23187 to measure and control cytoplasmic Ca^{2+} levels in intact red cells, *Cell Calcium* 1985; 6: 15–23.
78. **Sarkadi, B., Szasz, I., Gerlocyz, A., and Gardos, G.,** Transport parameters and stoichiometry of active calcium extrusion in intact human red cells, *Biochim. Biophys. Acta,* 1977; 464: 93–107.
79. **Diez, J., Hannaert, P., and Garay, R.,** Kinetic study of the Na^+-K^+ pump in erythrocytes from essential hypertensive patients, *Am. J. Physiol.,* 1987; 252: H1–H6.

Chapter 12

ION TRANSPORT AND LEFT VENTRICULAR HYPERTROPHY IN ESSENTIAL HYPERTENSION

Antonio Coca, Alejandro De la Sierra, and Alvaro Urbano-Márquez

TABLE OF CONTENTS

I. Introduction 248

II. Blood Pressure Overload and Left Ventricular Hypertrophy 249

III. Genetic Predisposition to Left Ventricular Hypertrophy in Arterial Hypertension 251

IV. Other Factors Involved in the Development of Left Ventricular Hypertrophy 252

V. Intracellular Signals of Myocardial Growth 254
- A. Ca^{2+} as Intracellular Messenger 254
- B. The Na^+,H^+ Exchanger 256
- C. The Phosphatidylinositol Turnover 258

VI. Intracellular Response to Initiating Signals and Development of Myocardial Hypertrophy 259
- A. Mechanisms of Mechanical, Neural, and Endocrine Control of Cardiac Hypertrophy 259
- B. Effect of Antihypertensive Therapy on Myocardial Signal Transducing Pathway and Reversal of Left Ventricular Hypertrophy 262

VII. Erythrocyte Ionic Transport Abnormalities and Left Ventricular Hypertrophy 263

VIII. Summary and Conclusions 266

Acknowledgments 268

References 268

0-8493-5474-9/94/$0.00 + $.50

I. INTRODUCTION

Cardiac morbidity and mortality in the shape of coronary artery disease (CAD), congestive heart failure (CHF), and sudden death still remain the most common and major complications of essential hypertension (EH) in developed countries.[1] The Framingham Heart Study[2,3] has demonstrated that in 75% of all patients in whom heart failure developed, EH was the underlying disease. Cardiomyopathies, inflammatory heart disease, CAD, and vascular defects were found in the remaining 25%. Moreover, though the mechanisms are not well understood, it is known that EH accelerates the process of coronary arteriosclerosis leading to myocardial ischemia in patients with genetic predisposition;[4] such a phenomenon exacerbates in the presence of left ventricular hypertrophy (LVH).

One of the most relevant findings in the Framingham study was the demonstration that patients with EH and definite electrocardiographic signs of LVH increased their mortality rates due to all cardiovascular diseases from three to ten times more than hypertensives without signs of cardiac hypertrophy. The incidence of CAD was 3.2-fold higher in the presence of LVH, while the incidence of CHF was approximately 8-fold as high. Of particular interest was the demonstration of a negative prognostic value of LVH even after adjustment for the severity of hypertension. This lends LVH the character of independent risk factor.[5] The confirmation of increased mortality rates due to all cardiovascular diseases among EH with LVH diagnosed by echocardiographic techniques[6] strengthens the important prognostic role of the development of LVH in the natural history of hypertensive disease.[7]

Indeed, LVH in hypertension modifies the equilibrium between the oxygen supply and demand by the myocardium. The coronary reserve, which represents the increment by which myocardial blood flow increases in response to maximum vasodilator stimuli, has been defined as the ratio of coronary resistance at rest to coronary resistance after maximal coronary vasodilation. It is appreciably reduced in hypertensives with LVH even in the absence of any stenosis of coronary arteries. Thus, in patients with hemodynamically controlled hypertension and normal coronary angiogram, a predisposition toward myocardial ischemia already exists. This process has been associated with the increased prevalence of both frequency and complexity of ventricular arrhythmias in essential hypertensives with LVH,[8,9] which could be linked to the increasing risk of sudden death in these patients. The relationship between the higher trend to ventricular ectopia and the risk of sudden death in hypertensives with normal coronary vessels is probably linked to the development of LVH (Figure 1).

The issue of whether reversal of LVH due to high blood pressure is a desirable therapeutic goal of antihypertensive therapy remains the subject of ongoing debate. Nevertheless, if LVH is judged to be a pathological process, reduction of myocardial hypertrophy would emerge as a desirable therapeutic goal. So far, only indirect evidence shows that reduction of LVH reverses the pathologic implications of cardiac hypertrophy in arterial hypertension.[10] Furthermore, clinical studies have shown

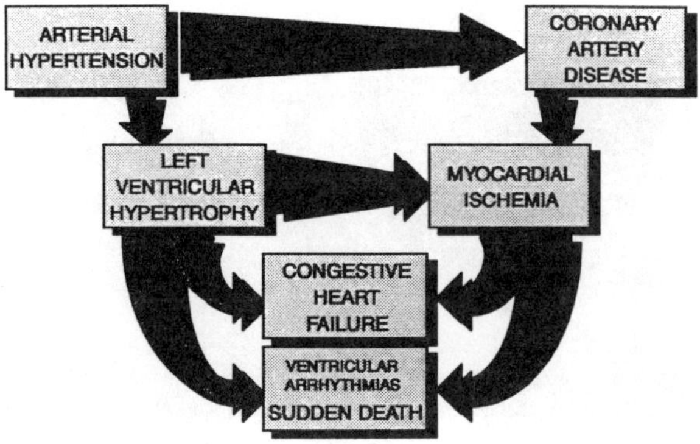

FIGURE 1. Interrelationships between arterial hypertension, LVH, and several manifestations of hypertensive heart disease. Hypertension accelerates coronary arteriosclerosis leading to myocardial ischemia in patients with genetic predisposition. This phenomenon is enhanced in the presence of LVH. The synergism between both processes leading to diastolic dysfunction is likely to be responsible for the development of congestive heart failure. Likewise, myocardial ischemia has been associated with the increased prevalence of both frequency and complexity of ventricular arrhythmias in essential hypertensives with LVH, which could be linked to the increasing risk of sudden death in these patients.

that not all forms of antihypertensive therapy lead to regression of myocardial hypertrophy, ranging from complete absence of effect, through a largely pressure-related decrease in muscle mass, to a unrelated to pressure reversal of LVH. The discrepancy between the extent of reduction in blood pressure and the regression of myocardial hypertrophy suggests that apart from arterial blood pressure, the degree of LVH is also determined by other factors. In this chapter, we review and discuss the molecular mechanisms determining myocardial growth in response to several stimuli on heart cells, and the relevance of sodium and calcium transport systems in this process.

II. BLOOD PRESSURE OVERLOAD AND LEFT VENTRICULAR HYPERTROPHY

The expected response of the heart when an increased workload is chronically imposed on the cardiac muscle is myocardial hypertrophy. Thus, it has been generally assumed that the development of LVH constitutes the main physiologic mechanism of adaptation in pressure overload secondary to the increase of peripheral resistance.[11] Although little is known about factors that influence the pattern of hypertrophy in either animals or humans, the classic study performed by Grossman et al.[12] provided data suggesting that the left ventricle response to a pressure overload was rather different from the observed after a volume overload. Left ventricular wall stress depends on the chamber size and configuration, the thickness of the ventricular wall, and intraventricular pressure. Thus, as seen in Figure 2, for either

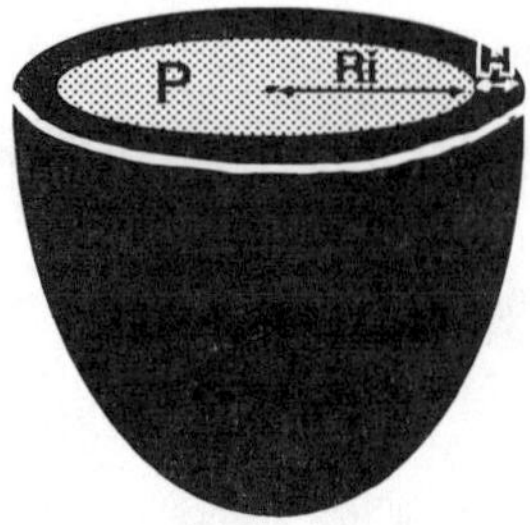

$$\sigma_m = \frac{P \cdot Ri}{2H\left(1 + \frac{H}{2Ri}\right)}$$

FIGURE 2. Diagrammatic representation of forces determining left ventricular wall stress. For either an ellipsoidal or spherical model, the average meridional systolic wall stress (σ_m) can be calculated by the Laplace law from the wall thickness (H), the inner chamber radius (R_i), and the intraventricular loading pressure (P).

an ellipsoidal or spherical model the average meridional systolic wall stress (σ_m) (wall tension supported by the ventricle during systolic ejection) can be calculated throughout the Laplace law from the wall thickness (H), inner chamber radius (R_i), and intraventricular pressure (P).

When the primary stimulus to hypertrophy is left ventricular pressure overload, the resultant rise in intracavitary pressure (P) leads to a progressive thickening of the ventricular wall (H). Grossman and co-workers[12] postulated that it was due to pressure overload resulting in increased peak systolic wall stress, which leads to a parallel replication of sarcomeres, wall thickening, and "concentric hypertrophy" (indicated by the enhanced H:R ratio). That is why the magnification of the numerator of the equation, determined by pressure overload, is compensated with the progressive rise of the denominator tending to return peak systolic stress to normal values without modifying the inner radius (R_i), thus acting as feedback inhibition.

Interestingly, a volume overload may be involved with the increase in arterial resistance in the pathogenetic mechanisms of some clinical forms of EH, such as primary hypertension in younger patients, hypertension in renal failure, and the severe and evolved forms of EH with nephroangiosclerosis. In this case, when the primary stimulus for hypertrophy is left ventricular volume overload, the enhancement of end left ventricular diastolic pressure results in myocardial fiber elongation and chamber enlargement, thus determining an increase of the internal ventricular diameter but a normal H:R ratio. Grossman and co-workers[12] postulated that it was due to the fact that volume overload resulting in increased end diastolic wall stress leads to a series replication of sarcomeres, fiber elongation, chamber enlargement, and "eccentric hypertrophy" (Figure 3).

The structural and morphological response of the myocardium to arterial hypertension is heterogeneous in clinical practice.[13] The Framingham study revealed an important variability in the morphologic patterns of LVH both in hypertensive patients and their normotensive relatives. On the other hand, LVH is a dynamic process which can develop in the short period of 1 to 2 weeks after experimental hypertension in animals.[14] Regression of LVH has been demonstrated within a few

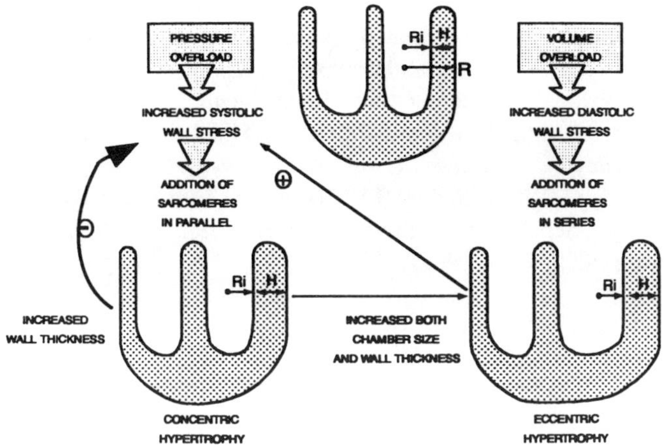

FIGURE 3. Mechanisms postulated by Grossman et al.[12] for the development of LVH as a result of pressure-overload or volume-overload, resulting in concentric or eccentric hypertrophy, respectively. H, wall thickness; R_i, inner chamber radius; R, outer left ventricular radius (R_i + H).

weeks of blood pressure control, both in experimental hypertension[15] and clinical practice.[16] Thus, contrary to classical thinking, LVH seems not to be a late and irreversible complication of EH, but an early phenomenon, subject to a dynamic modification in the evolution of the disease.[17]

III. GENETIC PREDISPOSITION TO LEFT VENTRICULAR HYPERTROPHY IN ARTERIAL HYPERTENSION

Because EH is genetically determined, the ability of the heart to respond with myocardial growth might also be, at least in part, genetically determined. Accordingly, every case of hypertensive cardiac hypertrophy could contain an individually varying genetic component that may help to explain the distinct morphologic patterns as well as the varying responses of the myocardium to antihypertensive treatment.

The variability in the morphologic patterns of LVH both in hypertensives and their normotensive relatives, the simultaneous enlargement of the right ventricle of some hypertensives without concomitant pulmonary hypertension,[18] the observation that LVH is more severe in black hypertensives than in whites, and the detection of LVH in animals[19] and in their normotensive relatives of hypertensives even in the "prehypertensive phase"[20] support the existence of a genetic predisposition to myocardial growth in EH. In the same way, demonstration of LVH in normotensive adolescents with a high risk for development of hypertension cannot be justified as a hemodynamic compensatory mechanism of adaptation to something that has not been established. In this context, the confluence of high blood pressure values in a subject with a special genetic substrate is what determines the morphological pattern and the magnitude of the myocardial hypertrophy. This confluence also can justify the observed findings of hypertensives with normal ventricular mass which are difficult to admit if we accept that the heart muscle responds to high blood pressure, always increasing the ventricular mass. As it happens with the distribution of blood pressure values, ventricular mass in the general population must be a continuous quantitative variable without a clearly defined level between normality and pathology. However, even considering the existence of a bias toward highest values of left ventricular mass index (LVMI) among hypertensives, there is an overlap between hypertensives exhibiting the lowest values of LVMI and normotensives displaying the highest values.

IV. OTHER FACTORS INVOLVED IN THE DEVELOPMENT OF LEFT VENTRICULAR HYPERTROPHY

As usually happens in biomedical research, analysis of the myocardial response after pharmacological antihypertensive treatment has allowed a better approach to the pathophysiologic mechanism of LVH. Clinical studies have shown that not all antihypertensive drugs have the same effect with respect to the reversal of LVH, even though blood pressure control to normotensive levels was achieved. These studies have strengthened the hypothesis that hemodynamic and genetic factors alone are not enough to explain the development of ventricular growth.[21,22]

Chronic treatment with diuretics[23] and vasodilators such as hydralazine[24] produces no regression of cardiac hypertrophy despite decreasing blood pressure. Conversely, methyldopa[25] is able to reduce LVH without further reduction of blood pressure. Between these extreme effects, treatment with angiotensin converting enzyme (ACE) inhibitors,[26] calcium-channel blockers,[27,28] prazosin and clonidin,[29] and several β-adrenergic blockers without intrinsic sympathicomimetic activity (ISA)[30,31] shows a regression of myocardial hypertrophy paralleled by the reduction of blood pressure. Thus, the spectrum of action of antihypertensive pharmacotherapy on cardiac hypertrophy ranges from complete absence of effect, through a largely pressure-related decrease in muscle mass, to a unrelated to pressure reversal of LVH (Figure 4).

As previously discussed, the discrepancy between the extent of reduction in blood pressure and the reversal of LVH implies that despite arterial pressure, other factors such as the sympathetic tone and the renin-angiotensin-aldosterone system are involved in the control of myocardial growth. Norepinephrine stimulates cell growth of isolated cultured myocardial cells.[32] Consequently, if catecholamines play a role in the development of LVH, it is possible that the stimulation of the adrenergic tone induced by diuretics and vasodilators have a trophic effect and may be responsible for the subsistence of an hypertrophied myocardium despite blood pressure reduction. Conversely, the ability of methyldopa to reduce circulating levels of norepinephrine may explain the reversal of cardiac hypertrophy independent of its antihypertensive efficacy.[25]

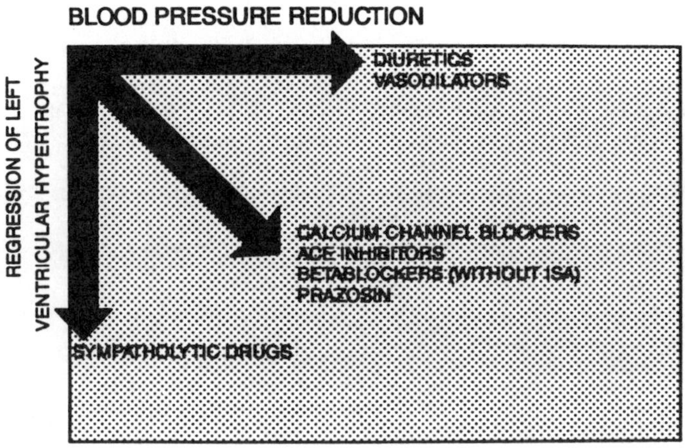

FIGURE 4. Schematic representation of the effect of antihypertensive pharmacotherapy on LVH. The spectrum of action ranges from complete absence of effect, through a largely pressure-related decrease in muscle mass, to an unrelated to pressure reversal of LVH.

It is well known that angiotensin II stimulates protein biosynthesis in the cardiac muscle[33] and may, in addition, enhance catecholamine secretion by the adrenal medulla.[34] It is also highly probable that the renin-angiotensin system of the myocardiocyte (cardiac RAS) play an important role in inducing cell growth independently of the hyperactivation of the systemic axis. It has been postulated that angiotensin II, synthesized in the myocardial cell, could interact with other humoral and growth factors, i.e., endothelium-derived growth factor (EDGF), platelet-derived growth factor (PDGF), epidermal growth factor (EGF), insulin, etc., to exert a paracrine or autocrine control on cell growth.[35] Thus, it seems that the ACE inhibitors reduce LVH through the inhibition of angiotensin II synthesis, particularly cardiac angiotensin. Conversely, the activation of the renin system after diuretic treatment also may contribute to the failure of these drugs in LVH reversal.

In summary, LVH would develop in subjects with a particular genetic substrate by the overlap of high blood pressure values and several factors linked to the adrenergic system, the RAS, other vasoactive substances, and growth factors (Table 1). Regardless, factors inducing myocardial growth activate myocardial membrane receptors responsible for a sequence of events, including initiating signals, coupling mechanisms, and the regulation of gene expression. As a result of these signals, membrane ion channels and ion transport systems are activated, leading to increased intracellular contents of Na^+, Ca^{2+}, inositol phosphates, and diacylglycerol (DAG), and to greater activity of protein kinases A (PKA) and C (PKC) with increased protein and DNA synthesis. Mechanisms of pathologic cardiac hypertrophy in hypertension could involve impaired function of any of these steps in this complex pathway.

TABLE 1
Factors Involved in the Development of Cardiac Hypertrophy

Genetic factors:	Genetic substrate predisposing to myocardial growth	
Hemodynamic factors:	Mechanical stretch on the left ventricle	
Other factors:	Sympathetic tone (catecholamines)	
	Renin-angiotensin-aldosterone axis (angiotensin II)	
	Cardiac angiotensin II	
	Proto-oncogenes (*c-myc, c-fos, c*-Ha-*ras*)	
	Growth factors:	EDGF
		PDGF
		EPGF
		Insulin-like growth factor (IGF-1)
		Fibroblast growth factors (aFGF, bFGF)
		Transforming growth factors (TGF-α, TGF-β)
	Growth hormone	
	Thyroid hormone	
	Insulin	
	Endothelin	
	Arginine-vasopressin	
	Bradykinin	
	Thrombin	
	Prostaglandins	
	Na^+ intake	
	Caloric intake	

V. INTRACELLULAR SIGNALS OF MYOCARDIAL GROWTH

A. Ca^{2+} AS INTRACELLULAR MESSENGER

A large number of cellular functions such as heart muscle contraction, arteriolar smooth muscle tone and contraction, norepinephrine release induced by acetylcholine, aldosterone secretion by the glomerulose cells of the adrenal gland, renin release by the juxtaglomerular cells, cell growth, and several membrane-linked processes are influenced by free cytosolic Ca^{2+} serving as a second messenger between the stimulus and the response.[36-38]

Cytosolic Ca^{2+} content is the result of the Ca^{2+} uptake from the extracellular medium through the plasma membrane and the Ca^{2+} released from the sarcoplasmic reticulum and the mitochondria through calcium channels. Calcium movements are controlled by specific receptors, intracellular messengers, and changes of the membrane potential, resulting in a transitory increase of free cytosolic Ca^{2+} concentration.[39] After exerting its action, Ca^{2+} is pumped out to the extracellular medium, the sarcoplasmic reticulum, and mitochondria by means of active transport systems (Figure 5).

The concentration of extracellular Ca^{2+} is approximately 1 mmol/l, whereas free cytosolic Ca^{2+} reaches concentrations 10,000-fold lower, 100 to 200 nmol/l. Consequently, there is an extraordinarily high transmembrane gradient.[39] Intracellular Ca^{2+} is not only regulated by the plasma membrane, but the mito-

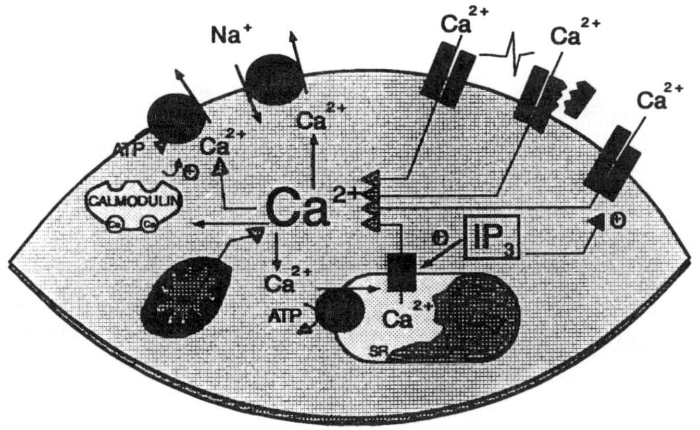

FIGURE 5. Ca^{2+} transport systems in plasma membrane, sarco(endo)plasmic reticulum (SR), and mitochondria (MIT) from eukaryotic cells. Cytosolic Ca^{2+} content is the result of the Ca^{2+} uptake from the extracellular medium through the plasma membrane and the Ca^{2+} released from the sarcoplasmic reticulum and the mitochondria through calcium channels. Calcium movements are controlled by specific receptors, intracellular messengers, or changes of the membrane potential, resulting in a transitory increase of free cytosolic Ca^{2+} concentration. After exerting its action, Ca^{2+} is pumped out to the extracellular medium, and to the sarcoplasmic reticulum and mitochondria by means of active transport systems. The systems in the Golgi membranes and in the lysosomes are still insufficiently characterized and have not been included in the figure. IP_3: inositol triphosphate.

chondria and the sarcoplasmic reticulum also play an important role in Ca^{2+} homeostasis.[39-41] Sarcoplasmic reticulum serves as the source of Ca^{2+} required to initiate any response depending on the cation, but it is not a compartment regulating the basal intracellular content. The plasma membrane is responsible for Ca^{2+} homeostasis by means of those transport systems moving calcium to the extracellular medium and maintaining transmembrane gradient. Two main transport pathways are involved in Ca^{2+} homeostasis. The Ca^{2+}-ATPase or Ca^{2+} pump is the main mechanism regulating the transmembrane Ca^{2+} gradient. The transport protein of this system is present in the plasma membrane and the sarcoplasmic reticulum membrane, and is composed of a polypeptide chain of 115,000 Da. Such a chain consists of a hydrophobic portion included within the thickness of the membrane lipid bilayer, and a hydrophilic portion that emerges on both sides.[42-44] The Ca^{2+} pump uses the energy produced by the hydrolysis of adenosine triphosphate (ATP) and each protein unit probably exhibits two binding sites for cytosolic Ca^{2+}. The Ca^{2+} pump is stimulated by the cytosolic protein, calmodulin.[37,38] This protein exhibits four binding sites for Ca^{2+}. When at least two Ca^{2+} molecules bind calmodulin, the protein forms a Ca^{2+}-ATPase-calmodulin complex that multiplies by a factor of 30 the affinity of the pump for calcium, thus simultaneously increasing the maximal rate.[45] The Ca^{2+}-ATPase determines both Ca^{2+} efflux through the cell membrane and Ca^{2+} influx to the sarcoplasmic reticulum. Nevertheless, despite its high affinity for cytosolic Ca^{2+} the pump is a low-capacity system, not being able to transport calcium in large amounts. Thus, it simply contributes to preserve low concentrations of this cation inside the cytosol.[39,44]

In 1968, Reuter and Seitz[46] reported the existence of another transport system of the cytoplasmic membrane from myocardial cells exchanging Na^+ by Ca^{2+}. This system has been characterized in several tissues and seems to play an important role in the cardiac muscle contraction.[39,47] The Na^+,Ca^{2+} exchanger, not exhibited by human erythrocytes, is located in the cytoplasmic membrane of several tissues, especially in excitable cells, but not in membranes of intracellular organelles.[39,44,48] It can exchange one cytosolic Ca^{2+} molecule for three extracellular Na^+ molecules, resulting in an electrochemical gradient at both sides of the membrane. This system can reverse the ionic flux depending on the intra- and extracellular Na^+ and Ca^{2+} concentrations. Contrary to what happens with the Ca^{2+} pump the Na^+,Ca^{2+} exchanger is a high-capacity, low-affinity system exhibiting low affinity for Ca^{2+} but high potency of stimulation. This property makes it the main mechanism for Ca^{2+} efflux after the massive cytosolic increase following depolarization in the excitable cells. To our knowledge, no physiologic mechanisms of regulation of this transport system have been identified, although it is well known that certain pharmacologic substances can inhibit the Na^+,Ca^{2+} exchanger, particularly some amiloride analogs.[49]

B. THE Na^+,H^+ EXCHANGER

This system was initially identified in 1976 by Murer et al.[50] in vesicles prepared from brush border membranes from the small intestine and the proximal tubule of the kidney. It is an electroneutral membrane transport system that exchanges one extracellular Na^+ for one intracellular H^+. The driving force for this antiport process seems to be the transmembrane gradient of sodium generated by the Na^+,K^+-ATPase. Consequently, the Na^+,H^+ exchanger can be considered a secondary active transport system coupling the hydrogen ion transport against its electrochemical gradient to the influx of sodium. The Na^+,H^+ exchanger can be inhibited competitively by amiloride and its analogs, such as ethylisopropyl-amiloride,[51-53] as well as the parathormone (PTH) and the atrial natriuretic peptide (ANP). The inhibitory effects of amiloride have been found to be competitive with respect to external Na^+, presumably resulting from binding amiloride to the externally exposed transport sites.

In the kidney, the Na^+,H^+ exchanger is present along the apical membrane of tubular cells in the proximal renal tubule. Other nephron segments such as the cortical part of the ascending branch of Henle's loop and the distal segments also possess this transport system in the apical membrane of the cells. The Na^+,H^+ exchanger is implicated in the regulation of acid-base metabolism, controlling urinary acidification and Na^+ reabsorption in the renal tubule.[51] The same exchanger or a very similar transport mechanism appears to be present in most, if not all, animal cells.[52,53] It has been involved in a variety of general functions such as (Figure 6):

1. Regulation of intracellular pH (pH_i): the Na^+,H^+ exchanger is activated by the decrease of pH_i,[54] reaching its maximal transport velocity (V_{max}) at 2 pH_i

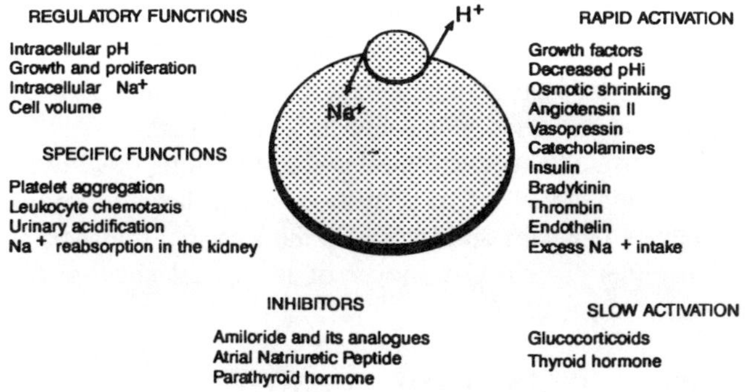

FIGURE 6. The Na^+,H^+ exchanger has been implicated in a variety of regulatory and specific functions. The rate of the Na^+,H^+ exchanger can be modulated in two different ways: a rapid activation pattern in which the effects are almost immediate, and a slow type of activation in which effects are apparent only after hours or days.

of approximately 6.0, whereas at pH_i near 7.4 the antiporter becomes virtually quiescent.[53]

2. Cell growth: this function is closely related to the regulation of pH_i because the cytoplasmic alkalinization has been claimed to be permissive for DNA and protein synthesis required for cellular proliferation and replication.[55]
3. Intracellular Na^+ concentration: up to 80% of the Na^+ that enters the cell can be mediated by this exchange,[56] this may be especially important in ischemic myocardial cells in which acidosis stimulates the antiport system and contributes to cytosolic Na^+ increase of the ischemic cells.[57]
4. Cell volume: in several cell types, a normally quiescent Na^+,H^+ exchanger can be activated by osmotically induced cell shrinking, thus promoting Na^+ and water entry into the cell;[51,58] moreover, in specific cells this antiporter is also involved in particular functions such as platelet aggregation, leukocyte chemotaxis, and proton secretion.[51,53]

The regulation of antiport activity has been reported in various tissues as well as in cultures of primary cells or established lines. The nature of the modulation can be placed in two categories: one in which the effects are almost immediate (seconds to minutes) and another in which activation is apparent only after many hours or even days. Although little is known about the specific molecular mechanism involved in the rapid activation of the antiport, it seems reasonable to hypothesize that the activation occurs via kinetic modifications such as an increase in the affinity of the transport protein for intracellular Na^+. Rapid activation that takes place after the agonist-induced phosphorylation of the antiport protein by PKC could probably result from a conformational change of the antiport, thus increasing the affinity of the Na^+,H^+ exchanger for intracellular H^+.[59] Several stimuli such as intracellular acid load, osmotic cell shrinking, growth factors (EGF, PDGF, EDGF), bradykinin, thrombin, catecholamines, insulin, angiotensin II, vasopressin (ADH), endothelin, and others can activate the antiport through this rapid pathway.[51,53] Conversely, thyroxine and glucocorticoids (dexamethasone) have been reported to modulate the Na^+,H^+ exchanger by a slow type of activation, which takes place over hours or days. Kinetic evidence indicates an increase in the maximal transport velocity that is consistent with either increased turnover of individual sites or with *de novo* synthesis of new exchanger units.[60]

C. THE PHOSPHATIDYLINOSITOL TURNOVER

A major recent advance in the understanding of how the Ca^{2+} messenger system operates followed the demonstration that receptor function in this system is linked to a specific enzyme, phospholipase C. This phosphodiesterase of the plasma membrane catalyzes the hydrolysis of a specific class of membrane phospholipids located in its inner leaflet, the phosphatidylinositols, thereby generating two intracellular messengers, inositol triphosphate (IP_3) and DAG. The phosphatidylinositides exist in three forms: phosphatidylinositol, phosphatidylinositol 4-phosphate, and phosphatidylinositol 4,5-bisphosphate, at a ratio of approximately 90:5:5. These forms are rapidly interconvertible by appropriate kinases and phosphatases.

When an appropriate agonist interacts with its plasma membrane receptor two events occur: an increase in the Ca^{2+} influx rate and the beginning of the phosphatidylinositol cycle inside the plasma membrane.[37,38] Stimulation of the membrane receptor determines that a group of coupled proteins, guanine nucleotide binding proteins (G proteins), activate phospholipase C which initiates the phosphatidylinositol turnover.[61] Within 15 s the enzyme catalyzes the hydrolysis of phosphatidylinositol 4,5-bisphosphate into two intracellular messengers: IP_3 and DAG.[62]

IP_3 is a water-soluble compound acting as a cytosolic signal to both sarcoplasmic reticulum and plasma membranes. This intermediate induces the opening of the so-called ''intracellular messenger operated Ca^{2+} channels'' and promotes the release of Ca^{2+} mainly from the sarcoplasmic reticulum, thereby causing a transient rise in the cytosolic free Ca^{2+} concentration. This rapid response, within less than 90 s, is followed by a Ca^{2+} reuptake to the sarcoplasmic reticulum by means of the Ca^{2+}-ATPase, and by the simultaneous calcium efflux to the extracellular medium mediated by both the Ca^{2+}-ATPase and the Na^+,Ca^{2+} exchanger. Within 3 to 5 min this pumping process returns cytosolic Ca^{2+} concentration ($Ca^{2+}{}_i$) to basal values. Ca^{2+} transients mediate the cellular response and are sufficient to activate a variety of enzyme systems (Figure 7).

DAG is not a water-soluble compound and remains in the plasma membrane. PKC is a calcium-activated, phospholipid-dependent enzyme of the plasma membrane that can exist in two forms: associated or unassociated with membrane phospholipids such as DAG.[63] In the nonassociated form it is relatively insensitive to activation by Ca^{2+}. When associated with DAG the enzymatic complex is highly sensitive to Ca^{2+}. The complex PKC-DAG-Ca^{2+} enhances its maximal velocity

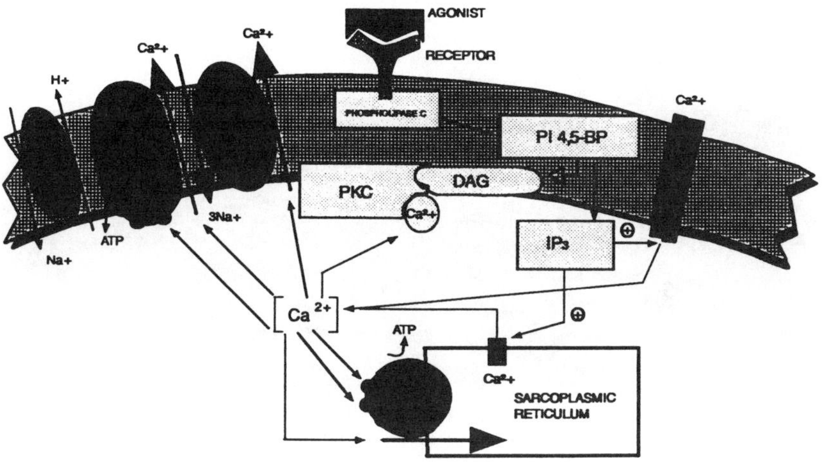

FIGURE 7. Signal transducing pathway of myocardial growth. Factors inducing myocardial hypertrophy activate membrane receptors responsible for a sequence of events, including initiating signals, coupling mechanisms, and regulation of gene expression. Stimulation of the membrane receptor activates phospholipase C and initiates the phosphatidylinositol turnover. The enzyme catalyzes the hydrolysis of phosphatidylinositol 4,5-bisphosphate (PI 4,5-BP) into two intracellular messengers: IP_3 and DAG. The former induces the opening of the so-called "intracellular messenger operated Ca^{2+} channels" and promotes the release of Ca^{2+} mainly from the sarcoplasmic reticulum, thereby causing a transient rise in the cytosolic free Ca^{2+} concentration. This rapid response is followed by Ca^{2+} reuptake to the sarcoplasmic reticulum by means of the Ca^{2+}-ATPase, and by a Ca^{2+} efflux to the extracellular medium mediated by both the Ca^{2+}-ATPase and the Na^+,Ca^{2+} exchanger. DAG remains within the plasma membrane and associates with PKC.

(V_{max}) 30 to 50 times. The activated enzymatic complex could lead phosphorylation of specific intracellular proteins and transcription factors (AP-1, AP-2) binding to a regulatory region, thereby activating RNA polymerase and cell growth.[64] Moreover, part of the cytosolic Ca^{2+} leads to an increase in the amount of Ca^{2+} within a submembrane cellular domain which regulates the activity of the calcium-sensitive form of PKC (Figure 8). The stretch of ventricular wall, several hormones, and vasoactive substances such as angiotensin II, norepinephrine, vasopressin, bradykinin, thrombin and endothelin, insulin, and growth factors act as initiating signals of myocardial hypertrophy (probably) using this signal transduction pathway.

VI. INTRACELLULAR RESPONSE TO INITIATING SIGNALS AND DEVELOPMENT OF MYOCARDIAL HYPERTROPHY

A. MECHANISMS OF MECHANICAL, NEURAL, AND ENDOCRINE CONTROL OF CARDIAC HYPERTROPHY

In subjects with a particular genetic substrate, the confluence of high blood pressure values together with the presence of several humoral agonists determines

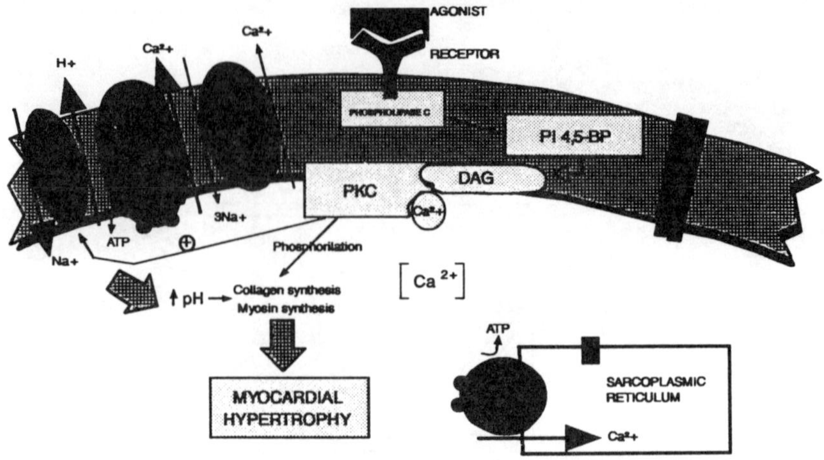

FIGURE 8. Signal transducing pathway of myocardial growth. When PKC associates DAG becomes highly sensitive to Ca^{2+}. The complex PKC-DAG-Ca^{2+} enhances its activity and initiates phosphorylation of specific intracellular proteins such as the Na^+,H^+ exchanger, myosin and collagen, and transcription factors, thereby activating RNA polymerase and promoting cell growth. Moreover, part of the cytosolic Ca^{2+} leads to an increase in the amount of Ca^{2+} within a submembrane cellular domain which regulates the activity of the calcium-sensitive form of the PKC.

the morphological patterns of myocardial growth in hypertensive patients. In any case, the response of the myocardiocyte to the different stimuli is the increase in cell size. Early morphologic abnormalities include enlarged cross-sectional areas due to the increased size of the myocardiocytes that exceed 12 μm in diameter. The roundness and basophilia of nuclei is more pronounced, and both nuclei and Golgi complexes exhibit an irregular shape. All these cellular events are due to the increased synthesis of myosin and the subsequent myofibrillar deposition.[65] In a more advanced step, the same initiating signals for myocardial growth also determine an increase in myocardial interstitial tissue and collagen content.[66,67]

The molecular mechanisms of pressure-overload LVH are not well understood.[64] An increase in intraventricular pressure from 0 to 25 mmHg has been proved to increase the rate of protein synthesis in rat hearts.[68] These and other related findings support the hypothesis that stretch of the ventricular wall initiates a signal transduction pathway that leads to enhanced protein synthesis. Mechanical stretch and cell deformation generate a wide range of intracellular signals that may modify rates of RNA and protein synthesis (Table 2). Cardiac muscle cell membranes contain nonselective mechanotransducer ion channels that are either activated or inactivated by stretch.[69] Thus, high blood pressure levels probably activate mechanoreceptors of the myocardial plasma membrane, inducing transmembrane ionic movements as effector mechanisms of hypertrophy.[69] Some studies have identified a deformation-dependent Na^+ influx and a Ca^{2+} stretch-dependent uptake in isolated perfused rat hearts as early signals of the protein synthetic pathway.[64]

TABLE 2
Effector Mechanisms and Intracellular Signals That May Be Induced by Mechanical Stretch Due to Left Ventricular Pressure Overload

Component	Intracellular signal
Stretch-sensitive channels	
Activated	
Cation channels	Na^+,K^+
Ca^{2+} channels	Ca^{2+}
Inactivated	
K^+ channels	K^+
Adenylyl cyclase	cAMP
Phospholipase C	Inositol phosphates
	Diacylglycerol
Na^+,H^+ exchange	Na^+,H^+

From Morgan, H. E. and Baker, K. M., *Circulation,* 83, 13, 1991. With permission.

Myocardial stretch increases the cytosolic Ca^{2+} and inositol triphosphate contents, as well as protein kinase activity, generating an intranuclear signal in the form of an enhanced expression of proto-oncogenes. Proto-oncogenes constitute DNA sequences of normal genes encoding several proteins involved in the regulation of cell growth: cytoplasmic protein kinases, membrane binding proteins, growth factors, growth factor receptors, and DNA binding proteins that modulate RNA transcription. At least three proto-oncogenes are expressed in pressure-overload hearts: *c-myc, c-fos,* and *c*-Ha-*ras*. The precise role of each of these proto-oncogenes in myocardial hypertrophy is not defined but they are probably necessary in order to orchestrate the important early changes in contractile protein synthesis.[70] In addition, stretch derived from the rise in blood pressure may also stimulate mechanoreceptors on the plasma membrane of endothelial cells leading to a signal pathway mediated through the endothelium.[71,72] Mechanical stimulation on the plasma membrane of endothelial cells may result in the release of either endothelin and endothelium-derived growth factors (EDGF), thus initiating the activation of phospholipase C.

The signal transduction generated by stretch or other types of cell deformation is complemented by transduction of neural and humoral signals of myocardial growth. Phospholipase C is simultaneously activated by neural and humoral agonists in several cell types, endothelial cells, platelets, fibroblasts, or myocardiocytes.[51,64] The endothelial release of EDGF or endothelin potentiate signals of the other agonists on plasma membrane receptors of myocardiocytes.[71,72] Platelet activation induced by increased cytosolic free Ca^{2+} may in turn release PDGF, acting as humoral agonists of phospholipase C activation both in endothelial cells and myocardiocytes. Angiotensin II, norepinephrine, vasopressin and other vasoactive substances, as well as insulin and several growth factors activate the same pathway when interacting with membrane receptors in endothelial cells, myocardiocytes, and fibroblasts.[64,73]

The activated complex PKC-DAG-Ca^{2+} leads to the phosphorylation of specific intracellular proteins, and results in the synthesis of myosin or collagen, as well as the activation of membrane proteins such as the Na^+,H^+ exchanger. Phosphorylation of this transport protein results in increased affinity for internal H^+ and higher rates of H^+ efflux which determine the alkalinization of the cytosol.[74] Therefore, the structural changes of the myocardial cells are not necessarily a direct consequence of the increase in blood pressure, but they can be the result of an excessive response to the agonists activating the Na^+,H^+ exchanger.[75]

The alkalinization of the cell interior is permissive for cell growth. In this sense, Ca^{2+} release from the sarcoplasmic reticulum mediated by IP_3 is pH dependent and decreases dramatically under pH_i values of 6.8.[73] Thus, cytosolic alkalinization due to Na^+,H^+ antiporter activation, which raises pH_i to values from 7.0 to 7.4 in cells stimulated by growth factors,[76] facilitates protein phosphorylation by PKC.

B. EFFECT OF ANTIHYPERTENSIVE THERAPY ON MYOCARDIAL SIGNAL TRANSDUCING PATHWAY AND REVERSAL OF LEFT VENTRICULAR HYPERTROPHY

Some of the nonpharmacologic measures as well as several drugs recommended for the pharmacologic treatment of arterial hypertension may reverse LVH interference in the intracellular signal transducing pathway. It is known that sodium chloride intake is one of the various factors that can contribute to left ventricular growth in both hypertensive rats[77] and EH patients.[78] In this sense, it has been reported that saline overload increases left ventricular mass, and a salt-restricted diet determines the regression of cardiac hypertrophy. Furthermore, LVH is more marked in salt-sensitive than in salt-resistant hypertensives.[79]

The mechanisms of cellular growth after sodium overload are not well understood, but it is known that high-salt ingestion activates the sympathetic nervous system and may raise the level of plasmatic catecholamines.[74,79] Furthermore, salt overload may lead to the stimulation of phospholipase C mediated by PDGF,[80] and the Na^+,H^+ exchanger has been observed to be more active in salt-sensitive hypertensives.[74] Therefore, low-salt diets could reduce the adrenergic activity, circulating catecholamines, and platelet activation, thus interfering in the signaling pathway that determines cardiac hypertrophy. On the other hand, because obesity is associated with LVH,[81] the decrease in caloric intake also contributes to the reversal of LVH, particularly if this measure is associated with saline restriction.[82]

Calcium-channel blockers reduce cardiac hypertrophy, and this interferes in the signal transducing pathway at several levels, particularly at the initiating signal level.[83] The control of blood pressure by these drugs and the subsequent reduction of this mechanical factor contributing to LVH may be important for the reversal of LVH induced by calcium-channel blocker treatment. Nevertheless, the inhibitory effect of these drugs on platelet activation may prevent the activation of plasma membrane receptors by PDGF and the stimulation of phospholipase C of the myocardiocytes.[84] Simultaneously, Ca^{2+} uptake mediated by voltage-sensitive calcium channels can be blocked by calcium antagonists. Thus, these drugs may also interfere in cell activation by vasoactive agonists and growth factors through the indirect decrease in the activity of the Na^+,H^+ and the Na^+,Ca^{2+} exchangers.[85]

ACE inhibitors constitute a group of drugs proven to have a remarkable effect on the regression of cardiac enlargement in hypertensives. They prevent not only the activation of phospholipase C by circulating angiotensin II but, most importantly, they inhibit the formation of angiotensin II inside the myocardial and endothelial cells. This characteristic has particular pathophysiological significance. On the other hand, insulin also activates the Na^+,H^+ exchanger[51] and is involved in the pathogenesis of cellular growth. The demonstration that EH is a clinical entity characterized by insulin peripheral resistance with hyperinsulinemia,[86] as well as the fact that ACE inhibitors have been reported to decrease such insulin resistance,[87] suggest that this mechanism may also contribute to the reduction of LVH in patients treated with these drugs. This hypothesis has not been proved.

Finally, treatment with β-adrenergic antagonists without ISA has been reported to promote the regression of cardiac hypertrophy, although results are controversial.[88] Even though the intrinsic sympathomimetic activity appears to play an important role, the controversial results of beta-blockers in the clinical therapeutical regression of LVH could have their origin in the fact that norepinephrine-mediated growth of isolated myocytes can be prevented by the blockade of α_1-receptors but not β-receptors.[32]

VII. ERYTHROCYTE IONIC TRANSPORT ABNORMALITIES AND LEFT VENTRICULAR HYPERTROPHY

As described in this chapter, intracellular Na^+, H^+, and Ca^{2+} contents are possible effector mechanisms of the signal transducing pathway involved in myocardiocyte growth. In recent years, evidence has emerged that alterations in the intracellular pool of ions, especially Na^+ and Ca^{2+}, may play a role not only in the pathogenesis of essential hypertension, but also in the myocardial growth of these patients. In this sense, we and others reported that patients with an increased maximal rate of Na^+,Li^+ countertransport exhibit some differences in severity of high blood pressure,[89] lipid profile,[90] plasma renin activity,[89,91] and left ventricular hypertrophy.[92,93] Moreover, Inoue et al.[94] recently reported that intraerythrocyte Na^+ content and intracellular concentration of Ca^{2+} in platelets were powerful determinants of the LVMI in essential hypertensives.

Therefore, it may be expected that the activity of several transmembrane transport systems responsible for Na^+ and Ca^{2+} movements should be modulated, activated, or depressed by mechanical, neural, and hormonal factors. In addition, kinetics of these transport pathways could be genetically modified resulting in increased cytosolic concentrations of those cations. These abnormalities also should be present in other cells not directly involved in the pathogenetic mechanism of high blood pressure or myocardial growth. Accordingly, it may be possible to detect abnormalities of several systems related to Na^+, H^+, and Ca^{2+} transport in erythrocytes of essential hypertensives and to try to investigate the relationship of these transport system abnormalities and the cardiac hypertrophy.

In order to test this hypothesis, we performed M-mode and bidimensional echocardiograms to a group of 40 untreated essential hypertensives, 27 men and 13 women, aged 23 to 56 years, for measuring interventricular septal thickness, posterior wall thickness, and left ventricular internal dimension at end diastole. Left ventricular mass was determined using the Penn convention criteria[95] and divided for the body surface area in order to calculate LVMI in grams per square meter. LVH was diagnosed if LVMI exceeded 110 g/m^2 in women and 130 g/m^2 in men.[97] The relative wall thickness ratio was obtained using the standardized formula: 2 × posterior wall thickness/left ventricular internal diastolic dimension.[96] Concentric hypertrophy was diagnosed if the patient had increased LVMI plus a relative wall thickness $\geqq 0.45$. Eccentric hypertrophy was considered if this ratio was lower than 0.45.[96]

In these patients we investigated the apparent dissociation constants (K50%) and maximal efflux rates (V_{max}) of erythrocyte Ca^{2+}-ATPase, Na^+,K^+-ATPase, Na^+,K^+,Cl^- cotransport and Na^+,Li^+ countertransport, the Na^+ influx rate which is dependent on Na^+,H^+ exchanger, and the rate constant of Na^+ leak by means of previously described methods.[98,99] Finally, several biochemical and hormonal determinations were also performed, including serum fasting glucose, lipid profile, plasma renin activity (PRA), both in basal conditions and after stimulation by furosemide and upstanding, basal aldosterone, plasma norepinephrine and epinephrine, and ANP.

Essential hypertensives were classified into two groups according to the presence or absence of LVH. Using the aforementioned criteria 26 (65%) hypertensives exhibited LVH and 14 (35%) patients did not. Among the 26 patients with LVH a morphological pattern of concentric hypertrophy was observed in 9 patients (35%), whereas the remaining 17 (65%) patients exhibited eccentric hypertrophy. As seen in Table 3, patients with cardiac enlargement showed a significantly higher intraerythrocyte Na^+ content (8.53 ± 0.26 vs. 7.43 ± 0.16 mmol/l cells; $p = 0.0012$), and a higher Na^+ influx rate dependent on the transmembrane erythrocyte Na^+,H^+ exchanger (10,177 ± 772 vs. 7460 ± 773 μmol/l cells h^{-1}; $p = 0.0182$). Both internal Na^+ content (8.54 ± 0.3 vs. 8.52 ± 0.1 mmol/l cells) and the activity of the Na^+,H^+ exchanger (11,837 ± 1252 vs. 9299 ± 933 μmol/l cells.h^{-1}) were identical in patients with concentric or eccentric hypertrophy. Although maximal velocities of the Na^+,K^+-ATPase and Na^+,K^+,Cl^- cotransport were slightly lower in patients with LVH, these differences were not significant. No differences were observed in the active Ca^{2+} transport system measured.

Table 4 shows that patients with LVH were slightly older than hypertensives without cardiac enlargement. Interestingly, no differences were observed in either systolic and diastolic blood pressure values or body mass index, which supports

TABLE 3
Different Erythrocyte Ionic Parameters in 40 Essential Hypertensives Classified According to the Presence or Absence of Left Ventricular Hypertrophy

Parameter	LVH (n = 26)	No LVH (n = 14)
Intraerythrocyte Na^+ content (mmol/l cells)	8.53 ± 0.26[a]	7.43 ± 0.16
Na^+,K^+-ATPase		
V_{max} (μmol/l cells h^{-1})	8751 ± 392	9334 ± 662
K50% (mmol/l cells)	18.52 ± 0.85	16.37 ± 1.33
Na^+,K^+,Cl^- contransport		
V_{max} (μmol/l cells h^{-1})	638 ± 65	760 ± 107
K50% (mmol/l cells)	13.12 ± 1.13	12.44 ± 1.75
Na^+,Li^+ countertransport		
V_{max} (μmol/l cells h^{-1})	326 ± 27	327 ± 39
K50% (mmol/l cells)	8.30 ± 1.17	7.23 ± 0.94
Na^+,H^+ exchanger		
Na^+ influx rate (μmol/l cells h^{-1})	10,177 ± 772[b]	7460 ± 773
Passive Na^+ leak		
Kp Na^+ (10^{-3} h^{-1})	19.47 ± 0.79	19.06 ± 1.19
Ca^{2+}-ATPase		
V_{max} (μmol/l cells h^{-1})	6618 ± 335	5703 ± 796
K50% (mmol/l cells)	80.04 ± 10.6	73.18 ± 16.0

Note: Values referred to as mean ± SEM.

[a] $p = 0.001$.
[b] $p = 0.0182$.

the hypothesis that mechanical and hemodynamic factors are not the major determinants of LVH. Among hypertensives with LVH a trend to higher values of serum glucose, cholesterol, low-density lipoprotein cholesterol and triglycerides was observed, but differences were not significant. Likewise, hormonal parameters did not show any statistical differences between groups.

All morphological parameters of cardiac enlargement, i.e., LVMI ($r = 0.46$; $p = 0.002$), interventricular septal thickness ($r = 0.35$; $p = 0.022$), and posterior wall thickness ($r = 0.53$; $p = 0.001$), and the relative wall thickness ratio ($r = 0.36$; $p = 0.021$) showed a positive correlation with the activity of the erythrocyte Na^+,H^+ exchanger. Nevertheless, despite the observation of higher intracellular Na^+ content in hypertensives with cardiac enlargement, those echocardiographic cardiac parameters did not show any correlation with intracellular Na^+. Finally, in a multiple stepwise regression analysis including age, intraerythrocyte Na^+ content, and the Na^+,H^+ exchanger activity, we found that only Na^+,H^+ antiport activity and age were independent determinants of the presence of LVH.

In summary, our results suggest that the increased intraerythrocyte Na^+ content observed in hypertensives exhibiting LVH could be related basically to the

TABLE 4
Clinical, Biochemical, and Hormonal Parameters in 40 Essential Hypertensive Patients Classified According to the Presence or Absence of Left Ventricular Hypertrophy

Parameter	LVH (n = 26)	No LVH (n = 14)
Age	44.7 ± 1.4[a]	37.3 ± 2.6
Systolic blood pressure (mmHg)	173.9 ± 2.7	165.7 ± 4.8
Diastolic blood pressure (mmHg)	103.5 ± 1.1	104.0 ± 2.3
Body mass index (kg/m^2)	28.1 ± 0.6	26.5 ± 1.1
Plasma glucose (mg/dl)	106.8 ± 5.7	94.9 ± 2.9
Cholesterol (mg/dl)	206.8 ± 8.4	198.2 ± 8.1
Triglycerides (mg/dl)	136.2 ± 31.5	117.1 ± 12.9
LDL cholesterol (mg/dl)	132.2 ± 7.7	125.6 ± 8.8
HDL cholesterol (mg/dl)	51.1 ± 2.3	50.6 ± 2.9
Basal PRA (ng/ml/h)	0.4 ± 0.1	0.5 ± 0.1
Stimulated PRA (ng/ml/h)	1.8 ± 0.3	2.6 ± 0.8
Aldosterone (ng/dl)	20.3 ± 2.1	14.6 ± 1.6
Epinephrine (pg/ml)	49.2 ± 9.0	33.6 ± 12.7
Norepinephrine (pg/ml)	222.8 ± 20.3	199.6 ± 29.9
Atrial natriuretic peptide (fmol/ml)	13.8 ± 1.2	11.0 ± 1.3

Note: Values referred to as mean ± SEM.

[a] $p = 0.024$.

hyperactivity of the Na^+, H^+ exchanger and, to a lesser extent, to the diminished activity of the sodium pump and cotransport system. The hyperactivity of the Na^+,H^+ exchanger is known to be responsible for a simultaneous net Na^+ influx and H^+ efflux from the cell. In myocardial cells, the transmembrane ionic movements could lead to either an increase in intracellular Na^+ content or to alkalinization of the intracellular medium, hence promoting protein synthesis. Whether this abnormality is primary and genetically determined, or is secondary to the prior activation of PKC remains to be elucidated. The apparent discordance between blood pressure values and left ventricular mass in hypertensives strengthens the hypothesis that factors other than blood pressure are also involved in the development of LVH in EH. In this sense, the enhancement of the Na^+,H^+ exchanger in erythrocytes of essential hypertensives seems to be a good biological marker of myocardial concentric or eccentric hypertrophy.

VIII. SUMMARY AND CONCLUSIONS

The Framingham Heart Study showed that essential hypertensives with definite electrocardiographic signs of LVH increased from three- to tenfold their mortality rates due to all cardiovascular diseases with respect to hypertensives without signs of cardiac hypertrophy. Of particular interest was the demonstration of a negative prognostic value of LVH even after adjustment for the severity of hypertension, which lends LVH the character of independent risk factor. Ventricular hypertrophy is a dynamic process that can develop and reverse in a period of a few weeks, both in experimental hypertension and clinical practice. Thus, contrary to the classic notion LVH seems not to be a late and irreversible pressure-related complication of EH, but an early phenomenon subject to a dynamic modification in the evolution of the disease.

Clinical studies have shown that not all forms of antihypertensive therapy lead to regression of myocardial hypertrophy, ranging from complete absence of effect, through a largely pressure-related decrease in muscle mass, to an unrelated to pressure reversal of LVH. The discrepancy between the extent of reduction in blood pressure and the regression of myocardial hypertrophy, as well as the simultaneous enlargement of the right ventricle observed in some hypertensives without concomitant pulmonary hypertension, suggests that apart from blood pressure values, the degree of LVH is also controlled by other factors. Likewise, detection of LVH in animals and normotensive relatives of hypertensives, even in the prehypertensive phase, and the substantial variability in morphologic patterns of LVH, both in hypertensives and their normotensive relatives, support a genetic predisposition to myocardial growth in EH. In this context, LVH would develop in subjects with a particular genetic substrate by the overlap of high blood pressure values and several factors linked to the adrenergic system, the renin-angiotensin-aldosterone system, other vasoactive substances, and growth factors.

Factors inducing myocardial growth activate membrane receptors responsible for a sequence of events, including initiating signals, coupling mechanisms, and regulation of gene expression. As a result of these signals, membrane ion channels and ion transport systems are activated, leading to increased intracellular contents of Na^+, H^+, Ca^{2+}, inositol phosphates, DAG, and to greater activity of PKA and PKC, with increased protein and DNA synthesis. Cardiac hypertrophy in hypertension could involve impaired function of any of these steps in this complex pathway. In this sense, we found that hypertensives with echocardiographic LVH exhibited several erythrocyte ion transport abnormalities such as a higher intracellular Na^+ content and enhanced ion translocation rates of the Na^+,H^+ exchanger, the former probably being secondary to the hyperactivation of the antiport. Moreover, the activity of the Na^+,H^+ exchanger positively correlated with the LVMI, interventricular septal thickness, posterior wall thickness, and the relative wall thickness ratio. Therefore, we speculate that hyperactivity of this antiport system detected in the erythrocytes of essential hypertensives is a good biological marker of myocardial growth. The issue of whether this abnormality is genetically determined or secondary to the prior activation of PKC remains to be elucidated. No doubt during the next few years research will be enlightening enough that we will understand perfectly the systems of transmission of intracellular signals involved in the etiopathogenia of the ventricular and arteriolar wall growth.

ACKNOWLEDGMENTS

Supported in part by Grant 90/0022 of the Fondo de Investigación Sanitaria (FIS), Ministerio de Sanidad y Consumo, Madrid, Spain, and by a grant from Laboratorios Prodes S.A., Barcelona, Spain.

REFERENCES

1. The 1988 Report of the Joint National Committee on Detection, Evaluation and Treatment of High Blood Pressure, *Arch. Intern. Med.*, 1988; 148: 1023–1038.
2. **Kannel, W. B.,** Some lessons in cardiovascular epidemiology from Framingham, *Am. J. Cardiol.*, 1976; 37: 269–282.
3. **Kannel, W. B., Castelli, W. P., Mellumara, A. M., McKee, P. H., and Fernleib, M.,** Role of blood pressure in the development of congestive heart failure, *N. Engl. J. Med.*, 1972; 287: 781–787.
4. **Chobanian, A. V., Brecher, P. I., and Haudenschild, C. C.,** Effects of hypertension and antihypertensive therapy on atherosclerosis: state of the art lecture, *Hypertension,* 1986; 8(Suppl. I): 15–21.
5. **Kannel, W. B.,** Prevalence and natural history of electrocardiographic left ventricular hypertrophy, *Am. J. Med.*, 1983; 75(Suppl. 3A): 4–11.
6. **Casalle, P. N., Devereux, R. B., Milner, M. et al.** Value of echocardiographic measurement of left ventricular mass predicting cardiovascular morbid events in hypertensive men, *Ann. Intern. Med.*, 1986; 105: 173–178.
7. **Massie, B. M., Tubau, J. F., Szlachcic, J., and O'Kelly, B. F.,** Hypertensive heart disease: the critical role of left ventricular hypertrophy, *J. Cardiovasc. Pharmacol.*, 1989; 13(Suppl. I): s18–s24.
8. **Messerli, F., Ventura, H. O., Elizardi, D. J., Dunn, F. G., and Frohlich, E. D.,** Hypertension and sudden death: increased ventricular ectopic activity in left ventricular hypertrophy, *Am. J. Med.*, 1984; 77: 18–22.
9. **McLenechan, J. M., Henderson, E., Morris, K. I. et al.,** Ventricular arrhythmias in patients with hypertensive left ventricular hypertrophy, *N. Engl. J. Med.*, 1987; 317: 787–792.
10. **Kannel, W. B., D'Agostino, R. B., Levy, D., and Belanger, A. J.,** Prognostic significance of regression of left ventricular hypertrophy, *Circulation,* 1988; 78(Suppl. II): 89 (Abstr.).
11. **Tarazi, R. C.,** The hemodynamics of hypertension, in *Hypertension: Physiopathology and Treatment,* Genest, J., Kuchel, O., Hamet, P., and Cantin, M., Eds., New York, McGraw-Hill, 1983; 15–42.
12. **Grossman, W., Jones, D., and McLaurin, L. P.,** Wall stress and patterns of hypertrophy in the human left ventricle, *J. Clin. Invest.*, 1975; 56: 56–64.
13. **Tarazi, R. C.,** Cardiovascular hypertrophy in hypertension, *Hypertension,* 1986; 8(Suppl. II): 187–190.
14. **Mulvany, M. J. and Korsgaard, N.,** Correlation and otherwise between blood pressure, cardiac mass and resistance vessel characteristics in hypertensive, normotensive and hypertensive/normotensive hybrid rats, *J. Hypertension,* 1983; 1: 235–244.
15. **Sen, S.,** Regression of cardiac hypertrophy: experimental animal model, *Am. J. Med.*, 1983; 75(Suppl. 3A): 87–93.
16. **Tarazi, R. C. and Fouad, F. M.,** Reversal of cardiac hypertrophy by medical treatment, *Annu. Rev. Med.*, 1985; 36: 407–414.

17. **Folkow, B.,** Cardiovascular structural adaptation: its role in the initiation and maintenance of primary hypertension, *Clin. Sci. Mol. Med.*, 1978; 55(Suppl.): 3s–22s.
18. **Nuñez, B. D., Messerli, F. H., Amadeo, C. et al.,** Biventricular cardiac hypertrophy in essential hypertension, *Am. Heart J.*, 1987; 114: 813–818.
19. **Yamori, Y., Mori, C., Nishio, T. et al.,** Cardiac hypertrophy in early hypertension, *Am. J. Cardiol.*, 1979; 44: 964–969.
20. **Radice, M., Alli, C., Avanzini, F. et al.,** Left ventricular structure and function in normotensive adolescents with a genetic predisposition to hypertension, *Am. Heart J.*, 1986; 111: 115–120.
21. **Frohlich, E. D. and Tarazi, R. C.,** Is arterial pressure the role factor responsible for hypertensive cardiac hypertrophy?, *Am. J. Cardiol.*, 1979; 44: 959–963.
22. **Frohlich, E. D.,** The heart in hypertension, in *Hypertension: Physiopathology and Treatment,* Genest, J., Kuchel, O., Hamet, P., and Cantin, M., Eds., New York, McGraw-Hill, 1983; 791–810.
23. **Wollam, G. L., Hall, D. W., Porter, V. D. et al.,** Time course of regression of left ventricular hypertrophy in treated hypertensive patients, *Am. J. Med.*, 1983; 75(Suppl.): 100A–110A.
24. **Drayer, J. I. M., Garding, J. M., Weber, M. S., and Aronow, W. S.,** Cardiac muscle mass during vasodilatation therapy of hypertension, *Clin. Pharmacol. Ther.*, 1983; 33: 727–732.
25. **Fouad, F. M., Nakashima, Y., Tarazi, R. C., and Salcedo, E. E.,** Reversal of left ventricular hypertrophy in hypertensive patients treated with methyldopa. Lack of association with blood pressure control, *Am. J. Cardiol.*, 1982; 49: 795–801.
26. **Nakashima, Y., Fouad, F. M., and Tarazi, R. C.,** Regression of left ventricular hypertrophy from systemic hypertension by enalapril, *Am. J. Cardiol.*, 1984; 53: 1044–1049.
27. **Schulman, S. P., Weis, J. L., Becker, L. C. et al.,** The effects of antihypertensive therapy on left ventricular mass in elderly patients, *N. Engl. J. Med.*, 1980; 322: 1350–1356.
28. **Strauer, B. E., Mahmoud, M. A., Bayer, F., Bohn, J., and Motz, U.,** Reversal of left ventricular hypertrophy and improvement of cardiac function in man by nifedipine, *Eur. Heart J.*, 1984; 5(Suppl. F): 53–60.
29. **Strauer, B. E., Bayer, F., Brecht, H. M., and Motz, W.,** The influence of sympathetic nervous activity on regression of cardiac hypertrophy, *J. Hypertension,* 1985; 3(Suppl. 4): s39–s44.
30. **Rowlands, D. B., Glover, D. R., Stallard, T. J., and Littler, W. A.,** Control of blood pressure and reduction of echocardiographically assessed left ventricular mass with once-daily timolol, *Br. J. Clin. Pharmacol.*, 1982; 14: 89–95.
31. **Allen, J. W., Kaiser, P. J., and Montenegro, A.,** Effects of atenolol on left ventricular hypertrophy and early left ventricular function in essential hypertension, *Am. J. Cardiol.*, 1989; 64: 1157–1161.
32. **Simpson, P.,** Norepinephrine-stimulated hypertrophy of cultured rat myocardial cell is an alpha-1-adrenergic response, *J. Clin. Invest.*, 1983; 72: 732–738.
33. **Schelling, P., Fischer, H., and Ganten, D.,** Angiotensin and cell growth: a link to cardiovascular hypertrophy?, *J. Hypertension,* 1991; 9: 3–15.
34. **Sen, S., Tarazi, R. C., and Bumpus, F. M.,** Cardiac effects of angiotensin-antagonists in normotensive rats, *Clin. Sci.*, 1979; 56: 439–444.
35. **Ferrario, C. M.,** Importance of the renin-angiotensin-aldosterone system (RAS) in the physiology and pathology of hypertension: an overview, *Drugs,* 1990; 39(Suppl. 2): 1–8.
36. **Rasmussen, H.,** Cellular calcium metabolism, *Ann. Intern. Med.*, 1983; 98: 809–816.
37. **Rasmussen, H.,** The calcium messenger system (first of two parts), *N. Engl. J. Med.*, 1986; 314: 1094–1101.
38. **Rasmussen, H.,** The calcium messenger system (second of two parts), *N. Engl. J. Med.*, 1986; 314: 1164–1170.
39. **Blaustein, M. P.,** Sodium/calcium exchange and the control of contractility in cardiac muscle and vascular smooth muscle, *J. Cardiovasc. Pharmacol.*, 1988; 12(Suppl. 5): s56–s68.
40. **Nicholls, D. G.,** The regulation of extramitochondrial free calcium ion concentration by rat liver mitochondria, *Biochem. J.*, 1978; 176: 511–522.

41. **Chapman, R. A.,** Excitation-contraction coupling in cardiac muscle, *Prog. Biophys. Mol. Biol.,* 1979; 35: 1–52.
42. **MacLennan, D.,** Purification and properties of the adenosine triphosphatase from sarcoplasmic reticulum, *J. Biol. Chem.,* 1970; 245: 4508–4518.
43. **Carafoli, E.,** Intracellular calcium homeostasis, *Annu. Rev. Biochem.,* 1987; 56: 395–433.
44. **Carafoli, E.,** Intracellular calcium regulation, with special attention to role of the plasma membrane calcium pump, *J. Cardiovasc. Pharmacol.,* 1988; 12(Suppl. 3): 77–84.
45. **Vincenzi, F. F. and Larsen, F. L.,** The plasma membrane calcium pump: regulation by a soluble Ca^{2+} binding protein, *Fed. Proc.,* 1980; 39: 2427–2431.
46. **Reuter, H. and Seitz, N.,** The dependence of calcium efflux from cardiac muscle on temperature and the external ion composition, *J. Physiol.,* 1968; 195: 451–470.
47. **Philipson, K. D.,** Sodium-calcium exchange in plasma membrane vesicles, *Annu. Rev. Physiol.,* 1985; 47: 561–571.
48. **Carafoli, E.,** The transport of calcium across the inner membrane of mitochondrial, in *Membrane Transport of Calcium,* Carafoli, E., Ed., London, Academic Press, 1982; 109–139.
49. **Siegel, P. K. S., Cragoe, E. J., Trumble, M. J., and Kaczorowski, G. J.,** Inhibition of Na^+/Ca^{2+} exchange in membrane vesicles and papillary muscle preparations from guinea pig hearts by analogues of amiloride, *Proc. Natl. Acad. Sci. U.S.A.,* 1984; 81: 3238–3242.
50. **Murer, H., Hopfer, U., and Kinne, R.,** Sodium/proton antiport in brush-border-membrane vesicles isolated from rat small intestine and kidney, *Biochem. J.,* 1976; 154: 597–604.
51. **Grinstein, S. and Rothstein, A.,** Mechanisms of regulation of the Na^+/H^+ exchanger, *J. Membr. Biol.,* 1986; 90: 1–12.
52. **Aronson, P. S.,** Kinetic properties of the plasma membrane Na^+-H^+ exchanger, *Annu. Rev. Physiol.,* 1985; 47: 545–560.
53. **Frighi, V. and Verna, R.,** The Na^+-H^+ antiport and its role in cell regulation, in *Bioengineered Molecules: Basic and Clinical Aspects,* Verna, R., Blumenthal, R., and Frati, L., Eds., New York, Raven Press, 1989; 97–107.
54. **Aronson, P. S., Nee, J., and Suhm, M. A.,** Modifier role of internal H^+ in activating the Na^+/H^+ exchanger in renal microvillous membrane vesicles, *Nature,* 1982; 299: 161–163.
55. **Madshus, I. H.,** Regulation of intracellular pH in eukaryotic cells, *Biochem. J.,* 1988; 250: 1–8.
56. **Frelin, C., Vigne, P., and Lazdunski, M.,** The role of the Na^+-H^+ exchange system in cardiac cells in relation to the control of the internal Na^+ concentration, *J. Biol. Chem.,* 1984; 259: 8880–8885.
57. **Tani, M. and Neely, J.,** Role of intracellular Na^+ in Ca^{2+} overload and depressed recovery of ventricular function of reperfused ischemic rat hearts. Possible involvement of H^+-Na^+ and Na^+-Ca^{2+} exchange, *Circ. Res.,* 1989; 65: 1045–1056.
58. **Grinstein, S., Clark, C. A., and Rothstein, A.,** Activation of Na^+-H^+ exchange in lymphocytes by osmotically induced volume changes and by cytoplasmic acidification, *J. Gen. Physiol.,* 1983; 82: 619–638.
59. **Frelin, C., Vigne, P., Barbry, P., and Lazdunski, M.,** Molecular properties of amiloride action and of its Na^+ transporting targets, *Kidney Int.,* 1987; 32: 785–793.
60. **Berk, B. C., Vallega, G., Griendling, K. K. et al.** Effects of glucocorticoids on Na^+-H^+ exchange and growth in cultured vascular smooth muscle cells, *J. Cell Physiol.,* 1988; 137: 391–401.
61. **Neer, E. J. and Clapham, D. E.,** Role of G protein subunits in transmembrane signalling, *Nature,* 1988; 333: 129–133.
62. **Berridge, M. J.,** Inositol triphosphate and diacylglycerol as second messenger, *Biochem. J.,* 1984; 220: 345–360.
63. **Takai, Y., Kishimoto, A., Iwasa, Y. et al.,** Calcium-dependent activation of a multifunctional protein kinase by membrane phospholipids, *J. Biol. Chem.,* 1979; 254: 3692–3695.
64. **Morgan, H. E. and Baker, K. M.,** Cardiac hypertrophy. Mechanical, neural and endocrine dependence, *Circulation,* 1991; 83: 13–25.

65. **Ferrans, V. J. and Rodriguez, E. R.,** Morphology of the heart in left ventricular hypertrophy, in *The Heart and Hypertension,* Messerli, F. H., Ed., New York, Yorke Medical Books, 1987; 75–86.
66. **Dawson, R., Milne, G., and Williams, R. B.,** Changes in the collagen of rat heart in copper-deficiency cardiac hypertrophy, *Cardiovasc. Res.,* 1982; 16: 559–565.
67. **Michel, J. B., Salzman, J. L., Ossondo, N. M. et al.,** Morphometric analysis of collagen network and plasma perfused capillary bed in the myocardium of rats during evolution of cardiac hypertrophy, *Basic Res. Cardiol.,* 1986; 81: 142–154.
68. **Xenophontos, X. P., Gordon, E. E., and Morgan, H. E.,** Effects of intraventricular pressure on protein synthesis in arrested rat hearts, *Am. J. Physiol.,* 1986; 251: C95–C98.
69. **Morris, C. E.,** Mechanosensitive ion channels, *J. Membr. Biol.,* 1990; 113: 93–107.
70. **Marban, E. and Koretsune, Y.,** Cell calcium, oncogenes, and hypertrophy, *Hypertension,* 1990; 15: 652–658.
71. **Lüscher, T. F.,** Imbalance of endothelium-derived relaxing and contracting factors. A new concept in hypertension?, *Am. J. Hypertension,* 1990; 3: 317–330.
72. **Simonson, M. S. and Dunn, M. J.,** Endothelin pathways of transmembrane signalling, *Hypertension,* 1990; 15(Suppl. I): 5–12.
73. **Maly, K., Hochleitner, B. W., and Grunicke, U.,** Interrelationship between growth factor-induced activation of the Na^+/H^+ antiporter and mobilization of intracellular Ca^{2+} in NIH3T3-fibroblasts, *Biochem. Biophys. Res. Commun.,* 1990; 167: 1206–1213.
74. **Aviv, A.,** Prospective review: the link between cytosolic Ca^{2+} and the Na^+-H^+ antiport: a unifying factor for essential hypertension, *J. Hypertension,* 1988; 6: 685–691.
75. **Lever, A. F.,** Slow pressor mechanisms and smooth muscle mitogens in hypertension, *J. Clin. Hypertension,* 1987; 3: 323–327.
76. **Siffert, W. and Akkerman, J. W. N.,** Na^+/H^+ exchange and Ca^{2+} influx, *Fed. Eur. Biochem. Soc.,* 1989; 259: 1–4.
77. **Meggs, L. G., Ben-Ari, J., Gummon, D., and Gordman, A. A.,** Myocardial hypertrophy: the effect of sodium and the role of sympathetic nervous activity, *Am. J. Hypertension,* 1988; 1: 11–15.
78. **Schmieder, R. E., Messerli, F. H., Garaveglia, G. E., and Nuñez, B. E.,** Dietary salt intake: a determinant of cardiac involvement in essential hypertension, *Circulation,* 1988; 78: 951–956.
79. **Heimann, J. C., Drumond, S., Rodrigues, A. T., Guedes, A. J., Dichtchekenian, V., and Marcondes, M.,** Left ventricular hypertrophy is more marked in salt-sensitive than in salt-resistant hypertensive patients, *J. Cardiovasc. Pharmacol.,* 1991; 17(Suppl. 2): 122–124.
80. **Limon, I., Blanc, J., Koutouzov, S., Knorr, A., Meyer, P., and Marche, P.,** Platelet phospholipase C activity in salt-dependent hypertension, *Hypertension,* 1990; 15: 381–387.
81. **Messerli, F. H., Sundgaard-Riise, K., Reisen, E. D. et al.,** Dimorphic cardiac adaptation to obesity and arterial hypertension, *Ann. Intern. Med.,* 1983; 99: 757–761.
82. **Reisin, E.,** Weight reduction as a therapeutic modality in hypertension. The influence of concurrent sodium deprivation, in *Hypertension: Pathophysiology, Diagnosis and Management,* Laragh, J. H. and Brenner, B. M. Eds., New York, Raven Press, 1990; 2025–2035.
83. **Struyker-Boudier, H. A. J., Smits, J. F. M., and De Mey, J. G. R.,** The pharmacology of calcium antagonists: a review, *J. Cardiovasc. Pharmacol.,* 1990; 15(Suppl. 4): 1–10.
84. **Addonizio, V. P., Fisher, C. A., Strauss, J. F., Wachtfogel, Y. T., Colman, R. W., and Josephson, M. E.,** Effects of verapamil and diltiazem on human platelet function, *Am. J. Physiol.,* 1986; 250: H366–H371.
85. **Rabkin, S. W.,** The effect of alteration of extracellular Na^+ or Ca^{2+} and inhibition of Ca^{2+} entry, Na^+-H^+ exchange, and Na^+-Ca^{2+} exchange by diltiazem, amiloride and dichlorobenzamil on the response of cardiac cell aggregates to epidermal growth factor, *Exp. Cell. Res.,* 1990; 188: 262–266.
86. **Pollare, T., Lithell, H. O., and Berne, C.,** Insulin resistance is a characteristic feature of primary hypertension independent of obesity, *Metabolism,* 1990; 39: 167–174.

87. **Lithell, H. O., Pollare, T., and Berne, C.,** Insulin sensitivity in newly detected hypertensive patients: influence of captopril and other antihypertensive agents on insulin sensitivity and related biological parameters, *J. Cardiovasc. Pharmacol.,* 1990; 15(Suppl. 5): 46–52.
88. **Motz, W. H. and Strauer, B. E.,** Differential therapy of hypertensive heart disease, *Am. J. Cardiol.,* 1990; 65: 60G–64G.
89. **De la Sierra, A., Coca, A., Aguilera, M. T., and Urbano-Marquez, A.,** Na^+-Li^+ countertransport in essential hypertension, *J. Hypertension,* 1988; 6: 931–937.
90. **Hunt, S. C., Williams, R. R., Smith, J. B., and Ash, K. O.,** Associations of three erythrocyte cation transport systems with plasma lipids in Utah subjects, *Hypertension,* 1986; 8: 30–36.
91. **Brugnara, C., Corrocher, R., Foroni, L., Steinmayr, L., Bonfanti, F., and De Sandre, G.,** Lithium-sodium countertransport in erythrocytes of normal and hypertensive subjects. Relationship with age and plasma renin activity, *Hypertension,* 1983; 5: 529–534.
92. **Yap, L., Arrázola, A., Soria, F., and Diez, J.,** Is there increased cardiovascular risk in essential hypertensive patients with abnormal kinetics of red blood cell lithium-sodium countertransport system?, *J. Hypertension,* 1989; 7: 667–673.
93. **Nosadini, R., Semplicini, A., Fioretto, P. et al.,** Sodium-lithium countertransport and cardiorenal abnormalities in essential hypertension, *Hypertension,* 1991; 18: 191–198.
94. **Inoue, I., Matsuura, H., Shingu, T. et al.,** Role of intracellular cation abnormalities in development of left ventricular hypertrophy, *J. Cardiovasc. Pharmacol.,* 1991; 17(Suppl. 2): 107–109.
95. **Devereux, R. B. and Reichek, N.,** Echocardiographic determination of left ventricular mass in man. Anatomic validation of the method, *Circulation,* 1977; 55: 613–618.
96. **Savage, D. D., Garrison, R. J., Kannel, W. B. et al.** The spectrum of left ventricular hypertrophy in a general population sample: the Framingham study, *Circulation,* 1987; 75(Suppl. 1): 26–33.
97. **Devereux, R. B., Casale, P. N., Kligfield, P., Eisenberg, R. R., Miller, D., Campo, E., and Alonso, D. R.,** Performance of primary and derived M-mode echocardiographic measurements for detection of left ventricular hypertrophy in necropsied subjects and in patients with systemic hypertension, mitral regurgitation and dilated cardiomyopathy, *Am. J. Cardiol.,* 1986; 57: 1388–1393.
98. **De la Sierra, A., Coca, A., Aguilera, M. T., Ingelmo, M., and Urbano-Márquez, A.,** Clinical profiles and erythrocyte Na^+ transport abnormalities of four major types of primary hypertension in Spain, *Kidney Int.,* 1989; 36: 114–119.
99. **De la Sierra, A., Hannaert, P., Ollivier, J. P., Senn, N., and Garay, R. P.,** Kinetic study of the Ca^{2+} pump in erythrocytes from essential hypertensive patients, *J. Hypertension,* 1990; 8: 285–293.

Chapter 13

ABNORMALITIES OF ION TRANSPORT IN HYPERCHOLESTEROLEMIA AND HYPERTRIGLYCERIDEMIA: A LINK WITH ESSENTIAL HYPERTENSION?

Steven C. Hunt, Lily L. Wu, and Roger R. Williams

TABLE OF CONTENTS

I. Introduction 274

II. Association of Ion Transport With Lipids and Lipoproteins 274
- A. Cross-Sectional Studies 274
- B. Follow-Up Studies 279
- C. Intervention Studies 281
  - 1. Exercise Intervention 281
  - 2. Dietary Intervention 282
  - 3. Lipid-Lowering Intervention 283
- D. Genetic Studies 284

III. Possible Mechanisms Relating Ion Transport to Lipids and Hypertension 285
- A. Membrane Fluidity 285
  - 1. Association With Hypertension 285
  - 2. Association With Lipids 286
- B. Insulin Resistance 290

IV. Conclusions 292
- A. Is Ion Transport Linked to Hypertension or Blood Pressure? 292
- B. Are Lipids and Lipoproteins an Intermediate Link? 294

References 295

0-8493-5474-9/94/$0.00+$.50

I. INTRODUCTION

As the importance of sodium became appreciated for its possible involvement in blood pressure regulation and the development of hypertension, mechanisms of moving sodium and other associated ions in and out of cells were intensively studied. Na-K ouabain-sensitive transport was recognized as the major sodium transporter to maintain proper ionic gradients. Na-K cotransport was later recognized as another transport system that could either remove or increase cellular sodium content depending on the existing gradients that were present. Significant differences were found between hyper- and normotensive patients.[1,2] In 1980, the first report of a Na-Na transport system measured by using Li for Na-Li countertransport was published showing abnormalities of this system in hypertensive patients.[3] It was later suggested that this system may represent a Na-H antiport system known to be an important sodium transport mechanism that existed in the renal proximal tubules.[4,5]

These transport systems have been described in other chapters and this chapter focuses on the possible modification of the expression of these systems in patients with lipid or lipoprotein abnormalities. Evidence is weighed as to whether dyslipidemia may be an underlying cause of or an intermediate link between ion transport abnormalities and the development of hypertension. Insulin resistance resulting in hyperinsulinemia has been shown to be closely related to dyslipidemia[6] and hypertension[7] and may have important effects on ion transport.[8] Resistance to cellular membrane uptake of glucose may also be affected by cell membrane lipid or phospholipid content, which affects membrane fluidity and may alter the binding capacity or activity of ion transport proteins.

II. ASSOCIATION OF ION TRANSPORT WITH LIPIDS AND LIPOPROTEINS

A. CROSS-SECTIONAL STUDIES

After the first evidence that ion transport was associated with hypertension, investigations began to measure additional variables that could explain a mechanism for altered transport to cause hypertension. An early observation that Na-Li countertransport dramatically increased during pregnancy and only returned to normal levels 4 months postpartum suggested that the alterations in Na-Li countertransport during pregnancy were instigated during the formation of the erythrocyte which has an average 4-month life span.[9] Correlations of Na-Li countertransport with plasma cholesterol[10] suggested that cell membrane alterations may result from the large increase in lipid levels during pregnancy. Two interesting observations have come from studies on pregnancy. First, there was no difference in Na-Li countertransport between normotensive pregnant women and women who had hypertension develop during pregnancy.[9] Second, in spite of the significant increase in Na-Li countertransport level during pregnancy, the temperature dependence of Na-Li countertransport in pregnant women remained similar to normotensive women.[11] This suggests that lipids and other hormonal changes that occur during pregnancy may change the Na-Li countertransport level, but that the fluidity of the membrane (which is hypothesized to be associated with hypertension) does not change to resemble the membrane fluidity in hypertensive women.

A study of Na-Li countertransport in patients with hyperlipidemia showed positive correlations with total and free cholesterol, triglycerides, apolipoprotein A, acetylcholinesterase, and phospholipids.[12] Patients who had both hypertension and hyperlipidemia had Na-Li countertransport levels of 0.38 mmol/l red blood cells (RBC) per hour compared to hyperlipidemic patient levels of 0.28 and normolipidemic, normotensive patient levels of 0.19. The effects of hypertension on Na-Li countertransport appeared to be independent of and additive to the effects of hyperlipidemia. The authors noted that the largest correlation for Na-Li countertransport occurred with acetylcholinesterase ($r = 0.43$), which hydrolyzes acetylcholine to choline, and this in turn forms phosphatidylcholine, an important membrane component. See Table 1 for a list of other correlations from multiple studies.

In a large population study of high risk families, significant correlations of plasma cholesterol, triglyceride, and high-density lipoprotein (HDL) cholesterol were found for Na-Li countertransport, Li-K cotransport, and the passive lithium leak.[13] The correlations were similar within both hyper- and normotensive groups. In multivariate analysis, the difference between hyper- and normotensive patients remained after adjustment for these lipid correlations and weight, again suggesting the independence and additivity of lipids and hypertension to ion transport level. This study also found no relationship of blood pressure to ion transport after adjustment for weight, lipids, and hypertension status. Triglycerides had the strongest multivariate correlation of 0.28 for Na-Li countertransport, 0.22 for Li-K cotransport, and 0.23 for the Li leak. Body weight had its strongest correlation with Na-Li countertransport (0.22) and weaker correlations with Li-K cotransport (0.10) and the Li leak (0.11). These associations of ion transport with weight and lipids were not found in youths under age 18.

In a general population study, hypertensive and borderline hypertensive patients had increased triglyceride levels as compared to patients with normal blood pressures.[14] At most levels of triglyceride, hypertensive males had increased Na-Li countertransport levels compared to normotensive males. The relationship in females was not as consistent and appeared to be confined to triglyceride values below 250 mg/dl. The authors also suggested that the mean unadjusted Na-Li countertransport value in hypertensives is higher than in normotensives because the factors that cause increases in Na-Li countertransport are more prevalent in the hypertensive group, not because there is a clearly definable cutpoint for high Na-Li countertransport values.

A study in a general male population from Paris[15] measured lipids and five ionic parameters: erythrocytic Na and K passive permeability, Na-K cotransport, Na-Li countertransport, and Na,K-ATPase pump activity. Total cholesterol was not associated with any of the five ion measurements. The only associations found were for triglycerides with Na-K cotransport and Na passive permeability, and HDL

TABLE 1
Na-Li Countertransport Correlations from Multiple Studies

Study	Cholesterol	HDL-C	TG	VLDL-C	BMI	Insulin	DBP
Corrocher et al.[12]	0.38[a]	0.07	0.30[b]	0.28[b,d]	[e]	—	—
Hunt et al.[13]	0.08[b]	−0.19[c]	0.35[c]	—	0.28[c]	—	0.19[c,f]
Hunt et al.[23]	0.09[b]	−0.11	0.32[c]	—	0.24[c]	—	—
Hunt et al.,[20] Williams et al.[21]	—	—	—	0.26[a]	0.38[c]	0.24[a]	—
Turner and Michels[14]	—	[b]	[b,g]	—	[b]	—	—
Hajem et al.[15]	NS[h]	NS	NS	—	NS	—	NS
Laurenzi and Trevisan[16] (Males)	0.16[c]	−0.08[a]	—	—	0.19[c]	—	—
Laurenzi and Trevisan[16] (Females)	0.13[c]	−0.12[c]	—	—	0.23[c]	—	—
Carr et al.[18]	0.33[a]	−0.44[c]	0.55[c]	0.56[c]	—	—	0.38[c]
Bunker et al.[22]	0.17[b]	−0.34[c]	—	0.44[c]	—	0.37[e]	0.26[c]
Adranga et al.[26]	NS	—	0.30[b]	—	NS	—	0.25[b]
Hespel et al.[27]	0.10	−0.41[b,i]	0.44[b]	—	—	—	—
McDonald et al.[28]	−0.01	—	0.01	—	0.08	—	0.31
McDonald et al.[29]	[b]	—	[c]	—	0.05	—	—

Abbreviations: TG, triglycerides; BMI, body mass index; DBP, diastolic blood pressure.

[a] $p < 0.01$.
[b] $p < 0.05$.
[c] $p < 0.001$.
[d] Pre-beta lipoprotein.
[e] Not reported.
[f] Mean blood pressure rather than diastolic blood pressure.
[g] Interaction of triglycerides between hypertensive, borderline, and normotensive blood pressure groups.
[h] Not significant.
[i] HLD_2 subfraction; HDL_3 was not significant similar to what was found in Reference 13.

cholesterol inversely with Na-K cotransport. Adjustment for body mass index, age, and alcohol intake removed the HDL cholesterol significance, but did not affect the triglyceride significance.

In the Gubbio population study,[16,17] blood pressure was significantly related to Na-Li countertransport until adjustment for other variables, such as body mass index, uric acid, and total cholesterol. Univariate correlations of Na-Li countertransport with lipids are given in Table 1. Although triglycerides were not measured, the correlation of Na-Li countertransport with non-HDL cholesterol was 0.18 and 0.17 for males and females (both $p < 0.001$).

Similar to the study of Corrocher et al., Carr et al. studied Na-Li countertransport in both hyperlipidemic and hypertensive patients.[18] The normolipidemic hypertensive patients had Na-Li countertransport levels very similar to hyperlipidemic normotensive patients (0.32 and 0.34 mmol/l RBC per hour, respectively), while those with both hyperlipidemia and hypertension had much higher levels (0.48 mmol/l RBC per hour). Compared to the normotensive, normolipidemic group, these three groups had significantly elevated Na-Li countertransport. Hypertensive patients as a group had elevated total cholesterol, low-density lipoprotein (LDL) cholesterol, very low-density lipoprotein (VLDL) cholesterol, triglycerides, and decreased HDL cholesterol. Almost 50% of the family members of the hypertensive, dyslipidemic probands had increased Na-Li countertransport. These relatives had significantly different lipid levels than normolipidemic controls, while the family members who did not have elevated Na-Li countertransport had lipid levels similar to the normolipidemic controls. However, hyperlipidemia and hypertension appeared to have independent and additive effects on Na-Li countertransport.

The familial concordance of dyslipidemia resembled familial combined hyperlipidemia, which is a condition of elevated triglycerides and/or LDL cholesterol, usually accompanied by low HDL cholesterol, in multiple family members. This study also suggested that Na-Li countertransport correlations with blood pressure or dyslipidemia came from combining groups with different Na-Li countertransport levels rather than quantitative linear relationships within groups. While studies have suggested the lack of a quantitative relationship of Na-Li countertransport with blood pressure because of the large overlap in values between hyper- and normotensive patients,[13,14,19] the study by Hunt et al.[13] clearly showed significant lipid correlations with Na-Li countertransport within groups, especially for triglyceride levels.

In a study to characterize the associations of ion transport with two common familial dyslipidemic syndromes, 131 hypertensive siblings from 58 different families were studied.[20,21] Lipids, lipoproteins, fasting insulin, and ion transport systems were measured. Hypertensive sibships were classified into four groups: (1) sibships with familial combined hyperlipidemia (FCHL, the presence of elevated triglyceride and/or LDL cholesterol levels (≥90th percentile) in two or more siblings with both abnormalities being present in the sibship), (2) sibships with hypertriglyceridemia and decreased HDL cholesterol in the absence of elevated LDL cholesterol (non-FCHL), (3) hypertensive siblings with normal lipids, and (4) normotensive spouses.

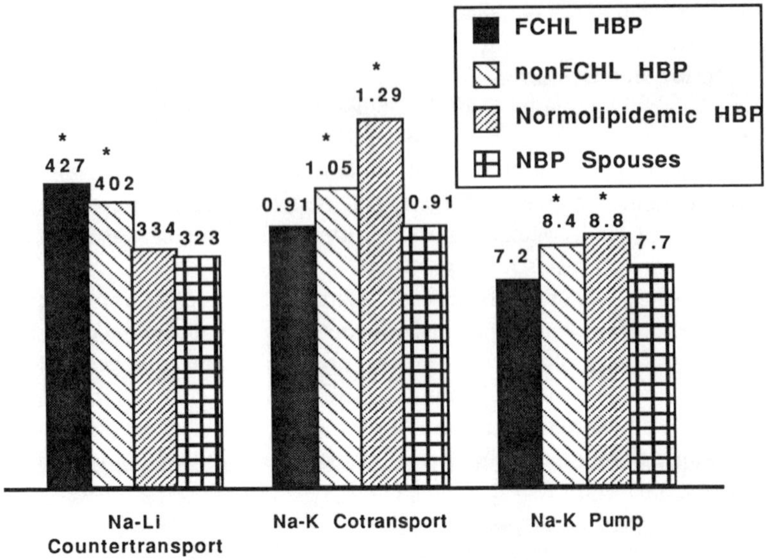

FIGURE 1. Comparison of ion transport means among four groups: hypertensive (HBP) patients with familial combined hyperlipidemia (FCHL), hypertensive patients with dyslipidemia not fitting the definition of FCHL (nonFCHL), normolipidemic hypertensive patients, and normotensive (NBP) spouses of the hypertensive patients. * Represents a significant difference compared to the normotensive spouses. Values for Na-Li countertransport are in μmol/l RBC/h; Na-K cotransport (furosemide-sensitive Na efflux) and Na-K pump V_{max} values (ouabain-sensitive Na efflux) are in mmol/l RBC/h.

The FCHL group had the highest Na-Li countertransport levels, followed by the dyslipidemic group without FCHL, the normolipidemic hypertensives, and the normotensive spouses (0.43, 0.40, 0.33, and 0.32 mmol/l RBC per hour, respectively) (Figure 1).

In this study, the hypertensive but normolipidemic patients had similar Na-Li countertransport levels to the normotensive spouses regardless of the variables used to adjust the data, including age, gender, body mass index, VLDL cholesterol, or fasting insulin levels. Na-Li countertransport levels in the FCHL group were most closely related to VLDL cholesterol and fasting insulin. Even after adjusting for obesity, fasting insulin levels and Na-Li countertransport were significantly higher in the FCHL group than the other groups, suggesting an insulin-resistant effect may elevate Na-Li countertransport independently of obesity. In the non-FCHL group (which had greater central obesity than the FCHL group) Na-Li countertransport correlated most strongly with body mass index and VLDL cholesterol. Adjustment for body mass index removed the significant insulin association in this group, suggesting that obesity-related insulin resistance may play an important role in elevating both Na-Li countertransport and the VLDL cholesterol. Therefore, although dyslipidemia and hyperinsulinemia were present in both FCHL and non-FCHL groups, they seem to have different reasons for the underlying insulin resistance: an obesity-independent mechanism in FCHL and an obesity-related mechanism in the non-FCHL group.

The correlation of Na-Li countertransport with fasting insulin and glucose across all groups was 0.24 and 0.21, respectively (both $p < 0.01$). Fasting plasma insulin also correlated with Na-K cotransport (0.19, $p < 0.05$) but not with the V_{max} for ouabain-sensitive Na efflux by way of the Na,K-ATPase pump (−0.11). In spite of these correlations, Na-K cotransport and ouabain-sensitive Na efflux were not elevated in the FCHL group, but were elevated in the non-FCHL and normal lipid hypertensive groups. Therefore, these two transport systems do not seem to be as strongly related to familial lipid abnormalities as Na-Li countertransport.

In summary, triglyceride levels seem to be consistently associated with ion transport even after adjustment for other variables. HDL cholesterol, which is often found to be reduced when triglycerides are elevated, has weaker correlations and may represent secondary effects of the elevated triglycerides. Total cholesterol or LDL cholesterol nearly always have weaker or nonsignificant correlations with ion transport. Na-Li countertransport appears to be related to both familial and non-familial lipid abnormalities and to two different types of insulin resistance, suggesting heterogeneity of this transport system.

B. FOLLOW-UP STUDIES

Follow-up studies provide the means to test whether abnormalities in ion transport precede the development of hypertension. Na-Li countertransport measured after a 2-year follow-up correlated with baseline Na-Li countertransport at 0.9 in one study[22] and 0.7 in another,[23] indicating that repeat measurements are fairly stable over time, but that environmental and experimental variation does exist. Coefficients of variation are usually in the 7 to 15% range in most studies. In the first study,[22] a 2 to 3 year follow-up of premenopausal women showed higher baseline Na-Li countertransport in those with elevated baseline triglycerides, fasting insulin, or diastolic blood pressure. The increase in fasting and 2-h insulin levels after 2 to 3 years was greater for those with the highest baseline Na-Li countertransport values, even after adjusting for change in body mass index. Systolic blood pressure increased more in those with the highest Na-Li countertransport values (5.6 mmHg) as compared to those with the lowest values (−2.2 mmHg). Change in Na-Li countertransport in a subset of the women correlated with changes in 2-h insulin and body mass index, but not with blood pressure. This suggests that Na-Li countertransport is responsive to changes in obesity, lipid, and insulin-related variables. Because blood pressure increased in those with the highest baseline Na-Li countertransport values but change in blood pressure did not correlate with change in Na-Li countertransport, the association of high Na-Li countertransport with those probably destined to become hypertensive is confirmed. A general association across all levels of blood pressure is not found, however. Only a particular subgroup of a more general population group appears to have a direct Na-Li countertransport and hypertension relationship.

In the second study with an average of 2.50 years of follow-up,[23] Na-Li countertransport increased about 0.02 mmol/l RBC per hour, $p < 0.0001$. During this time total cholesterol decreased, triglycerides increased, HDL cholesterol decreased, body mass index increased, and blood pressure increased. When these changes were correlated with each other, after adjustment for baseline values of these variables in addition to age, gender, and length of follow-up time, there were significant correlations between change in Na-Li countertransport and changes in total cholesterol (0.19), triglycerides (0.23), HDL cholesterol (0.07), body mass index (0.21), but not with systolic (−0.02) or diastolic (−0.01) blood pressure. The changes in lipids did correlate with changes in blood pressure, indicating a direct relationship between lipids and blood pressure and between lipids and Na-Li countertransport, but no direct correlation between blood pressure change and Na-Li countertransport change. The cross-sectional correlations for each of the two visits were very reproducible with the correlations for triglycerides and Na-Li countertransport of 0.34 and 0.32 for the first and second measurements, respectively.

The cross-sectional correlation of Na-Li countertransport with total cholesterol was significant only at the second visit of the families to the Cardiovascular Genetics Clinic. While the previous publication of data from the first visit showed a mild correlation using both hyper- and normotensive patients (0.08), it was reduced to 0.05 (not significant) when only analyzing the normotensives.[13] In the follow-up study, the change in Na-Li countertransport correlated with total cholesterol at 0.19, but was reduced when adjusted for body mass index changes to 0.10. For HDL cholesterol, the cross-sectional data showed inverse correlations with Na-Li countertransport, but the longitudinal data showed an increase in HDL cholesterol correlated with an increase in Na-Li countertransport, and this correlation was very weak at 0.08. This suggests that neither total cholesterol or HDL cholesterol were closely associated with Na-Li countertransport determination. Triglycerides, on the other hand, were consistently associated with Na-Li countertransport in the cross-sectional and prospective studies at much higher correlations (0.2 to 0.4) and were independent of body mass index levels or changes.

Finally, in a 7-year longitudinal study of 1458 adults from 98 pedigrees, the prospective development of hypertension was studied and related to baseline Na-Li countertransport[24] and other ion transport systems and cellular cation concentrations.[25] Baseline Na-Li countertransport did not predict the development of reported hypertension after 7 years of follow-up, with risk ratios of 1.02 before adjustment and 0.90 after adjustment for baseline age, diastolic blood pressure, body mass index, plasma triglycerides, HDL cholesterol, plasma glucose, and family history of hypertension. A relationship could not be found in any subgroup which might have been at higher risk, including a positive family history of hypertension or membership in a stroke or hypertension ascertained pedigree. However, as discussed in the section on the genetics of ion transport, the subgroup affected by genetic alterations in a particular transport system may be small enough that the effect may be masked when analyzing a larger subgroup where many patients will have hypertension due to other causes. No prospective relationship was found for Na-K cotransport [relative risks for a one standard deviation difference in means (RR) of 0.89], ouabain-sensitive Na efflux (RR = 1.05 for V_{max} or 0.83 for the rate constant), or altered plasma or intracellular levels of sodium, potassium, or magnesium (RR = 0.93 to 1.15). The passive lithium leak was significantly related to development of hypertension in a univariate model (RR = 1.26, p = 0.05) but was no longer significant after adjustment for baseline variables. Actual blood pressure measurement in this cohort after 10 years of follow-up is currently underway and will help determine if study deficiencies in the previous analysis may have masked a prospective relationship or whether the lack of a relationship is confirmed. Preliminary results using a very small sample size suggested that Na-Li countertransport genotype (rather than phenotype) may better define the subgroup at risk and be prospectively related to the development of hypertension, but this weak result will need confirmation using a much longer follow-up period to obtain a large number of individuals with the high Na-Li countertransport genotype who develop hypertension.

C. INTERVENTION STUDIES

1. Exercise Intervention

There have been a number of intervention studies to determine acute effects on ion transport, mostly on Na-Li countertransport, and whether changes in Na-Li countertransport parallel changes in blood pressure, lipids, and weight. Adragna et al.[26] employed an exercise intervention on males for 12 weeks. At baseline a significant correlation existed between Na-Li countertransport and triglycerides (0.30) of the same magnitude found in other studies (Table 1), but no correlation with total cholesterol. After 3 months of exercise, HDL cholesterol increased, weight, and heart rate decreased. Na-Li countertransport was significantly decreased by 0.05 mmol/l RBC per hour (15%) as compared to a nonsignificant increase in the controls of 0.02. The authors did not present the correlation of Na-Li countertransport and HDL cholesterol changes in this study, but did note that the Na-Li countertransport change occurred in the absence of a blood pressure change and did not correlate with total cholesterol change. None of the other ion transport measures changed, including measures of Na-K cotransport and Na-K pump activity.

In a 4-month exercise study on 27 men,[27] significant changes in Na-Li countertransport were again found, with reductions of 0.054 mmol/l RBC per hour (12%). Intracellular Na and weight also decreased while Na-K cotransport significantly increased by 13%. Although they found significant correlations of Na-Li countertransport with triglycerides (0.44) and HDL_2 cholesterol (−0.41) at baseline, the change in triglycerides or HDL_2 did not correlate with the change in Na-Li countertransport. Baseline triglycerides and phospholipids correlated with ouabain-sensitive Rb uptake and Na-K cotransport, but again, changes did not correlate with changes in ion transport.

The consistency between these two exercise studies in the amount of change in Na-Li countertransport after 4 months of exercise and the baseline correlations with lipids is remarkable. However, the absence of a correlation between changes in ion transport and lipids in these 4-month intervention studies contrast with the correlation found in the longitudinal study of 2.50 years without intervention. Exercise had its greatest effect on HDL_2 cholesterol with a 32% increase after only

2 months. Na-Li countertransport also had significantly decreased at the 2-month mark, while triglycerides and LDL cholesterol actually increased somewhat. Na-Li countertransport remained nearly constant in the following 2 months, while HDL_2 cholesterol increased slightly and LDL cholesterol decreased to baseline levels. Thus, it appears the exercise effect on Na-Li countertransport is a very acute effect that occurs in the first 2 months of exercise. It may be that exercise influences other parameters, such as hormone levels, that may affect Na-Li countertransport and prevent a simple correlation for change from being found.

In light of the fact that Na-Li countertransport only returned to normal in pregnant women 4 months postpartum, it may seem surprising that 2 months of exercise would be associated with the largest Na-Li countertransport change, with little further change. One half of the red cells would have turned over at this point, and the change in Na-Li countertransport would be expected to continue for the next 2 months unless the turnover was accelerated by the exercise. However, as Hespel et al.[27] point out, a large number of newly formed red cells would not be expected to have reduced Na content as was found, but should have increased K content, which was not found.

Other studies have found that other interventions may also cause short-term changes in Na-Li countertransport. A positive correlation between Na-Li countertransport and systolic blood pressure during a graded exercise tolerance test was found.[28] Both the maximum ($r = 0.56$) and the change ($r = 0.52$) in systolic blood pressure were significantly correlated with Na-Li countertransport. In this study of 22 men with borderline diastolic blood pressure there were no baseline correlations of Na-Li countertransport with triglycerides or total cholesterol. Therefore, the inconsistent results between shorter intervention studies and longer follow-up studies cannot be explained. Not enough is known about the mechanisms that alter ion transport and how the effects of altered transport are responded to physiologically. However, given the number of inconsistencies, one might hypothesize that the previously described relations of ion transport, weight, lipids, and blood pressure do exist, but have so many other control mechanisms that may be affected by different interventions that sometimes they are obscured or appear different depending on the intervention.

2. Dietary Intervention

In a 4-year nutrition intervention study by the same authors,[29] intervention using weight loss, sodium restriction, and reduction of alcohol intake showed significant correlations of Na-Li countertransport (measured during year 4) with 4-year weight gain and increase in body mass index. There were significant differences in Na-Li countertransport between those who were able to remain off medications over the 4 years with intervention (0.29 mmol/l RBC per hour) vs. those who were required to resume medications for hypertension (0.38 mmol/l RBC per hour). Higher Na-Li countertransport levels were associated with more severe hypertension which could not be controlled by the three interventions used in this study. Baseline serum triglycerides were significantly associated with Na-Li countertransport and the difference in Na-Li countertransport between those on and off medication, while total cholesterol was only associated with Na-Li countertransport in the overweight individuals.

A 3-week dietary intervention study of the effects of olive oil on ion transport and both serum and membrane lipids was performed on 11 normotensive males.[30] At the end of 3 weeks, triglycerides decreased from 84 to 62 mg/dl, $p < 0.005$, and total cholesterol decreased from 225 to 203 mg/dl, $p < 0.01$. HDL cholesterol, body weight, and blood pressure did not change. At the same time, erythrocyte membrane-saturated fatty acids significantly decreased and the cholesterol to phospholipid molar ratio increased. Na-K cotransport increased, with furosemide-sensitive Na efflux increasing from 0.53 to 0.91 mmol/l RBC per hour and a similar increase in K efflux. Na-Li countertransport decreased slightly but nonsignificantly. Therefore, dietary oleic acid, the primary monounsaturated fatty acid, is related to both cellular membrane changes, lipid level reductions, and alterations in ion transport.

3. Lipid-Lowering Intervention

Another intervention to test if changes in lipid levels are closely correlated with Na-Li countertransport changes is to reduce lipid levels by lipid-lowering medication. To study this, Carr et al.[31] measured lipids and Na-Li countertransport in seven patients with elevated cholesterol levels but normal triglycerides and nine patients with both elevated total cholesterol and triglyceride levels (combined hyperlipidemia) before and after diet or medication intervention. At baseline Na-Li countertransport was elevated only in the combined hyperlipidemia group as compared to normolipidemic controls. Diet ($N = 2$) or medication ($N = 7$) significantly reduced cholesterol and triglycerides in this group, with a reduction of Na-Li countertransport to normal levels. Na-Li countertransport was not reduced in the hypercholesterolemic group who had nonsignificant decreases in cholesterol and whose already low triglyceride levels remained constant. It is not known whether the lack of a Na-Li countertransport decrease in the hypercholesterolemic group may be attributable to the small cholesterol decrease induced by the intervention. The correlation between change in triglyceride levels and Na-Li countertransport levels for all 16 patients was $r = 0.64$, $p < 0.01$. Although there was also a significant correlation with change in cholesterol, it was only of borderline significance after adjusting for change in triglycerides ($p < 0.10$).

In a similar study, Weder et al.[32] used lovastatin to reduce cholesterol in patients with elevated cholesterol, but normal triglycerides. After 24 weeks in the double-blind, randomized trial, total cholesterol and LDL cholesterol were significantly decreased and HDL cholesterol was increased. Triglycerides were somewhat reduced ($p = 0.10$). However, there were no significant changes in Na-Li countertransport, Na-K cotransport, passive Li efflux, or cellular water content. Na content was reduced as was amiloride-sensitive platelet volume response to cellular acidification. This study tends to support the notion that changes in cholesterol are only mildly, if at all, related to changes in Na-Li countertransport. The change in triglycerides seems to be the most important controlling factor, and triglycerides were only somewhat reduced in this study.

D. GENETIC STUDIES

Initial analyses of Na-Li countertransport showed that there was a significant polygenic component of about 70% contributing to the variance of this measurement.[33] When subsequent analyses modeled a major gene effect in addition to a polygenic effect, a significant proportion of variance (34 to 53%) could be explained by the presence of a major gene that seemed to act in an autosomal recessive manner.[34-36] Three studies had similar results, further substantiating the bimodality of the Na-Li countertransport distribution suggested by epidemiological studies and suggesting that the subset of individuals homozygous for the underlying gene were at increased risk of hypertension.

Turner et al.[37] estimated that 3% of the variability in systolic blood pressure could be explained by Na-Li countertransport, half of which could be attributed to a major gene.[34] Motulsky et al.[35] found estimates of between 2.6 and 4.7% for systolic blood pressure. Estimates were smaller for diastolic blood pressure. The prevalence of the high Na-Li countertransport genotype was 6%. In the study of Hasstedt et al.,[36] 1 and 0.5% of the systolic and diastolic variance could be explained by Na-Li countertransport. The low percent of blood pressure variability explained by the major gene is partly a result of the low prevalence of the affected genotype (5%). However, the prevalence of hypertension in the high Na-Li countertransport genotype was double that found in the other two genotypes. The mean Na-Li countertransport separation between genotypes was consistent for all age groups and the gene for high Na-Li countertransport could be detected even in youths aged 5 to 9 years. Also, the mean values of triglycerides and weight were elevated in those with the high Na-Li countertransport genotype. In this cross-sectional study, higher body weight and triglyceride levels began to be apparent in the high Na-Li countertransport group beginning at age 10. Triglyceride, and to some extent, weight differences became progressively greater for the high Na-Li countertransport genotype in the older age groups.

While the initial study by Hasstedt et al. indicated some genetic heterogeneity because the major gene model did not fit all three type pedigrees ascertained by different criteria, subsequent analyses of Na-Li countertransport from either a repeat visit of the family cohort or of the original data, excluding a particular subset of pedigrees, showed that the major gene model fit all three groups of pedigrees and provided similar estimates to those found for the coronary heart disease (CHD) ascertained families.[109] Boerwinkle et al.[34] have also shown evidence for genetic heterogeneity, since the tau 2 transmission probability parameter was significantly different from that expected for a Mendelian trait. However, subsequent analysis of their data[38] showed not only a gender-specific effect on mean Na-Li countertransport levels within genotype, but also a proportion of pedigrees that had elevations of Na-Li countertransport without evidence for a single major gene. Therefore, only a portion of families with high Na-Li countertransport in a population will show segregation of Na-Li countertransport due to a major gene, and even these pedigrees may have specific gender and other covariate effects on Na-Li countertransport. An earlier study showed gender-specific heterogeneity, in that the relationship of plasma triglyceride levels with Na-Li countertransport was nonlinear and differed between males and females.[14] Hypertensive males had very high levels of Na-Li countertransport at high triglyceride concentrations, while hypertensive females had levels that were lower than the normotensive females when triglycerides were above 250 mg/dl. These nonlinear and gender-specific relationships will need to be included in the genetic models as they are identified to help better identify specific gene-environment associations and interactions. These more accurate models will increase the power of linkage analyses necessary to locate the responsible Na-Li countertransport gene.

Other ion transport systems have shown evidence for some genetic determination. A major gene has been intimated for intraerythrocytic sodium level[39] and the number of ouabain binding sites on the erythrocyte membrane.[40] However, neither of these variables seem to be closely associated with lipids or lipoproteins. Lipids can affect Na-K ATPase pump activity,[41,42] but this variable has the lowest estimate of genetic variability of any of the transport-related measurements.[43] While this does not rule out the presence of a single gene having an effect in a subset of the population, evidence has not been found for a single gene.

Total polygenic heritability for Li-K cotransport was 30% with no common environmental effect.[43] This transport system has significant bimodality, but does not fit a Mendelian transmission model.[110] Cusi et al.[44] have suggested a different pattern of inheritance in hypertensive vs. normotensive families for Na-K cotransport indicative of an underlying major gene. Even though cotransport seems to be associated with plasma triglyceride levels, the lack of a definitive major gene model has so far prevented examining the association between genotype and lipid concentrations.

III. POSSIBLE MECHANISMS RELATING ION TRANSPORT TO LIPIDS AND HYPERTENSION

A. MEMBRANE FLUIDITY

1. Association With Hypertension

Hypertension incidence increases with age, at least up to around age 60. In a study to assess cell membrane changes with age in patients with hypertension, electron spin resonance was used to measure membrane fluidity.[45] Intracellular calcium has important effects on reducing membrane fluidity.[46] Membrane fluidity decreased after calcium loading with ionophore A23187 and this decrease was greater in hypertensive than normotensive patients.[45] The change in fluidity was blocked by calcium antagonists.[47] This change was also correlated with age in the hypertensive patients, but not in the normotensive patients.[45] Because the normo- and hypertensive patients were approximately the same age, this finding may suggest age-related changes in membrane structure in persons being hypertensive, while those who remain normotensive experience little change. Another explanation suggested that a greater proportion of hypertensive patients had low renin hypertension. In these patients greater fluidity changes occur after calcium loading than in normal renin patients. Low renin has been associated with low Na-K cotransport in hypertension, while patients with elevated Na-Li countertransport had high renin levels.[48] Intracellular calcium levels also play an important role in renin release from the juxtaglomerular cells in the kidney. With increased calcium, renin release is reduced[49] and would present a low renin profile connected to decreased fluidity.

Fluidity has also been shown to be dependent on salt intake levels.[50] Low salt intake is associated with increased fluidity, while high salt intake slightly decreases fluidity compared to normal salt intake. Low-salt diets have the greatest blood pressure-reducing effects on individuals with decreased renin,[51] and perhaps change in membrane fluidity plays some role in the blood pressure change. As with ion transport systems, membrane fluidity in patients with secondary hypertension was not different from normotensive patients.[52] This was also confirmed by the study of Levy et al.,[11] in which the temperature-dependent breakpoint for Na-Li countertransport for secondary hypertensive patients was similar to the hypertensive patients.

Postnov et al.[53] have shown that in hypertension reduced calcium binding occurs in the inner surface of the erythrocyte, and suggested that this membrane defect was related to abnormalities in univalent cation transport. Decreased calmodulin-associated calcium efflux was noted in those patients with the calcium-binding defect in the absence of calmodulin content differences.[54] Acid phospholipids and unsaturated fatty acids decrease the sensitivity of calcium ATPase to calmodulin.[55] As previously mentioned, Levy et al.[11] have shown evidence for differences in membrane fluidity of hyper- and normotensive patients, and that this altered fluidity was associated with increased Na-Li countertransport. Studies in the spontaneously hypertensive rat (SHR) suggest that membrane abnormalities occur before the development of hypertension.[56] In humans, elevated levels of Na-Li countertransport and detection of the high Na-Li countertransport genotype could be inferred at young ages.[36]

Membrane fluidity is also decreased in insulin-dependent diabetes.[57] This decrease was associated with decreased Na,K-ATPase activity ($r = 0.83$) and an increase in acetylcholinesterase activity ($r = 0.70$). Other transport systems were not measured in this study, but we have previously mentioned the high correlation of acetylcholinesterase activity with Na-Li countertransport.[12] The possible involvement of acetylcholinesterase activity is described in the next section. Na-Li countertransport is altered in insulin-dependent diabetes and may help predict development of nephropathy.[58]

2. Association With Lipids

Although the previous section provided evidence that changes appear in membrane fluidity between essential hyper- and normotensive patients, the causes of fluidity change were not discussed. Altered plasma lipids, phospholipids, or lipoproteins may be the likely explanations. While an early report showed no difference in overall lipid composition of cells from hypertensive patients,[59] subsequent reports give an indication as to why no difference was found. When comparing rates of membrane incorporation of phosphatidylinositol species, no difference between hypertensive and control patients was found. However, there was a higher rate of phosphoinositide turnover in the cell membrane in normotensive individuals with a positive family history of hypertension as compared to matched controls.[60] The authors suggested that a defect exists before onset of hypertension which is lost or masked as compensation occurs for an existing hypertensive state. Another alternative is that amounts of specific phospholipid species may vary even though total amounts do not differ.

A study by Engelmann et al.[61] clearly showed differential effects of different species of phospholipids on Na-Li countertransport and Na-K cotransport. Phosphatidylcholine 16:0/18:1 had no effect on Na-Li countertransport but increased Na-K cotransport, while 16:0/18:2 decreased Na-K cotransport. Phosphatidylcholine 16:0/22:6 and di-16:0 increased both Na-Li countertransport and Na-K cotransport, although the increase in Na-Li countertransport lasted only until the phosphatidylcholine migrated from the outer to inner membrane leaflet. Marche et al.[62] have shown similar amounts of phosphoinositol in hyper- and normotensive patients, but greatly increased turnover rates. Furthermore, the turnover rates were not associated with increased blood pressure. Corrocher et al.[63] found an inverse correlation of Na-Li countertransport and polyunsaturated fatty acids and positive correlations with the oleic to linoleic acid ratio and monounsaturated to polyunsaturated fatty acid ratio. Significant differences took place in the membrane composition between normotensive hyperlipidemic and normolipidemic subjects. The lack of a correlation between the cholesterol to phospholipid ratio and Na-Li countertransport, in spite of the specific phospholipid alterations, again suggests that specific unsaturated fatty acid or phospholipid components may influence Na-Li countertransport, while others, which still affect the total cholesterol to phospholipid ratio, have no relationship.

Wiley and Cooper[64] have shown that increasing the cholesterol to phospholipid ratio by adding cholesterol to the medium will reduce the Na-K cotransport rate. The phospholipid concentration was not changed. Levy et al.[65] found that Na-Li countertransport was not changed after enriching the erythrocyte membrane with cholesteryl hemisuccinate, but they did find reductions in lithium efflux. Another study[41] found increased membrane fluidity in the livers of dietary obese rats due to a decreased saturated to unsaturated fatty acid ratio. These changes were associated with decreased Na,K-ATPase activity. These experiments suggest that the positive correlations found for Li-K cotransport, passive lithium efflux, and Na-Li countertransport with cholesterol[13] do not arise from alterations in membrane content of cholesterol because a decrease in transport with higher cholesterol would be predicted. Although correlations of cholesterol with ion transport have usually been weak or nonexistent, increased lipolysis of triglycerides result in increased cholesterol remnants that may be taken up by the cell membrane.[66] If a lipid effect is found on membrane structure, it is probably through a direct triglyceride pathway because triglycerides have the highest correlation with ion transport, both cross-sectionally and longitudinally. Bloj and Zilversmit[67] have presented evidence that unsaturated phosphatidylcholine content of the cell membrane determines the transport rate of cholesterol into and out of the cell membrane. If membrane fatty acid content, represented by plasma triglyceride or VLDL levels, were the rate limiting step for cholesterol incorporation, it may explain why correlations are higher for triglycerides than cholesterol with ion transport. The rate of phospholipid formation increases as more triglycerides are transported into the liver.[68]

An important paper by Vakakis et al.[69] shows that in patients with hypertriglyceridemia, red cell membranes and LDL have lower than normal ratios of cholesterol to phospholipid. The LDL is smaller and more dense, with only 45% of the normal cholesterol mass. Increased triglycerides reduce the ratio, allowing cholesterol to be transferred from the cell to lipoproteins, increasing membrane fluidity and possibly ion transport. FCHL is a clinical disorder that involves abnormalities in both triglycerides and cholesterol in multiple family members.[70] Low HDL cholesterol is also usually present.[71] One of the most striking features of FCHL is the presence of small, dense LDL which has a high correlation with serum triglyceride concentration.[72,73] Evidence for the association of small, dense LDL with increased risk of coronary heart disease has been published along with evidence for involvement of a major gene determining these levels.[74,75] FCHL was the most common familial syndrome in a series of siblings with onset of CHD before age 55.[71] It was also the most common syndrome in a study of hypertensive sib pairs with FCHL or dyslipidemia consisting of high triglycerides and low HDL cholesterol, which were found in about 15% of the sib pairs.[76] There was a striking coaggregation of hypertension and dyslipidemia. These sib pairs had small dense LDL, increased obesity, high fasting plasma insulin levels, and elevated Na-Li countertransport.[73] All of these characteristics would tend to provide conditions for a low cholesterol to phospholipid ratio, altered fluidity, and abnormal ion transport.

The clinical importance of this coaggregation is shown in a prospective study of twins, where CHD mortality rates were somewhat elevated for patients with either hypertension or dyslipidemia, but were dramatically elevated for patients with both hypertension and dyslipidemia.[77] The concordance of these two conditions seems to be very prevalent and could be directly related to an underlying abnormality which also alters ion transport. A recent abstract provided evidence for a familial trait involving increased insulin resistance and dyslipidemia in normotensive offspring of hypertensive parents as compared to offspring of normotensive parents and the familial abnormalities preceded the development of hypertension.[78] All of the above abnormalities of dyslipidemia, insulin resistance, and ion transport seem to be present before the onset of hypertension, suggesting that they may play an important role in the development of hypertension.

The lower cholesterol to phospholipid ratios found in hypertriglyceridemia contrast with higher ratios found in the LDL and normal ratios in RBC of familial hypercholesterolemia.[79,80] The high levels of serum cholesterol in these patients

TABLE 2
Comparison of Na-Li Countertransport Levels by Dyslipidemia Groups

Type of dyslipidemia	Age, gender, BMI adjusted Na-Li countertransport (mmol/l RBC/h)
Normolipidemic adults	
Normotensive (N = 487)	0.28
Hypertensive (N = 50)	0.34[a]
Familial hypercholesterolemia	
Normotensive (N = 29)	0.23[a]
Hypertensive (N = 2)	0.16[a]
Hyperapobetalipoproteinemia	
Normotensive (N = 4)	0.35
Familial combined hyperlipidemia	
Hypertensive (N = 17)	0.43[a]
Hypertriglyceridemia and hypoalphalipoproteinemia	
Hypertensive (N = 40)	0.37[a]

[a] Significantly different than normolipidemic normotensives, $p < 0.05$.

would increase cholesterol incorporation into the cell membrane, decrease fluidity, and decrease ion transport. Our own studies on familial hypercholesterolemia patients showed that they had lower Na-Li countertransport than all other normo- or hypertensive groups, with or without other forms of dyslipidemia (Table 2). This suggests two different mechanisms determining cholesterol to phospholipid ratios, one that increases the cholesterol content of the membrane through elevated serum cholesterol and one that reduces the ratio by way of increased triglycerides. Only the second pathway may be associated with hypertension because people with familial hypercholesterolemia do not tend to have increased incidence of hypertension. The incorporation or reduction of cholesterol may only have minimal effects on Na-Li countertransport, as suggested by Weder et al.,[31] while ratio changes due to changes in triglyceride levels may have greater Na-Li countertransport effects, as seen by Carr et al.[32]

A three-country dietary study showed significant plasma cholesterol and phospholipid differences as well as dietary-induced differences in erythrocyte phospholipid patterns.[81] The erythrocyte fatty acid composition was judged to be a better indicator of long-term dietary intake of fatty acids than plasma levels because the membrane amounts of fatty acids change slowly after abrupt dietary changes. Thus, constant exposure of erythrocyte, platelet, and presumably, smooth muscle cells to high levels of phospholipids and fatty acids would alter membrane composition and could easily affect transport activity. Lysophosphatidylcholine γ-stearoyl, a long-chain fatty acid, has been shown to inhibit Na,K-ATPase,[42] while dietary linoleic acid has been shown to alter membrane fluidity[82] and prevent the development of deoxycorticosterone acetate-salt hypertension in rats.[83] The prevention of hypertension in this study was supposedly due to decreased intracellular sodium and calcium concentration resulting from increased activity of the Na-K pump. As mentioned earlier, decreased calcium increases membrane fluidity.

Acetylcholinesterase (AchE) is an enzyme that converts acetylcholine to choline, which is used to form phosphatidylcholine. Correlations of acetylcholinesterase have been found for Na-Li countertransport[12] and Na,K-ATPase activity.[57] Its behavior is affected by changing dietary fat[84] or by changing the lipid content of the cell membrane.[85] If the membrane composition was changed so that a temperature breakpoint occurred in physiologic range, the activity would change in a nonlinear fashion on either side of that breakpoint. The correlation between acetylcholinesterase and membrane fluidity was -0.70.[57] Winegrad[86] has hypothesized that defects in Na,K-ATPase, acetylcholinesterase, and membrane fluidity in diabetes may arise from abnormal phospholipid metabolism. Because acetylcholinesterase had higher correlations with Na-Li countertransport than did triglycerides,[12] it may be that its activity is a more sensitive measure of the fluid state of the membrane.

B. INSULIN RESISTANCE

Insulin resistance and hyperinsulinemia have been recognized to be important in relating common metabolic and disease conditions, including CHD, noninsulin-dependent diabetes, obesity, dyslipidemia, and hypertension. At least three prospective studies have shown plasma insulin associated with CHD[87-89] and one with hypertension.[90] Kaplan[91] has described the relationship of insulin resistance, obesity, hypertension, and hypertriglyceridemia as "the deadly quartet", and suggested that prevention of obesity, especially upper body or central obesity, or the control of existing obesity, would reduce the incidence of the above disorders. Approximately 40% of hypertensives have lipid abnormalities and 46% of those with high cholesterol have hypertension, indicating a strong clustering of these disorders.[92] Hyperinsulinemia and insulin response has been strongly related in individuals who have multiple abnormalities in plasma VLDL, LDL, and HDL levels.[6] Insulin resistance has been shown to play an important role in hypertension, even in nonobese individuals.[7]

Increased insulin levels due to an underlying insulin resistance increase the synthesis and secretion of VLDL triglyceride by the liver resulting in the observed hypertriglyceridemia commonly seen in hypertension.[93] After weight loss, which increases the effectiveness of insulin, VLDL triglyceride secretion and plasma concentration decrease. In fructose-fed rats, blocking the production of insulin decreased the plasma triglyceride concentration and reduced blood pressure, indicating that the hypertension may be secondary to the insulin and/or lipid abnormalities.[94]

The underlying cause of insulin resistance is not yet known. It is not known whether lipid or lipoprotein abnormalities may themselves cause part of all of the insulin resistance in some individuals, especially those with primary genetic defects for abnormal lipids or lipoproteins. Free fatty acids are known to cause insulin resistance, suggesting that VLDL abnormalities may play a role in the development

TABLE 3
Correlations of Fasting Plasma Insulin Levels in 159 Hypertensive Individuals

Variable	Correlation
Na-Li countertransport	0.24
Na-K cotransport	0.19
Na-K ATPase pump rate constant	0.19
Plasma VLDL cholesterol	0.27
Body mass index	0.59

Note: All significant at $p < 0.05$.

From Williams, R. R., Hunt, S. C., Schumacher, M. C., et al., *Hypertension as an Insulin-Resistant Disorder. Genetic Factors and Cellular Mechanisms,* Elsevier, Amsterdam, 1991: 89-101.

of insulin resistance.[95] Resnick et al.[96] have proposed that intracellular cation imbalances may be responsible for the underlying insulin resistance, specifically, decreased cellular pH and Mg and increased Ca. If these ion concentrations were altered, compensatory mechanisms such as increased Na-H exchange, which increases the pH at the expense of possible further increases in intracellular Ca, may be activated. In addition, catecholamines, which reduce the effectiveness of insulin on glucose uptake, increase intracellular levels of calcium and may be synergistic with the above mechanisms.[97] Insulin can inhibit Ca-ATPase in erythrocytes which may further affect intracellular calcium and membrane fluidity.[98]

Insulin correlates with Na-Li countertransport, Na-K cotransport, and Na-K pump rate constant, as well as body mass index and plasma VLDL cholesterol (Table 3). In a another study, Na-Li countertransport also correlated with baseline fasting insulin and 2-h insulin.[22] Both baseline Na-Li countertransport and change in Na-Li countertransport over 2 to 4 years correlated with a change in 2-h insulin ($r = 0.35$ and 0.37, respectively). There are insulin receptors on the plasma membrane that cause stimulation of the Na-K pump and addition of insulin has been shown to stimulate the Na-K pump.[8] Moore has reviewed the mechanism of action of insulin on the Na-K pump and other transport systems and suggests that it may occur by way of changes in membrane fluidity. Any mechanisms by which insulin affects the membrane appear to be temperature dependent, because insulin inhibition of the Na-K pump disappears at 15°C, while ouabain continued to block the pump activity down to 1.5°C. Moore references two studies[99,100] to suggest that "insulin induces a localized lipid phase transition" and that "bilayer fluidity and glucose transport activity exhibit a parallel dependence on temperature". Therefore, at least four different variables, insulin, Na-K pump activity, Na-Li countertransport in hypertensive patients, and acetylcholinesterase activity seem to be temperature dependent and related to hypertension. Whether this is just a general phenomenon of membrane fluidity or whether a causal defect may relate these defects to hypertension will require further study.

Insulin has a number of other effects on transport including increasing the affinity for Na of the Na-K pump,[101] increasing reabsorption of Na in the kidney,[102] and increasing intracellular sodium[103] and pH.[104,105] The change in pH has been shown to be associated with insulin stimulation of Na-H exchange, as addition of amiloride blocks the insulin-stimulated pH change.[105] Insulin also decreases the affinity of calcium to bind with the cell membrane[106] and can inhibit the Ca-ATPase in fat cells[107] and erythrocytes.[98]

However, the above relationships are also not entirely consistent. A recent study of insulin and its effect on Na-Li countertransport in physiologic doses seems to conflict with the above experiments. Foyle and Drury[108] found that as insulin was added to the medium in doses ranging from 0 to 50 mU/l, Na-Li countertransport decreased rather than increased. If Na-Li countertransport is a mode of operation of the Na-H antiporter as some believe,[4] it would be expected to increase. It is not clear whether these results provide evidence that Na-Li countertransport is different *in vitro* than Na-H exchange or whether *in vivo* multiple effects of insulin on different transport systems produce secondary effects on Na-Li countertransport. It may also be that the inactivation of certain systems by the cellular washing process and use of an artificial medium needed to determine Na-Li countertransport alters ion concentrations that would react to the insulin in such a way as to increase Na-Li countertransport *in vivo*. Clearly, more research is needed into these areas before specific conclusions about the effects of insulin on Na-Li countertransport can be made.

IV. CONCLUSIONS

A. IS ION TRANSPORT LINKED TO HYPERTENSION OR BLOOD PRESSURE?

Many studies have not found significant quantitative associations of Na-Li countertransport with blood pressure itself, while finding significant results between normo- and hypertensive patients. These results would tend to indicate that as blood pressure progressively increases (associated with age or other factors) the activity of Na-Li countertransport is not altered. This should not be surprising because three genetic studies have shown that much of the variation of Na-Li countertransport in populations is determined by a major gene and other polygenes.[34-36] The proportion of variance explained by other environmental and measurement error effects may only be about 20%. Two other studies have shown that Na-Li countertransport remains fairly constant over time, as would be expected if it is mainly under genetic control,[22,23] although nongenetic factors certainly may significantly alter levels on an individual basis. These nongenetic influences on ion transport in the absence of related blood pressure changes strengthen the argument that ion transport may not directly affect blood pressure. More long-term studies will be needed to verify this.

The fairly consistent relationship of Na-Li countertransport with hypertension itself would seem contradictory to the above results. However, a number of possibilities could explain the results. Hypertension may be caused by some other independent abnormality which causes increased sodium retention, vascular volume or resistance, altered membrane fluidity, etc. As these abnormalities appear, ion transport mechanisms are activated to counteract these changes in order to maintain a more normal cellular environment. In other words, Na-Li countertransport may be a marker but not a cause of hypertension development.

After adjusting for the presence or absence of hypertension, no correlation of mean blood pressure with Na-Li countertransport, Li-K cotransport, or the Li leak was found.[13] Also no correlation was seen with blood pressure in the normotensive group after adjustment. This may imply that studies finding such a correlation with blood pressure in normotensive patients have either a greater number of individuals near the borderline blood pressure range where ion transport alterations associated with the primary cause(s) of the elevated blood pressure are beginning to be seen physiologically, or have a group of patients with increased prevalence of the primary cause of hypertension which is associated with Na-Li countertransport.

Alternatively, it is highly likely that ion transport defects account for only a proportion of hypertension; a direct relationship to blood pressure is found, but the varying results from study to study arise from the fact that different patient samples contain different proportions of individuals with the ion defect. From the genetic studies, it is estimated that only 5 to 6% of the population are homozygous for elevated Na-Li countertransport levels. In those studies with a high proportion of hypertension associated with ion transport defects, a correlation with blood pressure is seen. In those studies with a low proportion, the relationship is masked by a large proportion of individuals without an ion transport defect.

At least two of the genetic studies also suggest another interesting possibility.[34,36] Evidence was found for heterogeneity in the families studied because the transmission probabilities were not exactly at Mendelian expectations. Perhaps more than one gene may be involved which affects ion transport and which makes clearcut associations between ion transport and hypertension difficult. For example, two genes could be influencing ion transport, one for Na-K cotransport and one for Na-Li countertransport. The presence of one gene, such as for Na-K cotransport, may have significant impact on levels of Na-Li countertransport, even though the person does not have the gene for elevated Na-Li countertransport. Also, gene-gene interactions may be responsible for a certain amount of confounding, although the genes involved would have to be fairly common to have any impact on hypertension in the population.

Another alternative would be that two genes with major effects control the expression of a single ion transport system. One may envision a situation in which one gene controls the structure and activity of the actual transporter in the membrane independently of lipids, while another gene may control factors affecting ion transport activity by way of alterations in triglycerides, membrane fluidity and composition, altered intracellular ion content, insulin resistance, or obesity. This may be an explanation as to why the prospective study results showed no association of baseline ion transport with 7-year follow-up for hypertension.[24,25] The combination of a number of different causes of hypertension may make it so that no clearcut association with any one of them individually may be identified. It is indeed puzzling that a strong and consistent cross-sectional relationship of Na-Li countertransport with hypertension (but not blood pressure) was not verified by the prospective study. Longer follow-up time, using actual measured blood pressures rather than reported medication usage, and further understanding of the specifics of the ion transport mechanisms may be necessary to further resolve the conflicting results reported to date. However, one should not be discouraged by the conflicting evidence, because knowledge about ion transport continues to increase. Eventually, forthcoming molecular biology and biochemistry studies will help isolate the responsible genes and the transporters themselves.

B. ARE LIPIDS AND LIPOPROTEINS AN INTERMEDIATE LINK?

The literature reviewed in this chapter should make it clear that lipids and lipoproteins can have significant influence on ion transport. The research concerning the relationships between plasma and cellular membrane lipids, fatty acids, and phospholipids supports the hypothesis that plasma lipid concentrations influence membrane structure and function. What is not as clear is whether these functional changes are related to changes in ion transport and if they are, what is the mechanism? The research in this area, like that for the relationship of ion transport with blood pressure, is contradictory. The problem probably arises from the heterogeneity issue discussed above. Certain types of membrane components found in susceptible people may be related to ion transport, while others may be resistant to the same components. In some cases, dyslipidemia may have genetic origins that influence ion transport and blood pressure, while in other cases, abnormal metabolic effects from altered ion transport and concentration may raise lipid levels as a secondary phenomenon. Insulin resistance is known to elevate triglycerides, while increased triglyceride levels and free fatty acids increase insulin resistance. The key to unravel these circular pathways is to study homogeneous subsets of individuals and families. To do this may require the identification of new biochemical parameters to differentiate individuals with elevated ion transport levels into those with primary ion transport abnormalities and those with secondary abnormalities. Linkage to a genetic marker would greatly facilitate this process.

The epidemiologic studies discussed above on the common frequency of dyslipidemia and hypertension[70,73,74] suggest that ion transport, triglycerides, and hyperinsulinemia are closely associated with this syndrome. While it can be seen from previous discussions that the mechanism linking these three syndromes together is not completely understood, the evidence suggests that cellular membranes are involved. It may be that the structure of the membrane is altered or it may have different sensitivity to agonists, antagonists, intracellular ion concentration environment, or pH. The developing information about the role of insulin in hypertension, on ion transport, and on triglycerides provides an exciting possibility for further work in this area. As this work progresses, however, it should be remembered that even the insulin-resistance syndrome is not found in all hypertensive patients and is likely found in normotensive patients who will not ultimately develop hypertension. However, our own feeling is that understanding this syndrome will help us to ultimately more effectively treat and perhaps prevent hypertension in a sizable portion of those who have or are at risk of developing hypertension.

REFERENCES

1. **Garay, R. P. and Meyer, P.,** A new test showing abnormal net Na and K fluxes in erythrocytes of essential hypertensive patients, *Lancet,* 1, 349, 1979.
2. **Adragna, N. C., Canessa, M. L., Solomon, H., Slater, E., and Tosteson, D. C.,** Red cell sodium-lithium countertransport and sodium-potassium cotransport activity as a genetic marker in essential hypertension, *Br. Med. J.,* 284, 539, 1982.
3. **Canessa, M., Adragna, N., Solomon, H. S., Connolly, T. M., and Tosteson, D. C.,** Increased sodium-lithium countertransport in red cells of patients with essential hypertension, *N. Engl. J. Med.,* 302, 772, 1980.
4. **Canessa, M. L., Morgan, K., and Semplicini, A.,** Genetic differences in lithium-sodium exchange and regulation of the sodium-hydrogen exchanger in essential hypertension, *J. Cardiovasc. Pharmacol.,* 12, S92, 1988.
5. **Grinstein, S. and Rothstein, A.,** Mechanisms of regulation of the Na^+/H^+ exchanger, *J. Membr. Biol.,* 90, 1, 1986.
6. **Modan, M., Halkin, H., Lusky, A., Segal, P., Fuchs, Z., and Chetrit, A.,** Hyperinsulinemia is characterized by jointly disturbed plasma VLDL, LDL, and HDL levels, *Arteriosclerosis,* 8, 227, 1988.
7. **Ferrannini, E., Buzzigoli, G., Bonadonna, R., Giorico, M. A., Oleggini, M., Graziadei, L., Pedrinellia, R., Brandi, L., and Bevilacqua, S.,** Insulin resistance in essential hypertension, *N. Engl. J. Med.,* 317, 350, 1987.
8. **Moore, R. D.,** Effects of insulin upon ion transport, *Biochim. Biophys. Acta,* 737, 1, 1983.
9. **Worley, R. J., Hentschel, W. M., Cormier, C., Nutting, S., Pead, G., Zelenkov, K., Smith, J. B., Ash, K. O., Williams, R. R.,** Increased sodium-lithium countertransport in erythrocytes of pregnant women, *N. Engl. J. Med.,* 307, 412, 1982.
10. **Williams, R. R., Hunt, S. C., Dadone, M. M., Hasstedt, S., Smith, J. B., Ash, K. O., and Kuida, H.,** Preliminary analysis of sodium-lithium countertransport and blood pressure in Utah pedigrees, in *Topics in Pathophysiology of Hypertension,* Villarreal, H. and Sambhi, M. P., Eds., Martinus Nijhoff, Boston, 1984, 112.
11. **Levy, R., Paran, E., Keynan, A., and Livne, A.,** Essential hypertension: improved differentiation by the temperature dependence of Li efflux in erythrocytes, *Hypertension,* 5, 821, 1983.
12. **Corrocher, R., Steinmayr, M., Ruzzenente, O., Brugnara, C., Bertinato, L., Mazzi, M., Furri, C., Bonfanti, F., and De Sandr, G.,** Elevation of red cell sodium-lithium countertransport in hyperlipidemias, *Life Sci.,* 36, 649, 1985.
13. **Hunt, S. C., Williams, R. R., Smith, J. B., Ash, K. O.,** Associations of three erythrocyte cation transport systems with plasma lipids in Utah subjects, *Hypertension,* 8, 30, 1986.
14. **Turner, S. T. and Michels, V. V.,** Sodium-lithium countertransport and hypertension in Rochester, Minnesota, *Hypertension,* 18, 183, 1991.
15. **Hajem, S., Moreau, T., Hannaert, P., Lellouch, J., Orssaud, G., Huel, G., Claude, J. R., and Garay, R. P.,** Erythrocyte cation transport systems and plasma lipids in a general male population, *J. Hypertension,* 8, 891, 1990.
16. **Laurenzi, M. and Trevisan, M.,** Sodium-lithium countertransport and blood pressure: the Gubbio population study, *Hypertension,* 13, 408, 1989.
17. **Trevisan, M. and Laurenzi, M.,** Correlates of sodium-lithium countertransport: findings from the Gubbio epidemiological study, *Circulation,* 84, 2011, 1991.
18. **Carr, S. J., Thomas, T. H., Laker, M. F., and Wilkinson, R.,** Elevated sodium-lithium countertransport: a familial marker of hyperlipidaemia and hypertension?, *J. Hypertension,* 8, 139, 1990.
19. **Williams, R. R., Hunt, S. C., Kuida, H., Smith, J. B., and Ash, K. O.,** Sodium-lithium countertransport in erythrocytes of hypertension prone families in Utah, *Am. J. Epidemiol.,* 118, 338, 1983.

20. **Hunt, S. C., Wu, L. L., Hopkins, P. N., and Williams, R. R.,** Na-Li countertransport associations with plasma insulin and VLDL cholesterol in hypertensives with lipid abnormalities, *Hypertension,* 14, 356, 1989.
21. **Williams, R. R., Hunt, S. C., Schumacher, M. C., Hopkins, P. N., Wu, L. L., Barlow, G. K., Stults, B. M., Wilson, D. E., and Lalouel, J. M.,** Genes, hypertension and coronary heart disease: evidence for shared metabolic pathophysiology, in *Hypertension: An Insulin-Resistant Disorder. Genetic Factors and Cellular Mechanisms,* Smith et al., Eds., Elsevier, Amsterdam, 1991, 89.
22. **Bunker, C. H., Wing, R. R., Mallinger, A. G., Becker, D. J. et al.,** Cross-sectional and longitudinal relationship of sodium-lithium countertransport to insulin, obesity and blood pressure in healthy perimenopausal women, *J. Hum. Hypertension,* 5, 381, 1991.
23. **Hunt, S. C., Williams, R. R., and Ash, K. O.,** Changes in sodium-lithium countertransport correlate with changes in triglyceride levels and body mass index over 2 1/2 years of follow-up in Utah, *Cardiovasc. Drugs Ther.,* 4, 357, 1990.
24. **Hunt, S. C., Stephenson, S. H., Hopkins, P. N., Hasstedt, S. J., Williams, R. R.,** A prospective study of sodium-lithium countertransport and hypertension in Utah, *Hypertension,* 17, 1, 1991.
25. **Hunt, S. C., Stephenson, S. H., Hopkins, P. N., and Williams, R. R.,** Predictors of an increased risk of future hypertension in Utah pedigrees: a screening analysis, *Hypertension,* 17, 960, 1991.
26. **Adragna, N. C., Chang, J. L., Morey, M. C., and Williams, R. S.,** Effect of exercise on cation transport in human red cells, *Hypertension,* 7, 132, 1985.
27. **Hespel, P., Lijnen, P., Fagard, R. et al.,** Changes in erythrocyte sodium and plasma lipids associated with physical training, *J. Hypertension,* 6, 159, 1988.
28. **McDonald, A. M., Liao, Y., Trevisan, M., Dyer, A., Gosch, F. C., Stamler, R., and Stamler, J.,** Sodium-lithium countertransport and systolic blood pressure response to exercise, *J. Hypertension,* 8, 129, 1990.
29. **McDonald, A. M., Dyer, A. R., Liu, K., Stamler, R., Gosch, F. C., Grimm, R., Berman, R., and Stamler, J.,** Sodium, lithium-countertransport and blood pressure control by nutritional intervention in 'mild' hypertension, *J. Hypertension,* 6, 283, 1988.
30. **Pagnan, A., Corrocher, R., Ambrosio, G. B., Ferrari, S., Guarini, P., Piccolo, D., Brugnara, C., Opportuno, A., Bassi, A., Aprili, F., Bertinato, L., Olivieri, O., Baggio, G., Palu, C. D.,** Effects of olive-oil-rich diet on serum and membrane lipids and on cation transport in erythrocytes, *J. Hypertension,* 5(Suppl. 5), S247, 1987.
31. **Carr, S. J., Thomas, T. H., Laker, M. F., and Wilkinson, R.,** Lipid lowering therapy leads to a reduction in sodium-lithium countertransport activity, *Atherosclerosis,* 87, 103, 1991.
32. **Weder, A. B., Serr, C., Torretti, B. A., Bassett, D. R., and Zweifler, A. J.,** Effects of lovastatin treatment on red blood cell and platelet cation transport, *Hypertension,* 17, 203, 1991.
33. **Dadone, M. M., Hasstedt, S. J., Hunt, S. C., Smith, J. B., Ash, K. O., and Williams, R. R.,** Genetic analysis of sodium-lithium countertransport in 10 hypertension-prone kindreds, *Am. J. Med. Genet.,* 17, 565, 1984.
34. **Boerwinkle, E., Turner, S. T., Weinshilboum, R., Johnson, M., Richelson, E., and Sing, C. F.,** Genetic analysis of the distribution of sodium lithium countertransport in a sample representative of the general population, *Genet. Epidemiol.,* 3, 365, 1986.
35. **Motulsky, A. G., Burke, W., Billings, P. R., and Ward, R. H.,** Hypertension and the genetics of red cell membrane abnormalities, in *Molecular Approaches to Human Polygenic Disease,* Ciba Symposium 130, Bock G. and Collins, G., Eds., John Wiley & Sons, Chichester, 1987, 150.
36. **Hasstedt, S. J., Wu, L. L., Ash, K. O., Kuida, H., and Williams, R. R.,** Hypertension and sodium-lithium countertransport in Utah pedigrees: evidence for major locus inheritance, *Am. J. Hum. Genet.,* 43, 14, 1988.
37. **Turner, S. T., Johnson, M., Boerwinkle, E., Richelson, E., Taswell, H. F., and Sing, C. F.,** Distribution of sodium-lithium countertransport and its relationship to blood pressure in a large sample of blood donors, *Hypertension,* 7, 955, 1985.

38. **Rebbeck, T. R., Turner, S. T., Michels, V. V., and Moll, P. P.**, Genetic and environmental explanations for the distribution of sodium-lithium countertransport in pedigrees from Rochester, MN, *Am. J. Hum. Genet.*, 48, 1092, 1991.
39. **Hasstedt, S. J., Hunt, S. C., Wu, L. L., and Williams, R. R.**, The inheritance of intraerythrocytic sodium level, *Am. J. Med. Genet.*, 29, 193, 1988.
40. **Hasstedt, S. J., Wu, L. L., Kuida, H., and Williams, R. R.**, Recessive inheritance of a high number of sodium pump sites, *Am. J. Med. Genet.*, 34, 332, 1989.
41. **Izpisúa, J. C., Barber, T., Cabo, J., Hrelia, S., Rossi, C. A., Castelli, G. P., Lercker, G., Biagi, P. L., Bordoni, A., and Lenaz, G.**, Lipid composition, fluidity and enzymatic activities of rat liver plasma and mitochondrial membranes in dietary obese rats, *Int. J. Obesity*, 13, 531, 1989.
42. **Tamura, M., Inagami, T., Kinoshita, T., and Kuwano, H.**, A search for endogenous Na^+,K^+-ATPase inhibitor in acutely volume-expanded hog plasma led to lysophosphatidylcholine γ-stearoyl, *J. Hypertension*, 5, 219, 1987.
43. **Williams, R. R., Hasstedt, S. J., Hunt, S. C., Wu, L. L., Hopkins, P. N., Berry, T. D., Stults, B. M., Barlow, G. K., and Kuida, H.**, Genetic traits related to hypertension and electrolyte metabolism, *Hypertension*, 17(Suppl. 1), I69, 1991.
44. **Cusi, D., Stella, P., Pozzoli, E., Barlassina, C., Soldati, L., and Bianchi, G.**, Genetic polymorphism of Na-K countertransport in essential hypertension, *J. Hum. Hypertension*, 4, 307, 1990.
45. **Tsuda, K. and Masuyama, Y.**, Age-related changes in membrane fluidity of erythrocytes in essential hypertension, *Am. J. Hypertension*, 3, 714, 1990.
46. **Sauerheber, R. D., Lewis, U. J., Esgate, J. A., and Gordon, L. M.**, Effect of calcium, insulin and growth hormones on membrane fluidity: a spin label study of rat adipocytes and human erythrocyte ghosts, *Biochim. Biophys. Acta*, 597, 292, 1980.
47. **Tsuda, K., Tsuda, S., Minatogawa, Y., Iwahashi, H. et al.**, Effects of calcium antagonists on membrane fluidity in hypertension — an electron spin resonance study, *Am. J. Hypertension*, 1, 283, 1988.
48. **Arrázola, A. and Diez, J.**, Correspondences between the activity of the renin-angiotensin system and the erythrocyte Na^+ transport abnormalities in hypertension, *Am. J. Hypertension*, 3, 412, 1990.
49. **Fray, J. C. S., Park, C. S., and Valentine, A. N. D.**, Calcium and control of renin secretion, *Endocr. Rev.*, 8, 53, 1987.
50. **Masuyama, Y., Tsuda, K., Shima, H., Ura, M., Takeda, J., Kimura, K., and Nishio, I.**, Membrane abnormality of erythrocytes is highly dependent on salt intake and renin profile in essential hypertension: an electron spin resonance study, *J. Hypertension*, 6(Suppl. 4), S266, 1988.
51. **Longworth, D. L., Drayer, J. I. M., Weber, M. A., and Laragh, J. H.**, Divergent blood pressure responses during short-term sodium restriction in hypertension, *Clin. Pharmacol. Ther.*, 27, 544, 1980.
52. **Tsuda, K., Tsuda, S., Minatogawa, Y., Iwahashi, H. et al.**, Membrane fluidity of erythrocytes and its relevance to renin profile in essential hypertension, *Jpn. Circ. J.*, 52, 1301, 1988.
53. **Postnov, Y. V., Orlov, S. N., and Pokudin, N. I.**, Decrease of calcium binding by the red blood cell membrane in spontaneously hypertensive rats and in essential hypertension, *Pfluegers' Arch.*, 379, 191, 1979.
54. **Postnov, Y. V., Orlov, S. N., Reznikova, M. B., Rjazhsky, G. G., and Pokudin, N. I.**, Calmodulin distribution and Ca^{2+} transport in the erythrocytes of patients with essential hypertension, *Clin. Sci.*, 66, 479, 1984.
55. **Niggli, V. and Carafoli, E.**, Interaction of purified Ca^{2+},Mg^{2+}-ATPase from human erythrocytes with phospholipids and calmodulin, *Acta Biol. Med. Ger.*, 40, 437, 1981.
56. **Devynck, M. A., Pernollet, M. G., Nunez, A. M., and Meyer, P.**, Analysis of calcium handling in erythrocyte membranes of genetically hypertensive rates, *Hypertension*, 3, 379, 1981.

57. **Testa, I., Rabini, R. A., Fumelli, P., Bertoli, E., and Mazzanti, L.,** Abnormal membrane fluidity and acetylcholinesterase activity in erythrocytes from insulin-dependent diabetic patients, *J. Clin. Endocrinol. Metab.*, 67, 1129, 1988.
58. **Krolewski, A. S., Canessa, M., Warram, J. H., Laffel, L. B. M., Christlieb, A. R., Knowler, W. C., and Rand, L. L.,** Predisposition to hypertension and susceptibility to renal disease in insulin-dependent diabetes mellitus, *N. Engl. J. Med.*, 318, 140, 1988.
59. **Preiss, R., Prümke, H. J., Sohr, R., Müller, E., Schmeck, G., Bonaschak, H.,** Sodium flux and lipid spectrum in the erythrocyte membrane in essential hypertension, *Int. J. Clin. Pharmacol. Ther. Toxicol.*, 20, 105, 1982.
60. **Riozzi, A., Heagerty, A. M., Ollerenshaw, J. D., and Swales, J. D.,** Erythrocyte phosphoinositide metabolism in essential hypertensive patients and their normotensive offspring, *Clin. Sci.*, 73, 29, 1987.
61. **Engelmann, B., Op Den Kamp, J. A. F., and Roelofsen, B.,** Replacement of molecular species of phosphatidylcholine: influence on erythrocyte Na transport, *Am. J. Physiol.*, 258(Cell Physiol. 27), C682, 1990.
62. **Marche, P., Koutouzov, S., Girard, A., Elghozi, J. L., Meyer, P., and Ben-Ishay, D.,** Phosphoinositide turnover in erythrocyte membranes in human and experimental hypertension, *J. Hypertension,* 3, 25, 1985.
63. **Corrocher, R., Ferrari, S., Bassi, A., Guarini, P., Bertinato, L., Olivieri, O., Licia, G. M., Ruzzenente, O., Brugnara, C., and De Sandre, G.,** Membrane polyunsaturated fatty acids and lithium-sodium countertransport in human erythrocytes, *Life Sci.*, 41, 1171, 1987.
64. **Wiley, J. S. and Cooper, R. A.,** Inhibition of cation cotransport by cholesterol enrichment of human red cell membranes, *Biochim. Biophys. Acta,* 413, 425, 1975.
65. **Levy, R., Hevroni, D., Cabantchik, Z. I., and Livne, A.,** Li_i-Na_o countertransport and Li leak in erythrocytes are differentially affected by membrane enrichment with cholesteryl hemisuccinate, *Biochim. Biophys. Acta,* 854, 325, 1986.
66. **Zilversmit, D. B.,** A proposal linking atherogenesis to the interaction of endothelial lipoprotein lipase with triglyceride-rich lipoproteins, *Circ. Res.*, 33, 633, 1973.
67. **Bloj, B. and Zilversmit, D. B.,** Complete exchangeability of cholesterol in phosphatidylcholine/cholesterol vesicles of different degrees of unsaturation, *Biochemistry,* 16, 3943, 1977.
68. **Guyton, A. C.,** *Textbook of Medical Physiology,* 5th ed., W. B. Saunders, Philadelphia, 1976, 924.
69. **Vakakis, N., Redgrave, T. G., Small, D. M., and Castelli, W. P.,** Cholesterol content of red blood cells and low-density lipoproteins in hypertriglyceridemia, *Biochim. Biophys. Acta,* 751, 280, 1983.
70. **Goldstein, J. L., Schrott, H. G., Hazzard, W. R., Bierman, E. L., and Motulsky, A. G.,** Hyperlipidemia in coronary heart disease. II. Genetic analysis of lipid levels in 176 families and delineation of a new inherited disorder, combined hyperlipidemia, *J. Clin. Invest.*, 52, 1544, 1973.
71. **Williams, R. R., Hopkins, P. N., Hunt, S. C., Wu, L. L., Hasstedt, S. J., Lalouel, J. M., Ash, K. O., Stults, B. M., and Kuida, H.,** Population-based frequency of dyslipidemia syndromes in coronary-prone families in Utah, *Arch. Intern. Med.*, 150, 582, 1990.
72. **McNamara, J. R., Campos, H., Ordovas, J. M., Peterson, J., Wilson, P. W. F., and Schaefer, E. J.,** Effect of gender, age, and lipid status on low density lipoprotein subfraction distribution: results from the Framingham offspring study, *Arteriosclerosis,* 7, 483, 1987.
73. **Hunt, S. C., Wu, L. L., Hopkins, P. N., Stults, B. M., Kuida, H., Ramirez, M. E., Lalouel, J. M., and Williams, R. R.,** Apolipoprotein, low density lipoprotein subfraction, and insulin associations with familial combined hyperlipidemia: study of Utah patients with familial dyslipidemic hypertension, *Arteriosclerosis,* 9, 335, 1989.
74. **Austin, M. A., Breslow, J. L., Hennekens, C. H., Buring, J. E., Willett, W. C., and Krauss, R. M.,** Low-density lipoprotein subclass patterns and risk of myocardial infarction, *JAMA,* 260, 1917, 1988.

75. **Austin, M. A., Brunzell, J. D., Fitch, W. L., and Krauss, R. M.,** Inheritance of low density lipoprotein subclass patterns in familial combined hyperlipidemia, *Arteriosclerosis,* 10, 520, 1990.
76. **Williams, R. R., Hunt, S. C., Hopkins, P. N., Stults, B. M., Wu, L. L., Hasstedt, S. J., Barlow, G. K., Stephenson, S. H., Lalouel, J. M., and Kuida, H.,** Familial dyslipidemic hypertension: evidence from 58 Utah families for a syndrome present in approximately 12% of patients with essential hypertension, *JAMA,* 259, 3579, 1988.
77. **Selby, J. V., Newman, B., Quiroga, J., Christian, J. C., Austin, M. A., and Fabsitz, R. R.,** Concordance for dyslipidemic hypertension in male twins, *JAMA,* 265, 2079, 1991.
78. **Ferrari, P., Weidmann, P., Shaw, S., Giachino, D., Riesen, W., Allemann, Y., and Heynen, G.,** Altered insulin sensitivity, hyperinsulinemia and dyslipidemia in hypertension-prone humans, *Clin. Res.,* 39, 351A, 1991.
79. **Mills, G. L., Taylaur, C. E., and Chapman, M. J.,** Low-density lipoproteins in patients homozygous for familial hyperbetalipoproteinaemia, *Clin. Sci. Mol. Med.,* 51, 221, 1976.
80. **Shattil, S. J., Bennett, J. S., Colman, R. W., and Cooper, R. A.,** Abnormalities of cholesterol-phospholipid composition in platelets and low-density lipoproteins of human hyperbetalipoproteinemia, *J. Lab. Clin. Med.,* 89, 341, 1977.
81. **Dougherty, R. M., Galli, C., Ferro-Luzzi, A., and Iacono, J. M.,** Lipid and phospholipid fatty acid composition of plasma, red blood cells, and platelets and how they are affected by dietary lipids: a study of normal subjects from Italy, Finland, and the USA, *Am. J. Clin. Nutr.,* 45, 443, 1987.
82. **Devynck, M. A., Pernollet, M. G., Nunez, F. V., Monteray-Garestier, T., Helene, C., and Meyer, P.,** Diffuse structural alterations in cell membranes of spontaneously hypertensive rats, *Proc. Natl. Acad. Sci. U.S.A.,* 79, 5057, 1982.
83. **Kawahara, J., Sano, H., Kubota, Y., Hattori, K., Miki, T., Suzuki, H., and Fukuzaki, H.,** Dietary linoleic acid prevents the development of deoxycorticosterone acetate-salt hypertension, *Hypertension,* 15 (Suppl. 2), I 81, 1990.
84. **Bloj, B., Moreno, R. D., Farias, R. N., and Trucco, R. E.,** Membrane lipid fatty acids and regulation of membrane-bound enzymes. Allosteric behaviour of erythrocyte Mg^{2+}-ATPase, $(Na^+$-$K^+)$-ATPase and acetylcholinesterase from rats fed different fat-supplemented diets, *Biochim. Biophys. Acta,* 311, 67, 1973.
85. **Frenkel, E. J., Roelofsen, B., Brodbeck, U., Van Deenen, L. L. M., and Ott, P.,** Lipid-protein interactions in human erythrocyte membrane acetylcholinesterase. Modulation of enzyme activity by lipids, *Eur. J. Biochem.,* 109, 377, 1980.
86. **Winegrad, A. I.,** Does a common mechanism induce the diverse complications of diabetes?, *Diabetes,* 36, 396, 1987.
87. **Pyörälä, K.,** Relationship of glucose tolerance and plasma insulin to the incidence of coronary heart disease: results from two population studies in Finland, *Diabetes Care,* 2, 131, 1979.
88. **Ducimetiere, P., Eschwege, L., Papoz, J. L., Claude, R. J. R., and Rosselin, G.,** Relationship of plasma insulin levels to the incidence of myocardial infarction and coronary heart disease mortality in a middle-aged population, *Diabetologia,* 19, 205, 1980.
89. **Welborn, T. A. and Wearne, K.,** Coronary heart disease incidence and cardiovascular mortality in Busselton with reference to glucose and insulin concentrations, *Diabetes Care,* 2, 154, 1979.
90. **Skarfors, E. T., Lithell, H. O., and Selinus, I.,** Risk factors for the development of hypertension: a 10-year longitudinal study in middle-aged men, *J. Hypertension,* 9, 217, 1991.
91. **Kaplan, N. M.,** Upper-body obesity, glucose intolerance, hypertriglyceridemia, and hypertension, *Arch. Intern. Med.,* 149, 1514, 1989.
92. Working Group Report on Management of Patients with Hypertension and High Blood Cholesterol, NIH Publ. No. 90-2361, U.S. Department of Health and Human Services, Washington, DC, August, 1990.
93. **Reaven, G. M.,** Insulin resistance, hyperinsulinemia, hypertriglyceridemia, and hypertension: parallels between human disease and rodent models, *Diabetes Care,* 14, 195, 1991.

94. **Reaven, G. M., Ho, H., and Hoffman, B. B.,** Somatostatin inhibition of fructose induced hypertension, *Hypertension,* 14, 117, 1989.
95. **Kissebah, A. H., Adams, P. W., and Wynn, V.,** Interrelationship between insulin secretion and plasma free fatty acid and triglyceride transport kinetics in maturity onset diabetes and the effect of phenethylbiguanide (Phenformin), *Diabetologia,* 10, 119, 1974.
96. **Resnick, L. N. M., Gupta, R. K., and Laragh, J. H.,** Intracellular free Mg in erythrocytes of essential HBP: relation to blood pressure and serum divalent cations, *Proc. Natl. Acad. Sci. U.S.A.,* 81, 6511, 1984.
97. **Landsberg, L. and Young, J. B.,** Catecholamines and the adrenal medulla, in *Williams Textbook of Endocrinology,* 7th ed., Wilson, J. D., and Foster, D. W., Eds., W. B. Saunders, Philadelphia, 1985, 891.
98. **Davis, F. B., Davis, P. J., Nat, G., Blas, S. D. et al.,** The effect of in vivo glucose administration on human erythrocyte Ca^2-ATPase activity and on enzyme responsiveness in vitro to thyroid hormone and calmodulin, *Diabetes,* 34, 639, 1985.
99. **Amatruda, J. M. and Finch, E. D.,** Modulation of hexose uptake and insulin action by cell membrane, *J. Biol. Chem.,* 254, 2619, 1979.
100. **Melchior, D. L. and Czech, M. P.,** Sensitivity of the adipocyte D-glucose transport system, *J. Biol. Chem.,* 254, 8744, 1979.
101. **Moore, R. D.,** Effect of insulin upon the sodium pump in frog skeletal muscle, *J. Physiol.,* 232, 23, 1973.
102. **Nizet, A., Lefebvre, P., and Crabbe, J.,** Control by insulin of sodium potassium and water excretion, *Pfluegers' Arch.,* 323, 11, 1971.
103. **Moore, R. D., Munford, J. W., and Pillsworth, T. J.,** Effects of streptozotocin diabetes and fasting on intracellular sodium and adenosine triphosphate in rat soleus muscle, *J. Physiol. (London),* 338, 277, 1983.
104. **Fidelman, M. L., Seeholzer, S. H., Walsh, K. B., Moore, R. D.,** Intracellular pH mediates action of insulin on glycolysis, *Am. J. Physiol.,* 242, C87, 1982.
105. **Moore, R. D., Fidelman, M. L., and Seeholzer, S. H.,** Correlation between insulin action upon glycolysis and change in intracellular pH, *Biochem. Biophys, Res. Commun.,* 91(3), 905, 1979.
106. **Kissebah, A. H., Clarke, P., Vydelingum, N., Hope-Gill, H., Tulloch, B., and Fraser, T. R.,** The role of calcium in insulin action. III. Calcium distribution in fat cells; its kinetics and the effects of adrenaline, insulin and procaine-HCL, *Eur. J. Clin. Invest.,* 5, 339, 1975.
107. **Schoenle, E. and Froesch, E. R.,** In vivo control of the insulin-suppressible high-affinity Ca^{2+}-ATPase of fat cell membranes by growth hormone and its possible involvement in the regulation of glucose transport, *FEBS Lett.,* 123, 219, 1981.
108. **Foyle, W. J. and Drury, P. L.,** Reduction of Li^+-Na^+ countertransport by physiological levels of insulin *in vitro, J. Hypertension,* 9, 713, 1991.
109. **Hasstedt, S. J.,** unpublished results.
110. **Berry, T. D.,** unpublished results.

Chapter 14

ABNORMALITIES OF ION TRANSPORT AND THE PATHOPHYSIOLOGY OF ESSENTIAL HYPERTENSION: THERAPEUTIC IMPLICATIONS AND FUTURE PERSPECTIVES

Ricardo Garay, Nathalie Senn, and Jean-Pierre Ollivier

TABLE OF CONTENTS

I. Introduction 302

II. Red Blood Cell Ion Transport as an Indicator of Sensitivity to Diuretic Drugs 302

III. Centrally Acting Drugs 304

IV. Calcium Antagonists 305

V. Angiotensin Converting Enzyme Inhibitors 306

VI. Summary and Conclusions 306

References 308

0-8493-5474-9/94/$0.00 + $.50

I. INTRODUCTION

In infectious disease, detection of microorganisms and testing their antibiotic sensitivity has strongly improved the therapeutic management of patients. The same can be said for other common diseases such as diabetes, for which knowledge of insulin sensitivity improves therapeutic control. Conversely, essential hypertension lacks any biochemical means to predict drug sensitivity. This is an important problem because 30 to 50% of the patients are resistant to monotherapeutic treatment with any of the available antihypertensive drugs, and the physician has no choice but to follow a "trial and error" assay of one or more antihypertensive compounds.

Muller and Laragh[1] have tried to develop rational criteria to guide antihypertensive therapy. Thus, it has been suggested that diuretics are more efficient in patients with low renin activity and that vasorelaxants are more efficient in patients with normal or high renin. Bühler[2] has proposed the prescription of diuretics or calcium antagonists in aged patients and converting enzyme inhibitors or beta-blockers in young hypertensives. Unfortunately, these criteria proved to be insufficiently sophisticated for approaching the extraordinary etiological complexity underlying the sensitivity to antihypertensive drugs.

Over the last 12 or so years, multiple ion transport defects have been characterized in red blood cell (RBC) membranes from humans and rats with primary hypertension (see Chapter 1). It was suspected that these membrane abnormalities were "biochemical markers" of different types of essential hypertension, with different sensitivity to antihypertensive drugs, i.e., that "step-care" and other "blind" treatments could be avoided by selecting the antihypertensive drug as a function of the red cell ion transport abnormality.

Several investigators have recently attempted to use RBC ion transport in order to understand the action mechanism and therapeutical efficacy of antihypertensive drugs. We summarize here the relevant aspects of these studies, with a particular emphasis on the ion transport profile of responders and nonresponders to the different antihypertensive drugs.

II. RED BLOOD CELL ION TRANSPORT AS AN INDICATOR OF SENSITIVITY TO DIURETIC DRUGS

Some diuretic drugs, but not other antihypertensive compounds, can modify erythrocyte ion fluxes *in vitro,* i.e., they can directly inhibit membrane ion transport systems, particularly at chloride or bicarbonate sites. However, this seems not to be the case *in vivo* because, generally speaking, therapeutical plasma levels of diuretic drugs are not sufficiently high to inhibit erythrocyte ion fluxes. Indeed, most diuretic drugs are concentrated in the lumen of the nephron where they reach the high concentrations required to inhibit luminal sodium carriers.[3]

In vivo, diuretic drugs may affect erythrocyte ion carriers by indirect mechanisms. One important mechanism, particularly for loop diuretics, is hypokalemia. Thus, the appearance of hypokalemia during piretanide[4] or xipamide[5] administration

TABLE 1
Erythrocyte Na^+,K^+ Pump and $[Na^+,K^+,Cl^-]$ Cotransport Activities during Hydrochlorothiazide Administration in Essential Hypertensive Patients

	Na^+,K^+ pump (mmol/l cells/h)	$[Na^+,K^+,Cl^-]$ cotransport (μmol/l cells/h)
Before hydrochlorothiazide	1.73 ± 0.07	108 ± 22
After hydrochlorothiazide	1.91 ± 0.08	161 ± 29
p^a	0.041	0.014

Note: Values are given as mean ± SEM of 10 essential hypertensive patients who received 25 mg/d of hydrochlorothiazide for 45 d (8 d placebo washout pretherapy). Flux values were obtained in fresh cells according to previously published protocols.[3,29,30]

[a] Student *t*-test.

can reduce erythrocyte sodium pump activity and increase internal sodium contents. In the long-term, chronic hypokalemia may induce down-regulation of the membrane pump density with recovery of normal sodium contents.[6] The appearance of these compensatory phenomena coincides with the renewal time of erythrocytes (about 4 months).

Besides hypokalemia, another indirect modifier factor was clearly demonstrated by using potassium sparing diuretics. Thus, Niutta et al.[7] found that potassium canrenoate administration has the opposite effect of loop diuretics: it stimulates erythrocyte sodium pump activity and decreases internal sodium contents. Studies in rats with reduced renal mass treated with canrenone, the active metabolite of potassium canrenoate, have suggested that the sodium pump stimulation is due to a correction of volume expansion with reduced secretion of "endogenous ouabain-like factors".[8]

Discordant findings have been reported concerning the effect of thiazides on erythrocyte sodium contents.[9-11] This is probably due to the fact that thiazides can induce both hypokalemia and reduction of volume expansion. As a result, we investigated this latter action of hydrochlorothiazide on the sodium pump by incubating erythrocytes *ex vivo* at a fixed, constant external potassium concentration and by measuring pump-mediated sodium efflux. Table 1 shows the results obtained in essential hypertensive patients treated with hydrochlorothiazide for 45 d. It can be seen that hydrochlorothiazide administration induces a clear *ex vivo* stimulation of sodium pump activity. *In vivo,* this stimulatory action can be reduced and even inversed by the hypokalemia. Table 1 shows that besides sodium pump stimulation, hydrochlorothiazide administration induces an even more important stimulation of $[Na^+,K^+,Cl^-]$ cotransport activity.

The above studies suggested mechanisms by which diuretic drugs may act in low renin hypertensives: correction of volume expansion, reduced secretion of

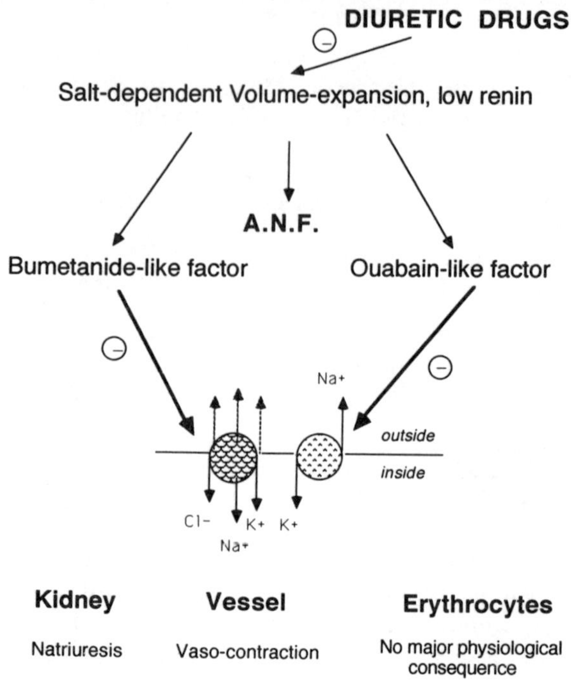

FIGURE 1. A model for the RBC as an indicator of sensitivity to diuretic drugs. Low pump, low cotransport hypertensives are similar to age-dependent, salt-sensitive hypertensives with low plasma renin activity. Diuretic drugs (and vasorelaxants with salidiuretic activity) reduce volume expansion, decrease the secretion of "ouabain-like" and "bumetanide-like" factors, and induce pump and cotransport restimulation. A.N.F., atrial natriuretic factor.

endogenous "ouabain-like" and "bumetanide-like" factors with restimulation of pump, and cotransport activity in vascular smooth muscle and vasorelaxation (Figure 1).

The present authors and associates[12] previously investigated hydrochlorothazide efficacy in essential hypertension as a function of kinetic parameters of erythrocyte ion transport pathways. Table 2 shows that hydrochlorotiazide responders have lower V_{max} for sodium pump than do nonresponders. V_{max} of cotransport was also lower than in nonresponders, but the difference was not statistically significant. Moreover, nonresponders exhibited significant increases in Na^+,Li^+ countertransport and membrane sodium leak (Table 2).

III. CENTRALLY ACTING DRUGS

A previous study investigated clonidine efficacy as a function of erythrocyte ion fluxes.[13] This study revealed that nonresponders had increased Na^+,Li^+ countertransport, [Na^+,K^+,Cl^-] cotransport, and membrane sodium leak.

TABLE 2
Hydrochlorothiazide Efficacy in Essential Hypertension as a Function of Erythrocyte Na^+ Transport Pathways

	Maximal rates (V_{max})			
	Na^+,K^+ pump (mmol/l cells/h)	$[Na^+,K^+,Cl^-]$ cotransport (μmol/l cells/h)	Na^+,Li^+ countertransport (μmol/l cells/h)	Na^+ leak ([1/h] × 10^3)
Responders (9)	6.42 ± 1.96	651 ± 196	202 ± 90	13.6 ± 2.4
Nonresponders (21)	8.83 ± 3.85	794 ± 349	313 ± 194	19.0 ± 5.6
p^a	<0.05	n.s.	0.057	<0.01
Normal range	5.5–9.5	450–750	80–260	10–17

Note: Values are given as mean ± SD. The number of subjects is indicated in parentheses. Patients received 25 mg/d of hydrochlorothiazide for 45 d. Responders were those hypertensives who normalized blood pressure with hydrochlorothiazide; i.e., systolic blood pressure ≤140 mmHg and diastolic blood pressure ≤90 mmHg (for details see Reference 12). Flux values were obtained in nystatine-treated cells according to previously published protocols.[29,30] n.s.: Nonsignificant.

[a] Student *t*-test

Increased sodium leak can be found in 15 to 30% of essential hypertensive patients and is frequently associated with increased $[Na^+,K^+,Cl^-]$ cotransport.[14] Moreover, increased Na^+,Li^+ countertransport is also frequently associated with increased $[Na^+,K^+,Cl^-]$ cotransport.[15,16] We reexamined our data on clonidine resistance and found that the correlation with the cotransport and countertransport systems disappeared after adjustment of the sodium leak.[13] Therefore, increased membrane sodium leak can be retained as a criteria of clonidine resistance.

IV. CALCIUM ANTAGONISTS

Dihydropyridine calcium antagonists are able to induce significant natriuresis in the first few days of treatment.[17-20] This seems to explain why calcium antagonists lower blood pressure more with high sodium intake, both acutely and chronically (for review see Reference 2). Moreover, similarly to diuretic drugs, calcium antagonists were reported to be more efficient in volume-expanded, low renin hypertensives, a prevalent pattern in older patients and black persons.[2]

A mechanistic explanation was suggested by studies in Dahl rats[21,22] and DOCA/salt rats,[23] showing that chronic nifedipine administration prevented increases in erythrocyte sodium contents and sodium pump inhibition.

However, the animal studies were only partially confirmed in humans. Thus, a fall in erythrocyte sodium content on treatment with nifedipine was found by Ericsson,[24] and Gray et al.[25] have found a decrease in leukocyte sodium and an increase in leukocyte sodium efflux rate constants after treatment with verapamil. However, Heagerty et al.[26] reported that nifedipine therapy was unable to modify the leukocyte sodium efflux rate constant.

TABLE 3
Antihypertensive Drug Response as a Function of Erythrocyte Ion Transport Abnormalities

	Type 1: low pump and cotransport	Type 2: high counter- and cotransport	Type 3: high Na^+ leak and cotransport
Diuretics	+ + + +	+	–
Calcium antagonists (dihydropyridines)	+ + +	+ + + +	–
ACE inhibitors	+ +	+ + +	–
Centrally acting drugs	+	+ + +	+

Note: The number of + signs indicates the magnitude of the antihypertensive response. These were roughly approximative values, estimated from the studies reviewed here.

With the exception of Heagerty et al.,[26] the above results suggest that similarly to hydrochlorothiazide, patients with low pump activity may be sensitive to dihydropyridine calcium antagonists. This hypothesis requires further investigation.

V. ANGIOTENSIN CONVERTING ENZYME INHIBITORS

Sanchez et al.[11] have recently reported that captopril is efficient in essential hypertensive patients with low cotransport activity. In these patients, captopril stimulates cotransport and pump fluxes and decreases erythrocyte sodium contents. Interestingly, this *in vivo* action on ion transport is similar to that of hydrochlorothiazide (Tables 1 and 2).

Sanchez et al.[11] found that in low cotransport hypertensives, captopril administration decreases exchangeable sodium. This suggests that the natriuretic action of angiotensin converting enzyme (ACE) inhibitors[27,28] may confer antihypertensive efficacy to these compounds in low renin (low pump and low cotransport) hypertensives.

In a previous study the authors[12] have found that as with clonidine, nonresponders to captopril tended to present an increased membrane sodium leak.

VI. SUMMARY AND CONCLUSIONS

The results reviewed here and in Chapter 1 suggest that at least three types of essential hypertension differ among others because of their sensitivity to antihypertensive drugs (Table 3). A first type of essential hypertension is characterized by low pump, low cotransport fluxes in erythrocytes and by its sensitivity to diuretic drugs (Figure 1). Vasorelaxants with salidiuretic activity (dihydropyridine calcium antagonists and ACE inhibitors) are also active in this type of hypertension.

Low erythrocyte pump and cotransport fluxes seem to be induced by the presence of endogenous "ouabain-like" and "bumetanide-like" factors in the plasma (Chapter 1). These were proposed to be endogenous "natriuretic factors" which are secreted in the circulation in order to compensate salt-dependent volume expansion (Chapter 1 and Figure 1). In vascular smooth muscle, low pump and low cotransport fluxes seem to be hypertensinogenic factors (Chapters 1 and 3).

Interestingly, the antihypertensive response to the above-mentioned drugs tends to be associated with erythrocyte pump and cotransport restimulation. This recovery of pump and cotransport activity is likely due to the reduction of volume expansion by diuretic drugs, with decreased secretion of endogenous "ouabain-like" and "bumetanide-like" factors.

The above arguments strongly suggest that low pump, low cotransport hypertensives are similar to age-dependent, salt-sensitive hypertensives with low plasma renin activity. Therefore, low pump, low cotransport, and low renin seem to be three biochemical markers of the same type of hypertension, salt-sensitive hypertension (Figure 1 and Chapter 1).

It is important to mention that over the long-term, the reduction in erythrocyte pump and cotransport activities may be compensated for by down-regulation of the membrane density of transport units. These compensatory mechanisms deserve further investigation.

A second type of essential hypertension is characterized by increased red cell Na^+,Li^+ countertransport and [Na^+,K^+,Cl^-] cotransport. Hypertensives belonging to this group seem to be resistant to diuretic drugs but sensitive to vasorelaxants (Table 3).

Hypertensives with high cotransport and countertransport fluxes tend to present normal or high plasma renin activity, disorders in lipid metabolism, and left ventricular hypertrophy (Chapter 1).

A third type of essential hypertension is characterized by both high membrane sodium leak and high [Na^+,K^+,Cl^-] cotransport in erythrocytes. Hypertensives belonging to this group are resistant to diuretics, ACE inhibitors, calcium antagonists, and centrally acting drugs (Table 3).

In conclusion, red cell studies are contributing to the further understanding of the mechanism of action of diuretic drugs and other antihypertensive compounds *in vivo*. Moreover, erythrocyte ion flux abnormalities seem to be biochemical markers of different types of essential hypertension with different sensitivity to antihypertensive drugs. Further studies are required in order to establish whether RBC ion fluxes may be useful for the therapeutical management of essential hypertensive patients.

REFERENCES

1. **Muller, F. B. and Laragh, J. H.,** Issues, goals, and guidelines for choosing first-line and combination antihypertensive drug therapy, in *Hypertension: Pathophysiology, Diagnosis, and Management,* Laragh, J. H. and Brenner, B. M., Eds., Raven Press, New York, 1990: 2107–2115.
2. **Bühler, F. R.,** Calcium antagonists, in *Hypertension: Pathophysiology, Diagnosis, and Management,* Laragh, J. H. and Brenner, B. M., Eds., Raven Press, New York, 1990: 2169–2179.
3. **Garay, R. P., Nazaret, C., Labaune, J. P., Mesangeau, D., and Moinet, G.,** CRE 10904 (2-(*p*-fluorophenoxy), 1-(*o*-hydroxyphenyl)-ethane: a new diuretic and antihypertensive drug acting by in vivo sulfation, *J. Pharmacol. Exp. Ther.,* 1990; 255: 415–422.
4. **Zidek, W., Baumgart, P., Karoff, C., Losse, H., and Vetter, H.,** Intracellular calcium in essential hypertension. A parameter for assessing effective antihypertensive treatment, *J. Hypertension,* 1984; 2(Suppl. 3): 495–497.
5. **Lijnen, P., Hespel, P., Fagard, R., Staessen, J., Goossens, W., Lissens, W., and Amery, A.,** Erythrocyte and leucocyte sodium and potassium transport systems during long-term diuretic administration in men, *J. Hypertension,* 1988; 6: 639–645.
6. **Beuckelmann, D. and Erdmann, E.,** Na^+,Li^+ countertransport and electrolyte composition in erythrocytes of patients with essential hypertension before and after antihypertensive treatment, *Klin. Wochenschr.,* 1986; 64: 1101–1105.
7. **Niutta, E., Cusi, D., Colombo, R., Tripodi, G., Pellizzoni, M., Pati, P., Cezana, B., Alberghini, E., Barlassina, C., and Bianchi, G.,** Antihypertensive effect of captopril, canrenoate potassium, and atenolol. Relations with red blood cell sodium transport and renin, *Am. J. Hypertension,* 1988; 1: 364–371.
8. **De Mendonça, M., Grichois, M. L., Pernollet, M. G., Wauquier, I., Trouillet-Thormann, B., Meyer, P., Devynck, M. A., and Garay, R.,** Antihypertensive effect of canrenone in a model where endogenous ouabain-like factors are present, *J. Cardiovasc. Pharmacol.,* 1988; 11: 75–83.
9. **Herlitz, H., Jonsonn, O., Elmfeldt, D., Nauclér, J., and Berglund, G.,** Intraerythrocyte sodium content and transmembrane sodium flux in hypertensive patients treated with diuretics or beta-adrenoceptor blockers, *Acta Pharmacol. Toxicol.,* 1984; 54: 37–42.
10. **Trevisan, M., Ostrow, D., Cooper, R., Liu, K., Sparks, S., Okonek, A., Stevens, E., Marquardt, J., and Stamler, J.,** Abnormal red blood cell ion transport and hypertension, *Hypertension,* 1983; 5: 363–367.
11. **Sanchez, R. A., Gimenez, M. I., Gilbert, B. H., Giannone, C., Marco, E., and Ramirez, A.,** Recovery of erythrocyte Na^+-K^+-Cl^- cotransport activity by enalapril. *Hypertension,* 1991; 17: 334–339.
12. **Senn, N., Ollivier, J. P., Abitbol, J. P., and Garay, R.,** Effect antihypertenseur du captopril, de l'hydrochlorothiazide, seuls ou en association, chez différentes catégories de malades hypertendus essentiels, *Arch. Mal. Coeur Vaiss.,* 1988; 81(Suppl. HTA): 155–158.
13. **Senn, N., Hajem, S., Frohly, P., Ollivier, J. P., and Garay, R. P.,** Clonidine sensitivity in hypertensive patients as a function of red cell ion transport, *J. Vasc. Med. Biol.,* 1991; 3: 285–289.
14. **Garay, R. P. and Nazaret, C.,** Na^+ leak in erythrocytes from essential hypertensive patients, *Clin. Sci.,* 1985; 69: 613–624.
15. **Adragna, N., Canessa, M., Solomon, H., Slater, E., and Tosteson, D. C.,** Red cell lithium-sodium countertransport and sodium-potassium cotransport in patients with essential hypertension, *Hypertension,* 1982; 4: 795–804.
16. **Garay, R. P., Nazaret, C., Hannaert, P., and Price, M.,** Abnormal Na^+,K^+ cotransport function in a group of patients with essential hypertension, *Eur. J. Clin. Invest.,* 1983; 13: 311–320.
17. **Garthoff, B., Kazda, S., Knorr, A., and Thomas, G.,** Factors involved in the antihypertensive action of calcium antagonists, *Hypertension,* 1982; 225: 263–270.

18. **Leonetti, G., Cuspidi, C., Sampieri, L., Terzoli, L., and Zanchetti, A.,** Comparison of cardiovascular, renal and humoral effects of acute administration of two calcium channel blockers in normotensive and hypertensive subjects, *J. Cardiovasc. Pharmacol.,* 1982; 4(Suppl. 3): S319–S324.
19. **Thananoparvan, C., Golub, M. S., Eggena, P., Barrett, J. D., and Shambi, M. P.,** Renal effects of nitrendipine monotherapy in essential hypertension, *J. Cardiovasc. Pharmacol.,* 1985; 6(Suppl. 7): S1040–S1044.
20. **Luft, F. C., Aronoff, G., Sloan, R., Fineberg, N., and Weinberger, M.,** Calcium channel blockade with nitrendipine, *Hypertension,* 1985; 7: 438–443.
21. **Knorr, A., De Mendonça, M., Garthoff, B., Morich, F., and Kazda, S.,** Chronic treatment with nifedipine prevents development of hypertension and abnormal red cell Na^+ transport in Dahl-S-rats, *Arch. Int. Pharmacodyn.,* 1985; 275: 248–258.
22. **Paschal, C., Hennessy, J., and Buckalew, V.,** Ion transport during hypertension (HT) development in Dahl (D) rats, *Fed. Proc.,* 1984; 43: 648–651.
23. **Knorr, A.,** Prevention by nifedipine of abnormal increase of cell sodium in experimental hypertension in rats, in *New Therapy of Ischaemic Heart Disease and Hypertension,* Lichtlen, P. R., Ed., Excerpta Medica, Amsterdam, 1986: 219–223.
24. **Ericsson, F.,** Effect of nifedipine on cellular electrolytes in fourteen patients with untreated primary hypertension, *Acta Med. Scand.,* 1985; 218: 69–72.
25. **Gray, H. H., Poston, L., Hilton, P. J., Smith, S. J., Markandu, S. J., and MacGregor, G. A.,** Reversal by verapamil of defect in sodium transport in leucocytes in essential hypertensives, *Br. Med. J.,* 1984; 288: 673–675.
26. **Heagerty, A. M., Bing, R. F., Thurston, H., and Swales, J. D.,** Calcium antagonists in hypertension: relation to abnormal sodium transport, *Br. Med. J.,* 1983; 287: 1405–1407.
27. **Brunner, H. R., Gavras, H., Waeber, B., Kershaw, G. R., Turini, G. A., Vukovich, R. A., McKinstry, D. N., and Gavras, I.,** Oral angiotensin converting enzyme inhibitor in long-term treatment of hypertensive patients, *Ann. Intern. Med.,* 1979; 90: 19–23.
28. **Navis, G. J., de Zeuw, D., and de Jong, P. E.,** Enalapril and the kidney: renal vasodilation and natriuresis due to the inhibition of angiotensin II formation, *J. Cardiovasc. Pharmacol.,* 1986; 8(Suppl. 1): 30–34.
29. **Diez, J., Hannaert, P., and Garay, R.,** A kinetic study of the Na^+,K^+ pump in erythrocytes from essential hypertensive patients, *Am. J. Physiol.,* 1987; 252: H1–H6.
30. **Garay, R.,** Kinetic aspects of red blood cell sodium transport systems in essential hypertension, *Hypertension,* 1987; 10(Suppl. 1): 11–14.

INDEX

A

Abnormalities of ionic transport systems, 273–294, see also specific types
- antihypertensives and, 306
- cross-sectional studies of, 274–279
- in erythrocytes, 16–17, 263–266
- essential hypertension pathophysiology and, 301–307
- follow-up studies of, 279–281
- genetic studies of, 284–285
- insulin resistance and, 290–292
- intervention studies of, 281–284
- membrane fluidity and, 275, 285–290
- pathophysiology of essential hypertension and, 301–307
- in primary hypertension, 3, 17

Absorptive epithelia, 5
ACE, see Angiotensin converting enzyme
Acetate, 232
Acetylcholinesterase, 275, 286, 290
Acid-base metabolism, 256
Acid-base transport, 121
ACTH, see Adrenocorticotrophic hormone
Adenosine diphosphate (ADP), 61, 63
Adenosine monophosphate (AMP), 27, 50, 124, 142, 144, 234
Adenosine triphosphatase (ATPase), 33, 59, 60, 61, 64, 187, 231
Adenosine triphosphate (ATP), 4, 60, 61
- adenosine diphosphate exchange with, 63
- depletion of, 239
- hydrolysis of, 255
- lithium-sodium countertransport system and, 91
- potassium channels dependent on, 74

Adipocytes, 235
ADP, see Adenosine diphosphate
Adrenal glands, 26
Adrenocorticotrophic hormone (ACTH), 174
Aging, 94
Alcohol, 69, 95, 100
Aldosterone, 148, 252, 264
Aldosteronism, 97
Alkaline shift, 124
Alkylating agents, 171, see also specific types
Alpha-adrenoceptor agonists, 208, see also specific types
Alpha-receptors, 263, see also specific types
Alzheimer's dementia, 98
Amiloride, 33, 91, 121, 145, 188, 190, 256
Amino acids, 235, see also specific types
Aminoglutathimide, 174
AMP, see Adenosine monophosphate
Anesthetics, 140, see also specific types
ANF, see Atrial natriuretic factor
Angiotensin, 102, 252
Angiotensin II, 8, 31, 102, 145, 219
Angiotension-converting enzyme (ACE) inhibitors, 39, 252, 253, 263, 306, see also specific types
Animal studies, 26, 70–71, 146, 305, see also specific animals; specific types
Anion exchange, 76
Ankyrin, 136
ANP, see Atrial natriuretic peptide
Antibodies, 159, 164, 165, 170, see also specific types
Antidigoxin antibodies, 159, 164, 165, 170
Antihypertensive agents, 301–307, see also specific types
- centrally acting, 304–305
- left ventricular hypertrophy reversal and, 262–263
- lithium-sodium countertransport system and, 101
- myocardial hypertrophy and, 249

Arginine-vasopressin (AVP), 142
Arrhenius plots, 96
Arterial hypertension, 251–252
Arterial membrane potential, 203–207
Aspartic acid, 235
Atenolol, 101
Aterial remodeling, 146
ATP, see Adenosine triphosphate
ATPase, see Adenosine triphosphatase
Atrial natriuretic factor (ANF), 13, 31, 50, 233, 234
Atrial natriuretic peptide (ANP), 183–191
- discovery of, 184
- in essential hypertension, 185–187, 190
- history of, 184–185
- in humans, 185
- intestinal cells and, 190
- kidney cells and, 187–188

left ventricular hypertrophy and, 256, 264
receptors of, 187
research on, 184–185
sodium transport and, 184, 187–189, 190
vascular smooth muscle cells and, 188–189
Atriopeptin III, 188
AVP, see Arginine-vasopressin

B

Band 3 proteins, 135–137, see also specific types
Bartter's syndrome, 98
Basolateral cell membranes, 13
Beta-adrenergic antagonists, 263, see also specific types
Beta-adrenergic blockers, 252, see also specific types
Beta-blockers, 234, 263, see also specific types
Beta-receptor agonists, 144, see also specific types
Beta-receptors, 263, see also specific types
Bicarbonate, 91, 134, see also Chlorine-bicarbonate exchange
Biological markers, 266
Birth control pills, 98
Blacks, 14, 15, 103, 127
Blood pressure overload, 249–251, 260
Body mass index, 75, 278, 280, 291
Body weight, 99, 275, 278, 282, 284
Bone marrow transplantation, 171
Bradykinin, 258, 259
Brain synaptosomes, 235, 236
Buffering capacity, 120
Bumetamide, 33, 51, 53, 140
Bumetamide-like factors, 14, 304

C

CAD, see Coronary artery disease
Cadmium, 234
Calcium
active transport of, 242
affinity to, 232
alkaline shift and, 124
in blacks, 127
cytosolic, 4, 7, 13, 16, 230, 242
myocardial growth and, 254
sodium-hydrogen antiport and, 125–127
efflux of, 256
extracellular, 8, 142
extrusion of, 4, 5, 73
influx of, 74, 231
intracellular, 73, 74, 231, 233, 239, 241
left ventricular hypertrophy and, 253, 263
membrane fluidity and, 285
as intracellular messenger, 254–256, 258
movements of, 254
myocardial growth and efflux of, 256
passive influx of, 231
release of, 73
sodium-hydrogen antiport and, 125–127
sodium pump and, 63
uptake of, 7, 263
Calcium antagonists, 74, 263, 305–306, see also specific types
Calcium binding capacity, 234–235
Calcium-binding sites, 235
Calcium channels, 5
agonists of, 207
blockers of, 199, 200, 205, 212, 252, 262
intracellular messenger operated, 258
myocardial growth and, 254
opening of, 242
receptor-operated, 8
vascular muscle, see Vascular muscle calcium channels
voltage-dependent, see Voltage-dependent calcium channels (VDCCs)
Calcium-dependent ATPase, see Calcium pump
Calcium-dependent protease, 34
Calcium dissipators, 5
Calcium ionophores, 234, 237, 239
Calcium pump, 4, 7, 9, 16, 229–242
calmodulin and, 232–233, 235, 238
disorders of, 234–242
calcium binding capacity and, 234–235
in essential hypertension, 238–242
in experimental hypertension, 235–237
in erythrocytes, 231, 237, 239
essential aspects of, 230–234
in essential hypertension, 234, 238–242
function of, 230–232
myocardial growth and, 255
physiological role of, 233
regulation of, 233–234
of sarcoplasmic reticulum, 234, 235
structure of, 230–232
Calmodulin, 231, 234
calcium pump and, 232–233, 235, 238
in essential hypertension, 238
inhibitors of reactions mediated by, 237
in platelets, 238

Calnaktin, 63
Calpain, 34
Canrenone, 75, 101, 303
Captopril, 101, 306
Carbon dioxide, 138
Cardiac contractility, 106
Cardiac glycosides, 158, 159, 166, see also specific types
Cardiac muscle membranes, 203
Cardiac output, 16
Cardiocytes, 16
Cardiomyocytes, 234–235
Cardiovascular function, 168–172, see also specific types
Cardiovascular remodeling, 104–106
Catecholamines, 18, 252, 258, see also specific types
Cationic transport, 140
Cell dehydration, 17
Cell growth, 257, 259, 261
Cell membranes, 4–10, 13
Cell replication, 16
Cell swelling, 17
Cellular buffering capacity, 120
Cellular growth, 104
Cellular pH, 291
Cell volume, 10, 17, 59, 257
Centrally acting antihypertensives, 304–305, see also specific types
Cerebrospinal fluid (CSF), 52, 175
CHF, see Congestive heart failure
Chloride channels, 50
Chloride removal, 91
Chlorine-bicarbonate exchange, 133–149
  abnormalities of, 146–148
  animal studies of, 146
  membrane distribution of, 135–138
  in nonerythroid cells, 141–142
  regulation of, 142
  in regulation of blood pressure, 143–146
  structure of, 135–138
  transport activity and, 138–142
  in vascular smooth muscle cell growth regulation, 145–146
  in vascular tone regulation, 144–145
Chlorine channels, 6, 8
Chlorine exchange, 7, 9, 15
2,5-P-Chloromercuribenzenesulforic acid, 91
2,5-Chloromercuribenzoate, 30
Cholesterol, 18, 64, 68, 275, 277, 278
  free, 99
  left ventricular hypertrophy and, 265
  plasma, 69
  serum, 99, 127
  sodium-hydrogen antiport and, 127
  total, 99, 127, 280, 283
Cholesterol lowering agents, 69, see also specific types
Choroid plexus, 7, 15
Chromatography, 159, 162, 166, 168, see also specific types
Chronic glomerulonephritis, 97
Cirrhosis, 167, 168
Clonidin, 252
Clonidine, 304, 305
Cobalt chloride, 237
Collagen, 260, 262
Compensatory response to excess sodium, 12–14
Concentric hypertrophy, 250, 264, 266
Congestive heart failure (CHF), 159, 248
Contraceptives, 98
Cooperativity coefficients, 2
Coronary artery disease (CAD), 248
Corticosterone, 174
Cotransport systems, see also specific types
  lithium-potassium, 275, 285
  potassium-chlorine, 5, 10, 17
  sodium-potassium, 169, 279, 280, 287, 291
  sodium-potassium-chlorine, see Sodium-potassium-chlorine cotransport system
Countertransport systems, 5, 236, see also specific types
Cross-sectional studies, 274–279
CSF, see Cerebrospinal fluid
Cyclic AMP, 27, 50, 124, 142, 144, 234
Cyclic GMP, 13, 124, 184, 188, 233, 234
Cytoplasmic alkalinization, 257
Cytoplasmic protein kinases, 261
Cytoskeleton, 136
Cytosolic calcium, 7, 13, 16, 230, 242
  concentration of, 233
  myocardial growth and, 254
  sodium-hydrogen antiport and, 125–127
Cytosolic pH, 120

D

DAG, see Diacylglycerol
Dahl rats, 27, 31–32, 68
  calcium antagonists and, 305
  calcium pump in, 237
  sodium-hydrogen antiport in, 120
  vascular muscle calcium channels in, 209, 212

voltage-dependent calcium channels in, 209, 212
Deoxycortisone (DOCA), 209, 212
Deoxycosterone acetate, 97
Dephosphorylation, 62, 232
Depolarization, 74, 205, 214–215
Dexamethasone, 174, 258
Diabetes, 100, 101, 102–103, 104, 107, 286
Diabetic nephropathy, 103
Diacylglycerol (DAG), 8, 258, 262
Diagnosis of essential hypertension, 3
DIDS, see 4,4′-Diisothiocyanatostilbene-2,2′-disulfonic acid
Digitalis, 13, 69
Digitalis-like factors, 14, 69, 157–176
  cardiovascular function and, 168–172
  cerebrospinal fluid sources of, 175
  hypertensive factor hypothesis and, 159–162
  natriuretic hormones and, 158–159, 161–162, 167, 171, 173
  plasma sources of, 165–172
  sources of, 164–175
    cerebrospinal fluid, 175
    plasma, 165–172
    tissue, 172–175
    urine, 164–165
  tissue sources of, 172–175
  urine sources of, 164–165
Digitalis-like hormone, 173
Digoxin, 159
  endogenous, 167, 170, 171
  immunoactivity of, 165, 169, 170, 174
Digoxin-like activities, 167, 170
Digoxin-like factors, 159
Digoxin-like immunoactivity, 162, 163, 167, 168, 174
Digoxin-like immunological activity, 166
Dihydropyridines, 200–201, 203, 210, 211, 305, 306, see also specific types
4,4′-Diisothiocyanatostilbene-2,2′-disulfonic acid (DIDS), 91, 121, 137, 144, 232
Dissociation constants, 64, 239, 241, 264
Diuretic-like factors, 14
Diuretics, 101, 252, 302–304, see also specific types
DNA binding proteins, 261, see also specific types
DNA synthesis, 145, 253
DOCA, see Deoxycortisone
Doman equilibrium, 141
Dyslipidemic syndromes, 277

E

Eccentric hypertrophy, 250, 264, 266
Echocardiography, 104, 106, 190, 248
EDGF, see Endothelium-derived growth factor
EDRF, see Endothelium-derived relaxing factor
EGF, see Epidermal growth factor
EH, see Essential hypertension
Electrical activity, 4
Electrolyte transport, 11
Endocrine control of hypertrophy, 259–262
Endogenous digitalis-like factors, 14, 69
Endogenous ouabain-like factor (EOLF), 13, 14
Endogenous ouabain-like substances, 71
Endothelial cells, 189
Endothelin, 8, 258, 259
Endothelium, 205, 218–219
Endothelium-derived growth factor (EDGF), 253, 258, 261
Endothelium-derived relaxing factor (EDRF), 73, 233, 234
Endoxin, 159
End stage kidney disease, 97
Enzymes, 39, 136, 233, 252, 253, 263, see also specific types
EOLF, see Endogenous ouabain-like factor
Epidermal growth factor (EGF), 142, 253, 258
Epinephrine, 63, 264
Epithelial cells, 47–48, 51–52
Epithelial tissue, 5–7
Erythrocytes, 26
  adenosine triphosphatase in, 33, 231
  age of, 93
  calcium binding capacity in, 234
  calcium pump in, 231, 237, 239
  cell membrane ionic transport systems in, 4–10
  chlorine-bicarbonate exchange in, 136, 139, 148
  cotransport rate for, 34
  digitalis-like factors and, 161, 172
  in essential hypertension investigation, 1–19
    clinical aspects of, 17–18
    ion flux studies and, 12
    kinetic studies and, 12–17
    perspectives on, 18
    rationale for use of, 10–11
  fatty acids in, 289
  ionic transport systems in, 9–10, 11
    abnormalities of, 3, 16–17, 263–266, 306

compensatory abnormalities of, 16–17
diuretic drug sensitivity and, 302–304
genetic changes in, 14–15, 16
lithium-sodium countertransport system in, 90, 93, 264
membrane-forming vesicles and, 235
sodium in, 59, 69
sodium-hydrogen exchange in, 264, 265
sodium-potassium-chlorine cotransport system in, 48, 50–51, 264
sodium-potassium pump in, 61, 71
sodium transport in, 2
Essential hypertension (EH), 230
atrial natriuretic peptide in, 185–187, 190
calcium binding capacity in, 234
calcium pump in, 234, 238–242
calmodulin in, 238
diagnosis of, 3
erythrocytes in investigation of, 1–19
clinical aspects of, 17–18
ion flux studies and, 12
kinetic flux studies and, 12–17
perspectives on, 18
rationale for use of, 10–11
left ventricular hypertrophy in, 247–267
antihypertensive agents in reversal of, 262–263
blood pressure overload and, 249–251, 260
erythrocyte ionic transport abnormalities and, 263–266
factors in development of, 252–253
genetic predisposition to, 251–252
intracellular response to, 259–263
myocardial growth and, 252, 254–259
reversal of, 262–263
lithium-sodium countertransport system in, 96
pathophysiology of, 120, 301–307
sodium and, 10
sodium-hydrogen antiport in, 125–127
sodium-potassium-chlorine cotransport system in, 26, 45–54
physiological role of, 46–50
sodium-potassium pump in, 57–80
altering of, 64–65
animal studies of, 70–71
general aspects of, 59–64
genetic factor in, 66–68
kinetic abnormalities of, 64–75
clinical aspects of, 74–75
critical analysis of, 76–79
in vitro, 77–78
pathophysiological aspects of, 72–74
pharmacological aspects of, 74–75
nongenetic factor in, 68–70
sodium transport and, 190
treatment of, 3
Estrogen-induced hypertension, 97
Ethylisopropyl-amiloride, 256
Etiological factors, 17
Exercise, 281–282
Experimental hypertension, 36, 212–214, 235–237
Extracellular calcium, 8, 142

F

Familial combined hyperlipidemia, 277
Familial dyslipidemic syndromes, 277
Familial hypercholesterolemia, 288
Familial hypertrophic cardiomyopathy, 104
Fasting glucose, 264
Fatty acids, 99, 283, 286, 287, 289, 290, see also specific types
Follow-up studies, 279–281
Free fatty acids, 290, see also specific types
Functional units, 60–61
Furosemide, 91, 140

G

Genetically hypertensive rats, 2, 15
Genetic animal models, 26
Genetic factor in sodium-potassium pump, 66–68
Genetic markers, 2, 26
Genetic predisposition to left ventricular hypertrophy, 251–252
Genetic studies, 26, 284–285
Glomerular filtration rate, 15, 184
Glomerular hyperfiltration, 103, 143
Glomerulonephritis, 97
Glomerulosclerosis, 103
Glucocorticoids, 258, see also specific types
Glucose, 264, 265
Glucose tolerance, 100, 102–103
Glutamic acid, 235
Glycolytic enzymes, 136, see also specific types
Glycosides, 158, 159, 166, see also specific types
GMP, see Guanosine monophosphate
G proteins, 8, 234, 258

Growth factor receptors, 261, see also specific types
Growth factors, 134, see also specific types
  endothelium-derived, 253, 258, 261
  epidermal, 142, 253, 258
  left ventricular hypertrophy and, 258, 259, 261
  platelet-derived, 142, 219, 253, 258, 261, 263
Growth hormone, 145
Guanosine monophosphate (GMP), 13, 50, 124, 184, 188, 233, 234
Guanylate cyclase, 13, 184, 188

H

HDLs, see High-density lipoproteins
Heart failure, 159, 248
HeLa cells, 60
Hemodialysis, 98
Hemodynamics, 101
Henle's loop, 6, 7, 15
Hepatocytes, 235
High-density lipoproteins (HDLs), 127, 148, 275–278, 280, 290
High performance liquid chromatography (HPLC), 159, 162, 166, 168
Hill's number, 108
HMGCoA, see 3-Hydroxy-3-methylgutoryl coenzyme A
Hormones, 134, 135, see also specific types
  adrenocorticotrophic, 174
  atrial natriuretic, see Atrial natriuretic peptide (ANP)
  digitalis-like, 173
  growth, 145
  myocardial growth and, 259
  natriuretic, see Natriuretic hormones
  parathyroid, 256
  putative, 158
  steroid, 174
  thyroid, 64, 234
HPLC, see High performance liquid chromatography
HPS, see Hypertension-prone substrain
Human studies
  of atrial natriuretic peptide, 185
  of calcium antagonists, 305
  of chlorine-bicarbonate exchange, 146–148
  of lithium-sodium countertransport system, 93–95
  of sodium-potassium-chlorine cotransport system, 37–39
Hydralazine, 252
Hydrochlorothiazide, 33, 303, 304, 306
Hydrogen, 5, 70, 258
Hydrogen pump, 4
Hydrolysis, 4, 255
6-Hydroxydopamine, 217
3-Hydroxy-3-methylglutoryl coenzyme A (HMGCoA) reductase inhibitors, 99, see also specific types
1,25-Hydroxyvitamin D, 234
Hypercholesterolemia, 288
Hyperinsulinemia, 100, 107, 263
Hyperlipidemia, 99, 100, 277
Hyperpolarization, 74
Hypertension-prone substrain (HPS) of Sabra rats, 16
Hypertensive factor hypothesis, 159–162
Hyperthyroidism, 98
Hypertriglyceridemia, 288
Hypertrophy, see also specific types
  concentric, 250, 264, 266
  eccentric, 250, 264, 266
  endocrine control of, 259–262
  left ventricular, see Left ventricular hypertrophy (LVH)
  mechanical control of, 259–262
  myocardial, 249, 259–263
  neural control of, 259–262
  vascular, 16
Hypokalemia, 101, 302, 303
Hypothyroidism, 98

I

IDDM, see Insulin-dependent diabetes mellitus
IMCD, see Inner medullary collecting duct
Inner medullary collecting duct (IMCD), 188
Inositol triphosphate, 8, 258, 262
Insulin, 63, 253, 258, 259, 263
  fasting, 278, 279
  lithium-sodium countertransport system and, 291, 292
  resistance to, 100, 102, 263, 290–292
  sensitivity to, 102–103
Insulin-dependent diabetes mellitus (IDDM), 101, 103, 104, 107, 286
Intervention studies, 281–284
Interventricular septal thickness, 265
Intestinal cells, 190
Intracellular calcium, 73, 74, 231, 233, 239, 241
  left ventricular hypertrophy and, 253, 263

membrane fluidity and, 285
Intracellular hydrogen, 258
Intracellular messengers, 254–256, 258, see also specific types
Intracellular pH, 134, 256
Intracellular proteins, 259, 262, see also specific types
Intracellular signals of myocardial growth, 254–259
Intracellular sodium, 171, 236, 253, 257
Intraerythrocytic sodium, 263, 285
Ion affinities, 2
Ion flux studies, 12
Ion transport proteins, 4

K

Ketanserin, 101
Kidney, 26, 106
acidification of, 143
arteries in, 11
atrial natriuretic peptide and cells in, 187–188
function of, 15, 166–168
sodium reabsorption in, 14, 101, 143, 292
transplantation of, 14
Kidney disease, 97, see also specific types
Kidney stones, 98
Kinetic abnormalities, see also specific types
of sodium-hydrogen exchange, 107–108
of sodium-potassium pump, 64–75
clinical aspects of, 74–75
critical analysis of, 76–79
in vitro, 77–78
pathophysiological aspects of, 72–74
pharmacological aspects of, 74–75
Kinetic properties, 91–93, 106, see also specific types
Kinetic studies, 2, 12–17, see also specific types
of sodium-potassium-chlorine cotransport system, 50
of sodium-potassium pump, 64

L

LDLs, see Low-density lipoproteins
Left ventricular hypertrophy (LVH), 18, 104, 247–267
angiotensin II and, 253, 258, 259
antihypertensive agents in reversal of, 262–263
blood pressure overload and, 249–251, 260
erythrocyte ionic transport abnormalities and, 263–266
factors in development of, 252–253
genetic predisposition to, 251–252
intracellular response to, 259–263
myocardial growth and, 252, 254–259
protein kinase C (PKC) and, 253, 257–259, 263, 266
reversal of, 252, 262–263
Left ventricular mass index (LVMI), 252, 264
Leukocytes, 305
Linoleic acid, 99, 287
Lipids, 68–69, 263, 264, 274–292, see also specific types
cross-sectional studies of, 274–279
follow-up studies of, 279–281
genetic studies of, 284–285
intervention studies of, 281–284
ionic transport systems and, 285–292
lithium-sodium countertransport system and, 99–100
lowering of, 283–284
membrane, 283
serum, 283
Lipolysis, 287
Lipoproteins, 274–292, see also specific types
cross-sectional studies of, 274–279
follow-up studies of, 279–281
genetic studies of, 284–285
high-density, 127, 148, 275–278, 280, 290
intervention studies of, 281–284
low-density, 18, 99, 127, 265, 277, 290
very low-density, 277, 278, 290, 291
Lithium, 90
Lithium fractional reabsorption, 15
Lithium leaks, 275, 281
Lithium-potassium cotransport system, 275, 285
Lithium-sodium antiport, 90
Lithium-sodium countertransport system, 2, 9, 15, 16, 17, 89–109
antihypertensives and, 101, 304
assays of, 91–93
body weight and, 99
cardiovascular remodeling and, 104–106
clinical assays of, 91–93
diabetes and, 100, 101, 102–103, 104, 107
in erythrocytes, 264
in essential hypertension, 96
genetic studies of, 284
glucose tolerance and, 100, 102–103
heritability of, 96

increased maximal rate of, 263
insulin and, 102–103, 291, 292
intervention studies of, 281
ionic transport abnormalities and, 275, 278, 279, 280
kidney sodium reabsorption and, 101
kinetic properties of, 91–93
left ventricular hypertrophy and, 263
lipids and, 99–100
maximal rate of, 263
membrane fluidity and, 286, 287, 290
peripheral hemodynamics and, 101
personality and, 100–101
physical activity and, 100
population studies of, 93–95
renin angiotensin system and, 102
in secondary hypertension, 97–98
sodium-hydrogen exchange and, 106–108
uric acid and, 100
variables in, 98–101
Lithium-sodium exchange, 90
Liver disease, 167, 168, see also specific types
Local anesthetics, 140, see also specific types
Longitudinal studies, 280
Lovastatin, 69, 99
Low-density lipoproteins (LDLs), 18, 99, 127, 265, 277, 290, see also specific types
Lupus erythematosus, 97
LVH, see Left ventricular hypertrophy
LVMI, see Left ventricular mass index
Lysophosphatidylcholine, 289

M

Magnesium, 5, 231, 232, 291
Magnesium-sodium exchange, 9
Manic-depressive disorder, 90
Maximal translocation rates, 2, 12
Mechanoreceptors, 260
Mechanotransducer ion channels, 260
Membrane abnormalities, 2
Membrane binding proteins, 261, see also specific types
Membrane depolarization, 214–215
Membrane electrolyte transport, 11
Membrane fluidity, 70, 275, 285–291
Membrane permeability, 211
Membrane potentials, 199, 203–207, 209, 212, 215, 217
Membrane sodium leak, 16
Membrane transport proteins, 11
Mesangial cells, 13
Metabolic acidosis, 143
Metabolic dissipators, 5
Methyldopa, 252
Michaelis-Menten activation, 139
Milan normotensive strain (MNS) of rats, 32, 33, 34, 35
Milan strain of spontaneously hypertensive (MSH) rats, 15, 17
calcium pump in, 236
sodium-potassium-chlorine cotransport system in, 27, 32–36, 51
Mineralocorticoids, 170, see also specific types
Minimal vascular resistance, 104
MNS, see Milan normotensive strain
Molecular biology of band 3-related anion exchange, 137–138
Molecular structure of sodium-potassium pump, 60–61
Molecular studies, 11
MSH, see Milan strain of spontaneously hypertensive
Myocardial cells, 236
Myocardial growth, 252, 254–259
Myocardial hypertrophy, 249, 259–263
Myocardial interstitial tissue, 260
Myocardial ischemia, 248
Myocardial plasma membrane, 260
Myocytes, 212–214
Myofibrillar deposition, 260
Myometrial cells, 234
Myosin, 260, 262
Myosin light-chain kinase, 233

N

Natriuresis, 184
Natriuretic hormones, 158–159, 161–162, 167, 171, 173, see also specific types
mechanism of action of, 159
physiological evidence of, 158
sodium-potassium pump and, 69
Natriuretic response, 12
Nephrons, 6, 13
Neural control of hypertrophy, 259–262
Neurons, 16
Neurotransmission, 215–217
NIDDM, see Noninsulin-dependent diabetes mellitus
Nifedipine, 208, 305
Nitroprusside, 212

Nonerythroid cells, 141–142
Noninsulin-dependent diabetes mellitus (NIDDM), 102, 103
Noradrenaline, 8, 73, 144, 145
Noradrenergic neurons, 16
Noradrenergic output, 16
Norepinephrine, 63, 204, 216, 217, 252, 259, 264
Nucleotides, 124, see also specific types
Nystatin, 93

O

Obesity, 99, 278
Oleic acid, 99, 287
Oral contraceptives, 98
Osmotic cell shrinking, 258
Ouabain, 68, 69, 73, 78
  atrial natriuretic peptide and, 189
  binding of, 64, 70, 71, 285
  depressant action of, 73
  digitalis-like factors and, 160, 165, 175
  hydrogen binding to, 70
  potassium channels and, 74
  sodium efflux and, 64, 70, 78, 280
  sodium-potassium pump and, 6, 9, 73
Ouabain-like factors, 13, 14, 187, 303, 304, see also specific types
Ouabain-like substances, 69–70, 71, 72, 74, 75, 77, see also specific types
Ouabain-resistant HeLa cells, 60
Oxytocin, 234

P

Paracrine factors, 218–219
Parathyroid hormone (PTH), 256
Parvalbumins, 235
Passive permeability, 16
Patch-clamp methods, 200, 203, 206, 207, 212, 215, 216
Pathophysiology, 3
  of essential hypertension, 120, 301–307
  of sodium-potassium pump activity, 72–74
PCR, see Polymerase chain reaction
PDGF, see Platelet-derived growth factor
Peripheral hemodynamics, 101
Peripheral resistances, 13, 72, 73, 242
Personality, 100–101
pH
  cellular, 291
  chlorine-bicarbonate exchange and, 134–135
  cytosolic, 120
  intracellular, 134, 256
  regulation of, 120–122, 134–135
  resting, 121
  sodium-hydrogen antiport and, 120–122, 123
Phenylalanine, 35
Phloretin, 93, 140
Phorbol esters, 145, 146, see also specific types
Phorbol-12-myristate-13-acetate, 142
Phosphatidylcholine, 233, 290
Phosphatidylethanolamine, 235
Phosphatidylinositol, 234, 235, 258–259
Phosphatidylinositol-biphosphate, 233
Phosphatidylinositol 4,5-bisphosphate, 258
Phosphatidylinositol-monophosphate, 233
Phosphatidylinositol 4-phosphate, 258
Phosphatidylserine, 235
Phosphoinositol, 287
Phospholipase C (PLC), 8, 122, 258, 261, 262, 263
Phospholipids, 69, 233, 275, 286, 288, 289, see also specific types
Phospholomban, 234
Phosphorylation, 62, 126, 232, 259, 262
Physical activity, 100, 281–282
Ping-pong model, 92, 139
Piretanide, 302
PKA, see Protein kinase A
PKC, see Protein kinase C
Plasma membranes, 122, 135, 136, 235, 260
Plasma renin activity (PRA), 14, 18, 190, 264
Platelet-derived growth factor (PDGF), 142, 219, 253, 258, 261, 263
Platelet hyperactivity, 127
Platelets, 238
PLC, see Phospholipase C
Plethysmography, 105
Plurimetabolic syndrome, 100
Polycystic kidney disease, 97
Polymerase chain reaction (PCR), 35
Polyunsaturated fatty acids, 99, 287, see also specific types
Posterior wall thickness, 265
Postischemic vascular resistance, 106
Potassium, 5, 62, 78, 303
Potassium channels, 4, 74
Potassium chloride, 17
Potassium-chlorine cotransport system, 5, 10, 17
Potassium electrochemical gradients, 4–5
Potassium-potassium exchange, 63

Potassium-sodium exchange, 61–62
Potassium sparing diuretics, 303, see also specific types
Potential-dependent channels, 74
PRA, see Plasma renin activity
Prazosin, 252
Pregnancy, 98, 168, 274, 282
Pressure-induced membrane depolarization, 214–215
Pressurization, 205, 215
Primary hypertension, 3, 11, 17, 50–53
Progesterone, 174
Proteases, 34, see also specific types
Protein kinase A (PKA), 253
Protein kinase C (PKC), 122, 124, 126, 127, 142
Proteins, see also specific types
  band 3, 135–137
  dephosphorylation of, 232
  DNA binding, 261
  G, 8, 234, 258
  intracellular, 259, 262
  ionic transport, 4
  membrane binding, 261
  membrane transport, 11
  phosphorylation of, 232, 259, 262
  synthesis of, 253, 260
Protons, 107, 139–140, 231
Proto-oncogenes, 261
Proximal sodium reabsorption, 15
Psoriasis, 98
PTH, see Parathyroid hormone
Putative hormone, 158

Q

Quin-2, 237

R

Race studies, 14, 15, 67, 103, 127
Rats, see also specific types
  Dahl, see Dahl rats
  genetically hypertensive, 2, 15
  hypertension-prone substrain of Sabra, 16
  Milan normotensive strain of, 32, 33, 34, 35
  Milan strain of spontaneously hypertensive, see Milan strain of spontaneously hypertensive rats
  Sabra, 16
  sodium and, 10
  sodium-potassium-chlorine cotransport system in, 28–36
  spontaneously hypertensive, see Spontaneously hypertensive rats (SHR)
  Sprague-Dawley, 10
  Wistar Kyoto normotensive, see Wistar Kyoto normotensive (WKY) rats
Receptor-operated calcium channels, 8
Red blood cells, see Erythrocytes
Relaxing factors, 73, 233, 234, see also specific types
Renal, see Kidney
Renin, 14, 190, 263, 264, 286
Renin-angiotensin system, 102, 253
Renin-angiotensin-aldosterone system, 252
Renovascular hypertension, 97
Resting pH, 121
Restriction fragment length polymorphism (RFLP), 68
RFLP, see Restriction fragment length polymorphism
Rhesus monkeys, 168, 169, 170
RNA polymerase, 259
RNA synthesis, 260

S

Sabra rats, 16
Salicylates, 140, see also specific types
Saline overload, 236, 237, 262
Salt, see Sodium
Sarcoplasmic reticulum, 7, 230, 234, 235
Saturated fatty acids, 99, see also specific types
Secondary hypertension, 97–98, 286
Secretive epithelia, 5
Self-inhibition, 139
SHR, see Spontaneously hypertensive rats
Skeletal muscle, 234
Smooth muscle cells, 5, 7–8, 16, 230, 234, see also Vascular smooth muscle cells (VSMCs)
Sodium, 2, 5, 10
  absorption of, 143
  compensatory response to excess intake of, 12–14
  digitalis-like factors and, 170
  dissociation constant for, 64
  efflux of, 63, 64, 70, 78, 280, 305
  in erythrocytes, 59, 69
  essential hypertension and, 10
  excess intake of, 12–14

intake of, 262, 286
internal content of, 13
intracellular, 171, 236, 253, 257
intraerythrocytic, 263, 285
in kidney arteries, 11
kidney reabsorption of, 14, 101, 143, 256, 292
leukocytes and efflux of, 305
loading of, 13
maximal rate of efflux of, 64
ouabain-sensitive efflux of, 64, 70, 78, 280
overload of, 262
phosphorylation dependent on, 62
in primary hypertension, 11
proximal, 143
reabsorption of, 14, 15, 27, 101, 143, 256, 292
restriction of, 96, 262, 282
retention of, 106
sensitivity to, 10, 14, 50, 51, 52, 77
chlorine-bicarbonate exchange and, 143
left ventricular hypertrophy and, 262
race studies of, 67
transmembrane gradient of, 256
transport of, 5, 33, 159
atrial natriuretic peptide and, 184, 187–189, 190
in erythrocytes, 2
essential hypertension and, 190
inhibitors of, 166, 172
washout of, 53
Sodium antiports, 5
Sodium-calcium countertransport system, 236
Sodium-calcium exchange, 5, 13, 18, 73, 74, 145, 230
decrease in activity of, 263
myocardial growth and, 256, 258
Sodium channels, 4, 188
Sodium-dependent chlorine exchange, 7, 9
Sodium dissipators, 5
Sodium electrochemical gradients, 4–5
Sodium exchange, 5, see also specific types
Sodium-hydrogen antiport, 119–128
amiloride-sensitive, 121
description of, 122–125
in essential hypertension, 125–127
pH and, 120–122, 123
Sodium-hydrogen exchange, 7, 9, 15, 16, 134, 264, 291
amiloride-sensitive, 190
atrial natriuretic peptide and, 188
decrease in activity of, 263
in erythrocytes, 264, 265
kinetic abnormalities of, 107–108
kinetic properties of, 107–108
left ventricular hypertrophy and, 256–258, 262
lithium-sodium countertransport system and, 106–108
myocardial growth and, 256–258
Sodium leaks, 16, 66, 71, 264, 304, 305
Sodium-lithium countertransport system, see Lithium-sodium countertransport system
Sodium-magnesium exchange, 9
Sodium-potassium cotransport system, 169, 279, 280, 287, 291
Sodium-potassium-chlorine cotransport system, 2, 6, 7, 8, 15, 16, 25–40
antihypertensives and, 304, 305
atrial natriuretic peptide and, 188, 189
calcium pump and, 236
characteristics of, 27–28
in epithelial cells, 47–48, 51–52
in erythrocytes, 48, 50–51, 264
in essential hypertension, 45–54
physiological role of, 46–50
in experimental hypertension, 36
in humans, 37–39
physiological role of, 46–50
in primary hypertension, 50–53
in rats, 28–36
in vascular smooth muscle cells, 49–50, 52–53
Sodium-potassium exchange, 61–62
Sodium-potassium pump, 13, 57–80
altering of, 64–65
animal studies of, 70–71
clinical aspects of, 74–75
density of, 66
diminished activity of, 73–74
enzymatic aspects of, 61–63
in erythrocytes, 61, 71
functional aspects of, 61–63
general aspects of, 59–64
genetic factor in, 66–68
hemodynamic effects of, 73
inhibitors of, 66, 69, 71
kinetic abnormalities of, 64–75
clinical aspects of, 74–75
critical analysis of, 76–79
in vitro, 77–78
pathophysiological aspects of, 72–74
pharmacological aspects of, 74–75
kinetic studies of, 64

molecular structure of, 60–61
nongenetic factor in, 68–70
ouabain-sensitive, 6, 9
pharmacological aspects of, 74–75
regulation of, 63–64
transport modes of, 61–63
Sodium pump, 16, 63
digitalis-like factors and, 160, 161, 168, 172, 175
diuretics and, 303
inhibitors of, 162
stimulation of, 303
Sodium-sodium exchange, 62–63
Spectrin-actin cytoskeleton, 136
Spontaneously hypertensive rats (SHR), 14, 17
brain synaptosomes in, 236
calcium binding capacity in, 234, 235
calcium pump in, 239
chlorine-bicarbonate exchange in, 146
membrane fluidity and, 286
Milan strain of, see Milan strain of spontaneously hypertensive (MSH) rats
myocardial cells in, 236
sodium-hydrogen antiport in, 120
sodium-potassium-chlorine cotransport system and, 27, 28–31, 50, 53
sodium-potassium pump in, 68, 71, 78
stroke-prone, 210
vascular muscle calcium channels in, 208, 209, 210, 211
voltage-dependent calcium channels in, 208, 209, 210, 211
Sprague-Dawley rats, 10
Steroid hormones, 174, see also specific types
Stilbenes, 140, 143, see also specific types
Substrates, 63, 139, see also specific types
Sudden death, 248
Sympathetic nervous system, 216
Sympathominetic activity, 263
Synaptosomes, 235, 236
Syndrome X, 100

T

TGF, see Tubuloglomerular feedback
Therapeutic index, 166
Thiazides, 140, 303, see also specific types
Thrombin, 258, 259
Thyocianate, 232
Thyroid hormones, 64, 234, see also specific types
Thyroxine, 258
Transcription factors, 259
Translocation rates, 2, 12
Transplantations, 14, 171
Trial and error assays, 302
Trifluorperazine, 239
Triglycerides, 68, 99, 265, see also specific types
genetic studies of, 284
ionic transport abnormalities and, 275, 279, 280, 281, 282
lipolysis of, 287
Troponins, 235, see also specific types
Tubuloglomerular feedback (TGF), 33
"Type A" behavior, 100–101
Tyrosine, 35

U

Uric acid, 100

V

Vascular hypertrophy, 16
Vascular muscle calcium channels, 197–220
abnormal current in, 207–214
arterial membrane potential and, 203–207
background on, 198–199, 207–208
endothelium factors in regulation of, 218–219
in experimental hypertension, 212–214
in myocytes, 212–214
neurotransmission and, 215–217
paracrine factors in regulation of, 218–219
regulation of, 214–219
Vascular resistances, 104, 106, 242
Vascular smooth muscle cells (VSMCs), 13, 31
atrial natriuretic peptide and, 188–189
calcium binding capacity in, 234
calcium pump in, 242
chlorine-bicarbonate exchange and, 144, 145–146
contractility of, 16
growth regulation of, 145–146
ionic transport systems in, 7–8
lithium-sodium countertransport system and, 106
sodium-potassium-chlorine cotransport system in, 49–50, 52–53
Vascular tone regulation, 144–145
Vasodilators, 252, see also specific types
Vasopressin, 142, 144, 145, 258, 259

VDCCs, see Voltage-dependent calcium channels
Ventricular arrhythmias, 248
Ventricular hypertrophy, 18, 104, see also Left ventricular hypertrophy (LVH)
Verapamil, 211
Very low-density lipoproteins (VLDLs), 277, 278, 290, 291
Vitamin D, 234
VLDLs, see Very low-density lipoproteins
Voltage-dependent calcium channels (VDCCs), 198–207
  abnormal current in, 207–214
  background on, 198–199, 207–208
  calcium pump and, 230
  endothelium factors in regulation of, 218–219
  in experimental hypertension, 212–214
  intrinsic regulation of, 203–207
  left ventricular hypertrophy and, 263
  long-lasting type, 199, 200, 201, 202, 203, 210, 211
    calcium inactivation of, 216
    enhanced, 208
    intrinsic regulation of, 203–207
    myocytes and, 212–214
    regulation of, 215, 216
  in myocytes, 212–214
  neurotransmission and, 215–217
  paracrine factors in regulation of, 218–219
  regulation of, 214–219
  subtypes of, 199–203
  transient-type, 199, 200, 201, 202, 203
    intrinsic regulation of, 203–207
    myocytes and, 212–214
    regulation of, 215, 216
VSMCs, see Vascular smooth muscle cells

W

Water retention, 106
Weight loss, 282
Wistar Kyoto (WKY) normotensive rats, 14, 28, 30, 31
  chlorine-bicarbonate exchange in, 146
  sodium-potassium pump in, 71
  vascular muscle calcium channels in, 208, 209, 210, 211
  voltage-dependent calcium channels in, 208, 209, 210, 211
WKY, see Wistar Kyoto

X

Xipamide, 140, 148, 302